Clinical Neurophysiology
of the Vestibular System

Contemporary Neurology Series available:

Fred Plum, M.D. and Fletcher H. McDowell, M.D., *Editors-in-Chief*

Clinical Neurophysiology of the Vestibular System

ROBERT W. BALOH, M.D.

Associate Professor
Department of Neurology and
Division of Head and Neck Surgery (Otolaryngology)
UCLA School of Medicine
Los Angeles, California

VINCENTE HONRUBIA, M.D.

Professor
Division of Head and Neck Surgery (Otolaryngology)
UCLA School of Medicine
Los Angeles, California

 F. A. DAVIS COMPANY, PHILADELPHIA

Library of Congress Cataloging in Publication Data

Baloh, Robert W.
  Clinical neurophysiology of the vestibular system.

  (Contemporary neurology series; 18)
  Includes bibliographies and index.
  1. Vestibular apparatus. 2. Vestibular function tests.
  3. Neurophysiology. I. Honrubia, Vincente, joint author.
  II. Title. II. Series.
  QP471.B34   612'.858   78-15467
  ISBN 0-8036-0580-3

*This book is dedicated
to our parents*

Foreword

Extensive research on human vestibular reflexes initiated by Robert Bárány in 1907 provided the foundation for clinical analysis of pathologic processes in the labyrinth of the ear or in the pathways and centers of the vestibular system.

In the early period of clinical research, knowledge of the anatomy and physiology of the vestibular system was rudimentary and the techniques for stimulation of the labyrinth and measurement of reflexes were crude. In the past 70 years, owing to significant technologic advances and an increase in the number of investigators entering the field, there has been a spectacular change. Abundant qualitative and quantitative information is now available on the structure and function of the peripheral and central vestibular systems with numerous reports on the symptoms and diagnoses of vestibular disfunction.

Drs. Baloh and Honrubia have met the need for a concise text that integrates the numerous advances in the field of vestibular research with clinical diagnoses. The authors have made noteworthy contributions to otoneurology and this book contains carefully prepared, concise explanations of what is known at present, and judicious treatment of areas of controversy. The simple and direct style of the first three chapters on neurophysiology will give the reader an excellent foundation for the discussion of clinical problems in later chapters. Extensive bibliographies at the end of each chapter supplement the text and are a valuable source of information on all aspects of vestibular function.

This book will be especially useful to students and residents as well as to neurologists, otologists, and ophthalmologists.

R. Lorente de Nó, M.D.

Contents

CHAPTER 1

Vestibular Function: An Overview

Expressed simply, the role of the vestibular sensory organs is to transduce the forces associated with head acceleration and gravity into a biologic signal. The control centers in the brain use this signal to develop a subjective awareness of head position in relation to the environment (orientation) and to produce motor reflexes for equilibrium and locomotion.

During head movement, the force (F) exerted upon the vestibular end organs (from Newton's second principle) is equal to the product of their mass (m) and their acceleration (a): $F = ma$.* Since the mass of the end organ is constant, the force associated with head acceleration generates a signal in the labyrinth that is proportional to the head acceleration. The mathematical operation required to convert an acceleration signal to a measure of head displacement involves two integrations, one to obtain head velocity from acceleration and the other to obtain head displacement from velocity. The central nervous system (CNS) computes head position by performing the equivalent of a mathematical integration on the labyrinthine signal.

Modern inertial guidance systems that control the trajectory of space vehicles include the same basic components: a monitor for displacement based on sensors for linear and angular acceleration and a central processor that integrates this information, computing the coordinates of the space position. The central processor also maintains a memory of the trajectory and can therefore make appropriate adjustments in course when necessary.[5]

BIOPHYSICAL BASIS OF RECEPTOR SPECIALIZATION

The vestibular system monitors the forces associated with angular and linear accelerations of the head by means of five organs located within the labyrinthine cavities of the temporal bones on each side of the skull.[10, 19, 29, 48] The saccular and utricular macules sense linear acceleration and the cristae of the three semicircular canals sense angular acceleration of the head. The capacity of the macules and cristae to function as sensors of linear and angular acceleration, respectively, rests on their anatomic configurations.

---

* If mass is in kilograms and acceleration in meters/second², then the unit of force is the newton (the force acting on a kilogram of mass to impart an acceleration of a meter per second per second).

1

Macules

Each macule consists of a sensory membrane with a surface area less than 1 mm² supporting a "heavy load," the otolith (specific gravity approximately 2.7), composed of calcareous material embedded in a gelatinous matrix, with a mean thickness of 50 μm (Fig. 1a). The position of the load on the receptor depends on the magnitude and direction of the force acting upon it (Fig. 1b, c).[10, 11, 69] Even when the head is at rest the calcareous material, because of its mass, exerts a force (F_g) upon the receptor equal to the product of its mass (m) and the acceleration due to the gravitational pull of the earth (g), which at sea level is 9.80 m/sec².

The distribution of F_g acting on the underlying sensory cells changes with different degrees of head tilt and can be represented by two vectors (Fig. 1b): one vector (F_t) tangential and the other (F_n) normal to the surface of the receptor. The value of the tangential vector is proportional to the sine of the angle θ made by F_g with F_n (i.e. the angle of tilt). As will be shown later, it is this tangential force (F_t) and the resulting otolith displacement that constitute the effective stimulus to the sensory cells.

During linear head acceleration tangential to the surface of the receptor (Fig. 1c), the instantaneous force (F'_g) acting upon the macules is also the result of two vector forces: one (F_t) in the opposite direction of the head displacement and the other (F_g) due to gravitational pull. Again the effective force producing otolith displacement is the tangential force (F_t). In both cases the sensory cells of the macules transmit information on the displacement of the otolith membrane to the

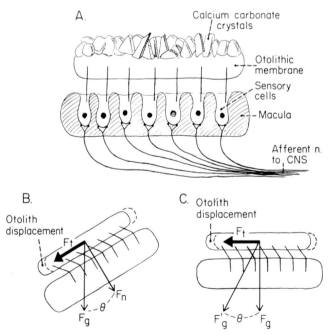

Figure 1. A graphic illustration of the main anatomical features of the macule (A) and the distribution of forces associated with static head tilt (B) and linear acceleration tangential to the surface (C) (for orientation of sensory cells in each macule, see Figure 20, Chapter 2).

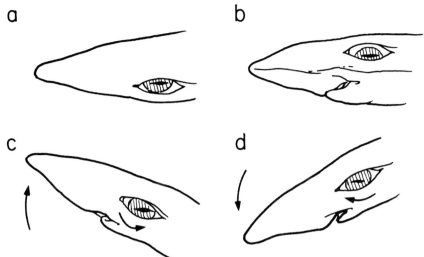

Figure 2. Compensatory eye deviations in the shark produced by static head tilt. (Adapted from Maxwell, S. S.: *Labyrinth and Equilibrium*. Lippincott, Philadelphia and London, 1923.)

CNS; here reflexes are initiated to contract muscles which dynamically oppose the force acting upon the head and thus maintain equilibrium.

A classic example of an otolithic reflex is the change in eye position of fish, amphibians and rodents when their heads and bodies are tilted from the horizontal and held in that position (Fig. 2). In such a condition the eyes align themselves in the orbits so as to maintain their normal relation parallel to the horizon.[54] To this goal the extraocular muscles of the eyes acquire a new level of contraction, or tone, that remains unchanged as long as the head is held in the new position. Because of the permanency of the muscle tone such reflexes are classically known as the static labyrinthine reflexes, and the macules are known as the static labyrinthine organs.

Cristae

Natural head movements consist of a combination of linear and rotational vectors, the latter acting upon a different set of sensors located in the semicircular canals.[19, 48] The latter are small rings approximately 0.65 cm in transverse diameter with an inner cross sectional diameter of 0.4 mm (Fig. 3). They are filled with fluid that has a density and viscosity slightly greater than water. The receptor organs, the cristae, are mounted in the wall of the rings where they sense the displacement of the fluid during head rotation.[19] The sensory epithelium of the cristae is covered by a bulbous, gelatinous mass called the cupula, whose specific gravity is the same as that of the surrounding fluid.[60] Therefore, unlike the otolith of the macules, the cupula does not exert a resting force on the underlying sensory epithelium. Because of the narrowness of the canals, the fluid can only move longitudinally along the tube. Angular acceleration of the head displaces the fluid relative to the wall of the canal. The cupula moves with the fluid, exerting a force on the underlying sensory epithelium.

The semicircular canal reflexes have been called phasic or kinetic, since they are thought to be primarily responsible for muscle contractions associated with

3

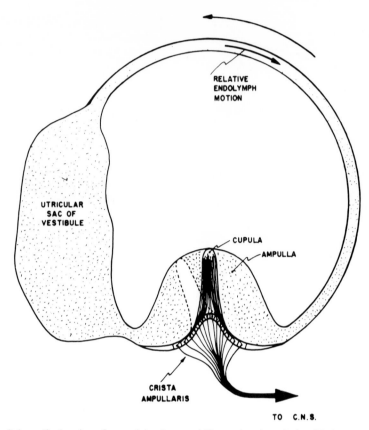

Figure 3. Schematic drawing of a semicircular canal illustrating the relationship between the direction of head rotation (large arrow), endolymph flow (small arrow) and cupular deviation. (From Melvill-Jones, G.: Organization of neural control in the vestibulo-ocular reflex arc. In Bach-Y-Rita, P., Collins, C. C. and Hyde, J. E. (eds.): *The Control of Eye Movements*. Academic Press, New York, 1971.

the maintenance of equilibrium during motion.[49] An example of a semicircular canal reflex is the compensatory eye movement associated with angular head rotation (Fig. 4). Head rotation to one side results in an eye movement in the opposite direction in order to maintain clear vision.[44, 61] If the head rotation exceeds that which can be compensated for by motion of the eye in the orbit (e.g. in Fig. 4d) the reflex takes the form of nystagmus. This is a back-and-forth eye movement in which a slow deviation lasting between 0.5 and 2 seconds is interrupted by a flick in the opposite direction lasting 0.1 to 0.2 seconds. If the fast components were removed from the tracing in Figure 4d and the slow components joined end to end, the resulting sinusoidal eye movement would continue to be approximately equal and opposite to the sinusoidal head movement seen in Figure 4a and b.

CLASSIFICATION OF VESTIBULAR REFLEXES

The rationale for classifying the cristae of the semicircular canals as kinetic receptors and the macules of the utricle and saccule as static receptors was based on a narrow view of their overall function. Both sets of receptor organs produce

4

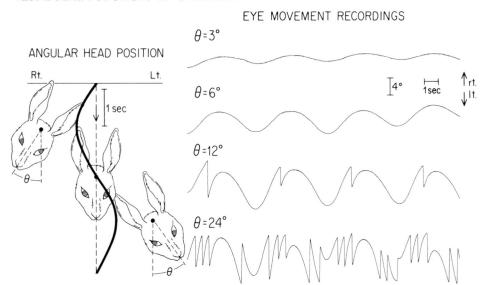

Figure 4. Compensatory eye movents in the rabbit produced by sinusoidal angular acceleration of the head (0.2 Hz) at four different peak angular displacements (θ).

motor reflexes that cannot be differentiated on the basis of the resulting movement. Therefore, it is more appropriate to divide the reflexes into categories based on their functional role rather than on the receptor from which they originate.

At least three major functional roles for vestibular reflexes can be identified. The first is to produce negative geotropic movement to compensate for changes in the direction of the force of gravity. If the pull of gravity on the body were unopposed by forces developed in the muscles, the body would collapse onto the ground. Reflexes in this category are initiated in the macules but not in the semicircular canals. The second role is to produce "kinetic" or transitory contractions of muscles for maintenance of equilibrium and ocular stability during movement. This category includes reflexes arising from both the semicircular canals during angular acceleration and the otolithic organs during linear acceleration. Most natural head movements contain both types of acceleration and the vestibular reflexes act in combination to maintain orientation. A third role of vestibular reflex activity is to help maintain posture and muscular tone.[49, 50, 51, 52] Both the macules and cristae participate in this role. The labyrinthine contribution to skeletal muscular tone can be demonstrated by the change in posture that follows unilateral labyrinthectomy in normal animals.[16, 23, 49] Tone is increased in the extensor muscles of the contralateral extremities and decreased in the ipsilateral extensor muscles. An even more striking demonstration of the vestibular role in maintenance of muscular tone is the removal of decerebrate rigidity after sectioning of both vestibular nerves or destruction of the vestibular nuclei.[4, 30] The extensor rigidity that results from transection of the nervous system at the caudal end of the mesencephalon is markedly decreased when the tonic labyrinthine input is removed.

PHYLOGENY OF THE VESTIBULAR SYSTEM

The role of the labyrinth in maintaining orientation has remained the same from the earliest organisms in the animal kingdom. But as with other sensory organs,

5

some changes, both functional and morphologic, have evolved. Only the most primitive forms of life, such as *Monera* (bacteria and blue-green algae) and *Protista,* which include many unicellular organisms (flagella), have been able to adapt to the environment without specialized receptors for the detection of gravitational force. In these animals, as well as in plants, geotropic motion is probably due to the difference in density of undifferentiated parts that "detect" the pull of gravity. For example, when the stem of the plant, *Bryophyllum calycinium,* is placed in a horizontal position, certain chemical substances gather in greater concentration on the lower side of the stem causing it to grow faster than the upper side. This forces the stem to grow in a vertical direction.[42]

The most primitive gravity receptor organ, the statocyst, appeared more than 600 million years ago, in the late Precambrian era.[33] It is present in the most developed phylum of the *Coelenterata,* beginning with some jellyfish, allowing the animal to orient itself in relation to the horizon by sensing the direction of the gravitational force of the earth. The statocyst is a fluid-filled invagination or sac containing a calcinous particle, the statolith, or multiple particles, the statoconia, of density greater than the fluid (Fig. 5). The particles, attracted by gravity, rest their weight differentially over special sensory cells in the wall of the cyst. The direction of the force on the underlying sensory cells therefore depends on the position of the animal in space.

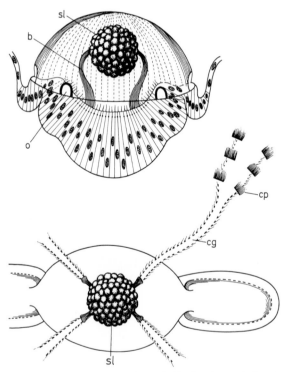

Figure 5. Diagram of the statocyst of the tenophore Collianira. Lateral view (top) and apical view (bottom). b, balancer cilia, cg, ciliated groove, cp, comb plate, o, opening of the translucid roof, sl, statolith. (From Markl, H.: The perception of gravity and of angular acceleration in invertebrates. In Kornhuber, H. H. (ed.): *Handbook of Sensory Physiology,* vol. VI, part 2. Springer-Verlag, New York, 1974, with permission.)

From this simple statocyst to the labyrinth of higher animals, a continuous increment in anatomic complexity occurs that accompanies the phylogenetic evolution of the taxa (Fig. 6). Next, phylogenetically, to the statocyst of medusae is that of mollusks (e.g. octopus, sepia). In addition to a statocyst containing multiple otoconia, the first crista appears in these primitive animals. The development of this new receptor, still in the same cavity as that of the otolith, accompanies the appearance of motor reflexes to angular acceleration, including nystagmus.[13, 17, 21] In primitive fish (cyclostomes) the statocyst cavity, previously open to the outside, is closed and filled by an endogenous secretion (endolymph).

Two surviving cyclostomes, the hagfish and lamprey, demonstrate an important step in the phylogenetic development of the vestibular labyrinth. In the hagfish a simple circular tube is interrupted anteriorly and posteriorly by bulbous enlargements, the ampullae, each containing a primitive crista (Fig. 6a). Between the ampullae in an intercommunicating channel lies the macule communis, the forerunner of the utricular and saccular macules. The labyrinth of the lamprey is

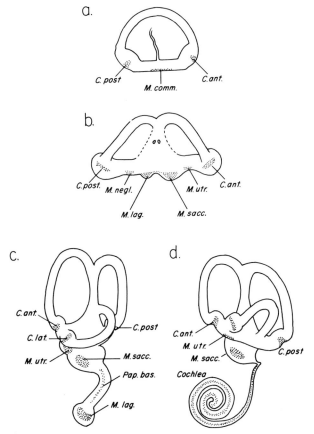

Figure 6. Phylogeny of the labyrinth. (a) myxine, (b) petromyzon, (c) bird, (d) mammal. C. post., posterior canal, M. comm., common macule, C. ant., anterior canal, M. negl., neglector macule, M. lag., lagenar macule, M. sacc., saccular macule, M. utr., utricular macule, C. lat., lateral or horizontal canal, Pap. bas., basilar papilla. (From Wersäll, D. J. and Bagger Sjöbäck, D.: Morphology of the vestibular sense organs. In Kornhuber, H. H. (ed.): *Handbook of Sensory Physiology.* Vol. VI, Part 2. Springer-Verlag, New York, 1974, with permission.)

more complex, consisting of an anterior and posterior canal communicating with a bilobulated sac containing separate utricular and saccular macules. The predecessor of the auditory organs appears after the development of a membranous labyrinth that is divided into two cavities. In the inferior of the two cavities (the saccule), two new receptor areas develop, the lagenar macule and the basilar papilla (Fig. 6b). In crocodiles, however, these receptors are contained in a cavity separate from the saccule, while in birds the basilar papilla is a long uncoiled organ, the predecessor of the coiled cochlea (Fig. 6c).[2]

With the advent of modern fish (about 100 million years ago) the vestibular labyrinth reached its peak of development and relatively little change has taken place since that time.[33] The basic structure of the three semicircular canals, and the utricle and saccule is similar in all higher vertebrates (Fig. 6d). Gray[33] considered the vestibular end organ of modern fish to represent the "highest perfection" of the vertebrate organ of equilibrium. The utricule and semicircular canals are relatively larger than those in other classes of vertebrates. Since fish do not have the highly developed afferent systems of proprioception, touch and vision that higher vertebrates possess, they are apparently more dependent on the labyrinth to provide orienting information.

The membranous labyrinths of modern fish lie in the bony chamber of the skull directly behind the orbits. In its subsequent evolution in amphibians, birds, and mammals, the membranous labyrinth is completely surrounded by a bony labyrinth enclosing the periotic space. This space is filled with perilymphatic fluid and suspensory connective tissue acting as a shock absorber. The planes of the three semicircular canals vary from species to species, although in primates they are approximately orthogonal to each other. The arc of the semicircular canals also varies considerably from that of a triangle in reptiles to an ellipse in birds to an almost true circle in mammals.[33]

Parallel to the separation of receptor organs, afferent nerve fibers differentiated into bundles that maintained independent identity in the internal auditory canal and at the entrance to the brain stem.[15, 43] The afferent nerve from the utricle and horizontal and anterior semicircular canals and some of the nerve fibers from the saccule formed the superior division of the vestibular nerve, while most nerve fibers from the saccule and the nerve from the posterior semicircular canal contributed to the inferior branch (Fig. 7). The afferent fibers from the auditory organ form a separate nerve anterior and inferior to the vestibular nerve. Together these two nerves constitute the eighth cranial nerve, and within them, a system of efferent fibers from the CNS gates or modulates the activity of the peripheral organs.[31, 62] Phylogenetically this neural feedback system is already present in gastropods in which action potentials directed from the brain to the receptors have been recorded.[73]

In comparison to the vestibular sensory organs, central vestibular connections became progressively more complex in higher vertebrates. This complexity accompanied the development of other afferent systems for the maintenance of equilibrium (vision, proprioception) and pathways for interaction of these systems with the vestibular system. The vestibular nuclei are one of the first supraspinal cell groups that differentiated themselves from the reticular formation.[39] Lampreys have two discernible vestibular nuclear groups, the dorsal and ventral, composed of granular and spindle-shaped cells. Modern fish (teleosts) have four discernible vestibular nuclei although the nuclei contain relatively few cells. This basic organization of four vestibular nuclear groups is maintained throughout the

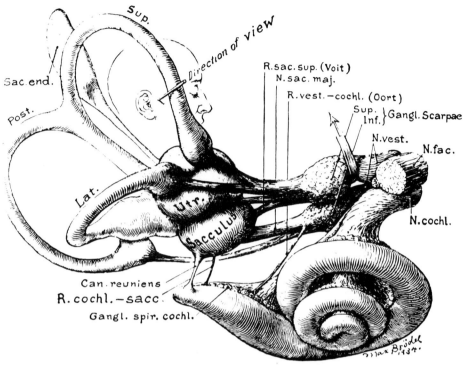

Figure 7. The afferent nerve supply to the labyrinthine end organs. (From Brodel, M.: *Three Unpublished Drawings of the Anatomy of the Human Ear.* W. B. Saunders Co., Philadelphia, 1946, with permission.)

higher vertebrates, although the relative size of each nuclear group varies from species to species. In invertebrates and early vertebrates secondary connections of the vestibular nuclei are primarily vestibulospinal in keeping with their major role in maintaining body orientation.[59] Vestibulocerebellar connections become progressively more prominent in higher vertebrates. The development of these "modern" vestibular pathways accompanies the development of increasingly complex somatic and ocular motor skills. In primates, vestibulocerebellar and vestibulo-ocular connections form a large part of the central vestibular pathways while vestibulospinal connections are less prominent.[41] The lateral vestibular nucleus (Deiters' nucleus), a major source of vestibulospinal fibers, is the most prominent nuclear group in lower mammals, while in man it is small and almost confined to the vestibular root entry zone. By comparison, the superior vestibular nucleus is barely detectable in lower vertebrates, but is prominent in man where it is the major source of vestibulo-ocular fibers. It extends rostrally from the root entry zone (at the medullopontine junction) to the midpontine region.[39]

FORCE TRANSDUCTION: THE HAIR CELL

Morphologic Characteristics

The basic element of the labyrinthine receptor organs that transduces mechanical force to nerve action potentials, the hair cell (Fig. 8), is already developed in

9

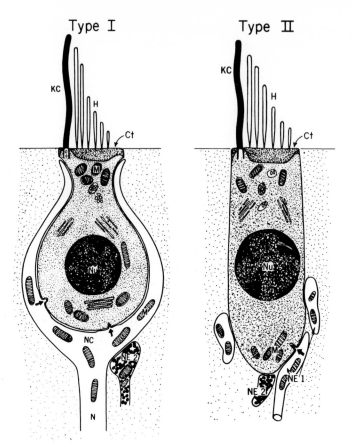

Figure 8. Schematic drawing of the two basic types of hair cells. KC, kinocilium, H, hairs, Ct, cuticular plate, M, mitochondria, Nu, nucleus, Nc, nerve chalice, NE, nerve ending. (Adapted from Ades, H. W. and Engstrom, H.: Form and innervation of the vestibular epithelia. In *Symposium on the Role of the Vestibular Organs in the Exploration of Space.* U.S. Naval School of Aviat. Med., Pensacola, Florida, 1965. NASA SP-77.)

the statocysts of invertebrates.[14, 74] Transducer cells are surrounded by supporting cells in specialized epithelial areas in the walls of the statocyst. In lower vertebrates a bundle of nonmobile cilia protrudes from the apical surface of the cylindrical hair cells. The basal portion of the cell makes contact with many terminals of afferent and efferent nerve fibers. The former carry information from the receptor to the CNS, and the latter provide feedback to the receptor cells from the CNS.

The increased complexity of the labyrinthine end organs from an evolutionary point of view is not limited to changes in gross anatomic features but is also expressed in the development of new structural details in the receptor cells.[47] Two types of hair cells occur in birds and mammals (Fig. 8). Type II cells are cylindrical with multiple nerve terminals at their base (as in lower vertebrates), while type I cells are globular or flask-shaped with a single large chalice-like nerve terminal surrounding the base.[70] The afferent fibers innervating type I hair cells are among the largest in the nervous system (up to 20 μm in diameter).

A bundle of nonmobile stereocilia protrudes from the cuticular plate on the apical end of each receptor cell. The height of the stereocilia increases stepwise from one side to the other and next to the tallest stereocilia a thicker, longer hair, the kinocilium protrudes from the cell's cytoplasm through a segment of cell membrane lacking the cuticular plate. The kinocilium is anchored to the cell by a structure called the basal body, closely resembling the centriole. The stereocilia vary in length in the two different sense organs, being shortest in the macules (a few microns) where they are embedded in the otolithic membrane. In the cristae they measure up to 36 microns in length and protrude into the gelatinous cupula.

Relationship between the Direction of Force and Hair Cell Activation

The adequate stimulus for hair cell activation is a force acting parallel to the top of the cell resulting in bending of the hairs (a shearing force).[8, 64] A force applied perpendicular to the cell surface (a compressional force) is ineffective in stimulating the hair cell.[6, 16, 25] The stimulus is maximal when the force is directed along an axis that bisects the bundle of stereocilia and goes through the kinocilium (Fig. 9). Deflection of the hairs toward the kinocilium decreases the resting membrane potential of the sensory cells (depolarization). Bending in the opposite direction

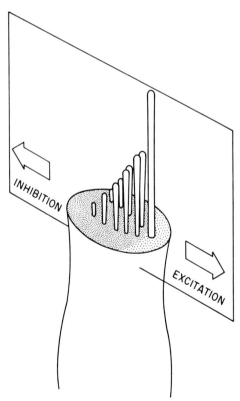

Figure 9. Relationship between the direction of force and hair cell activation. (From Flock, Å.: Sensory transduction in hair cells. In Lowenstein, W. R. (ed.): *Handbook of Sensory Physiology, Principles of Receptor Physiology*, vol. 1. Springer-Verlag, New York, 1971, with permission.)

produces the reverse effect (hyperpolarization).[27,28] The effect is minimal when the hair deflection is perpendicular to the axis of maximal excitation.

Physiologic Characteristics of Hair Cell Activation

The molecular process that produces excitation of the hair cell is believed to result from a change in electric conductance of the cell membrane produced by mechanical deformation of the surface of the cell during displacement of the hairs (Fig. 10).[20,37,66] The hair-bearing surface of the cell membrane is morphologically different from the rest, being thicker and more electron-dense. Its ohmic resistance changes in proportion to the magnitude of the hair deflection during physiologic stimulation, causing a modulated leakage of electric currents in a local circuit between other areas of the cell membrane and the top. The voltage drop produced in the vicinity of the hair cells by the changing current is known as the microphonic potential, the so-called generator potential of these receptor organs.[34,72] The generator potential follows the frequency of the stimulus and increases almost linearly with its magnitude. In contrast to nerve action potentials the microphonics have no refractory period (following the frequency of the stimulation above several thousand Hz), are highly resistant to anoxia, and may remain partially active after the animal's death. The electric current associated with the generator potentials acts upon the synaptic contacts between the hair cells and the nerve terminals either directly or by activating chemical transmitters to modulate the firing of action potentials by the afferent neurons.

Most of the basic information regarding the physiologic properties of hair cells and their afferent nerves has been obtained through a study of hair cell systems in nonmammalian species. Analysis of the lateral line organs of fish and amphibians

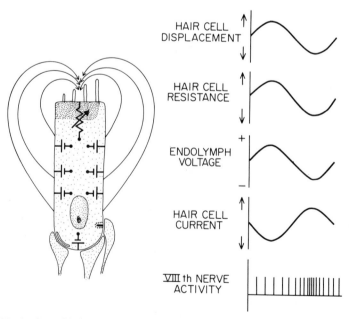

Figure 10. Mechanism of hair cell activation. Sinusoidal displacement of the stereocilia produces a sinusoidal modulation of the vestibular nerve firing rate. See text for details.

have been particularly useful. These organs consist of groups of hair cells, neuromasts, aligned in longitudinal rows on the side of the animal's body and head.[22] A free-standing gelatinous cupula covering the hairs transmits the force associated with water displacement into hair cell deflection that in turn results in a change in firing rate of the afferent nerve.

One of the most significant findings concerning hair cell function was the discovery by Hoagland in 1932 that the afferent nerves from lateral line organs generated continuous spontaneous activity.[36] This observation has subsequently been confirmed in all other hair cell systems and represents a fundamental discovery in sensory physiology. While the mechanism responsible for the spontaneous firing of action potentials in the afferent nerves has not been identified, depolarization and hyperpolarization of the hair cells' membrane potential result in a modulation of this spontaneous activity. Bending of the hairs toward the kinocilium results in an increase of the spontaneous firing rate and bending of the hairs away from the kinocilium results in a decrease.[46] The spontaneous firing rate varies among different animal species and among different sensory receptors. It is thought to be greatest in the afferent neurons of the semicircular canals of mammals (up to 90 spikes per second) and lowest in some of the acoustic nerve fibers innervating mammalian cochlear hair cells (1 to 2 spikes per second). [32, 40]

Basis for Stimulus Specificity of Inner Ear Receptor Organs

As suggested earlier, the density of the otolithic membrane overlying the hair cells of the macules is greater than that of the surrounding endolymph. The weight of this membrane produces a shearing force (F_t) on the underlying hair cells that is proportional to the sine of the angle between the line of resulting gravitational vector and a line perpendicular to the plane of the macule. The hair cell cilia in the cristae of the semicircular canals are embedded in the cupula, a jelly-like substance of the same specific gravity as that of the surrounding fluids. The cupula therefore does not exert a force on the underlying crista and is not subject to displacement by changes in the line of gravitational force. The forces associated with angular head acceleration, however, do result in a displacement of the cupula that stimulates the hair cells of the crista in the same way that displacement of the otoliths stimulates the macular hair cells.

In the cochlea the hair cells are mounted on the flexible basilar membrane in the organ of Corti. Covering the organ of Corti and resting over the hair cell is the tectorial membrane, a relatively rigid structure attached to the wall of the cochlea. A small acoustically induced pressure difference across the basilar membrane causes the organ of Corti and hair cells to vibrate at the frequency of sound. When the basilar membrane moves, the hair cells are displaced in relationship to the relatively fixed tectorial membrane (acting as a hinge).[7]

In all cases the effective stimulus to the sensory cells is the relative displacement of the cilia produced by application of mechanical force to their surroundings. Since the mechanical properties of the "supporting and coupling" structures are different the frequency ranges at which the cilia can be moved by the applied force are different. The otoconia are maximally displaced during accelerations such as those associated with steady head displacement, but their motion rapidly diminishes if the linear acceleration changes at a frequency greater than 0.5 Hz due to the characteristics of the restraining visco-elastic forces holding the otoliths to the macule.[69] The semicircular canals respond maximally to constant angular acceleration but their sensitivity diminishes when the head acceleration changes sinusoidally at increasing frequencies. At frequencies greater than 5 to 10 Hz, their sensitivity is minimal. This frequency limitation is due to the inertial and viscous forces restraining the displacement of fluid and cupula in the narrow semicircular canals. Because of the great flexibility of the basilar membrane the range of sound frequencies to which the hair cells in the cochlea are sensitive varies from 20 to 20,000 Hz.

ORGANIZATION OF CENTRAL VESTIBULAR PATHWAYS

Vestibular Reflexes

The basic elements of a simple vestibular reflex arc are the hair cell, an afferent bipolar neuron, an interneuron and an effector neuron.[45] The terminal fibers of the afferent neuron make synaptic contact with the hair cell and transmit nerve signals to the nervous system where, by means of the interneuron, a connection is made with the effector neuron. The effector neuron in turn controls the activity in an appropriate muscle or makes connections with neurons from other sensory reflex arcs (vision, proprioception) to coordinate orienting behavior.[38,45] This simple three neuron reflex arc is already developed in the phylum *Mollusca,* among which the class *Cephalopoda* has contributed to many classic anatomic and physiologic studies of gravitational reflexes.[13] An example of a three neuron vestibular reflex in man is the semicircular canal-ocular reflex. Angular acceleration to the right in the plane of the horizontal canals results in an increased firing of the afferent nerve from the ampulla of the right horizontal semicircular canal. This afferent signal is carried to the vestibular nucleus situated in the dorsolateral medulla. A neuron in the vestibular nucleus then transmits the signal to an effector neuron in the left abducens nucleus. Contraction of the left lateral rectus muscle initiates the compensatory deviation of the left eye to the left.

This simple example obviously does not provide the entire picture of the organization of the canal-ocular reflexes since it does not take into account the bilateral symmetrical canal system and the need for excitation and inhibition of four different horizontal ocular muscles. With head rotation to the right in the plane of the horizontal canals, an increase in firing of the right horizontal ampullary nerve is accompanied by a decrease in the corresponding left nerve. In addition, some of the interneurons are inhibitory and by means of these two classes of neurons the afferent signal coming from the ampullary nerve exerts a dual influence on the effector system: it excites the agonist group of muscles and inhibits the antagonist group of muscles.

The control of motor responses by the labyrinth is therefore a four-way mechanism (Fig. 11). Stimulation of a receptor in the right (R) labyrinth increases the output of the afferent neurons, exerting an increased excitatory influence on the agonist ($\uparrow$R$^+$) and inhibitory influence on the antagonist ($\uparrow$R$^-$) groups of muscles. Because of the symmetry between the two labyrinths, the same receptor in the other ear simultaneously diminishes its afferent output, thereby disfacilitating the excitatory influence ($\downarrow$L$^+$) in the antagonist muscle and disinhibiting the agonist muscle ($\downarrow$L$^-$). The end result in the horizontal canal-ocular reflex is contraction of the left lateral and right medial rectus muscles and relaxation of the left medial and right lateral rectus muscles. This general plan of organization applies to all labyrinthine-mediated reflexes.

14

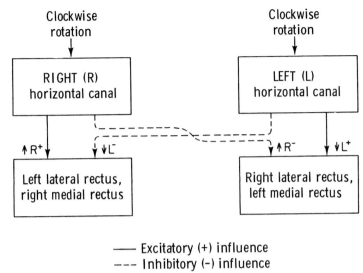

——— Excitatory (+) influence
– – – Inhibitory (–) influence

Figure 11. Organization of the horizontal semicircular canal-ocular reflex.

Interaction with Other Systems

The maintenance of body equilibrium and posture and appreciation of spatial orientation in everyday life are complex functions involving multiple receptor organs and neural centers in addition to the labyrinths. Visual and proprioceptive reflexes in particular must be integrated with vestibular reflexes to insure postural stability. For example, during most natural head movements, gaze stabilization is achieved by vestibular, neck proprioceptive and visual interaction. When the vestibularly induced eye movements lie in a direction opposite to that required to maintain the desired gaze position the visual reflexes override the vestibular reflex. The kind of head rotation that would produce compensatory eye movement in the dark does not do so in the light if the subject can fixate on a target moving in phase with his head (Fig. 12). The vestibulocerebellum (flocculonodular lobes) is important for mediating visual-vestibular interaction.[38, 63] Animals who have undergone cerebellectomy and humans with cerebellar lesions are unable to inhibit vestibular signals with visual fixation.[67, 68] Electrophysiologic studies in animals reveal that floccular Purkinje cells receive primary vestibular afferent signals and visual signals and in turn send out Purkinje cell impulses to second-order neurons of the vestibulo-ocular reflex arc.[3, 57] These cells apparently "compare" visual and vestibular signals and if the signals are in conflict with each other the characteristics of the vestibular response change at the level of the vestibular nucleus.[56]

The input from cervical proprioceptive receptors acts in combination with that from the labyrinth to maintain ocular stability during simultaneous head and neck movements.[9] The proprioceptive signals orginate from receptors deep in the ligaments and joints of the upper cervical vertebrae (C1 to C3) and interact at the vestibular nucleus with afferent vestibular signals.[18, 58] Stimulation of the neck joint receptors activates neurons in the contralateral vestibular nucleus that are

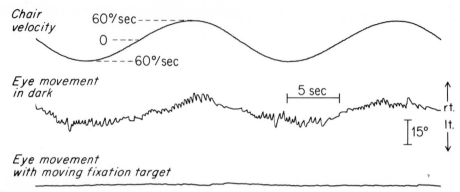

Figure 12. Eye movement induced in a normal human subject by sinusoidal angular acceleration (0.05 Hz, maximum velocity 60 deg/sec) in the dark and in the light with a target moving in phase with the subject.

part of the semicircular canal-ocular reflex pathway. Turning the head to the right stretches the joint ligaments and thereby activates receptors in the left side of the neck. This activity excites neurons in the right vestibular nucleus which in turn excites neurons in the left abducens nucleus.[35] The pathways responsible for vestibulocervical interaction are illustrated in Figure 13. In addition, inhibitory interneurons in the vestibular nuclei are stimulated by afferent nerve signals from the neck so as to maintain the necessary balance between excitation of agonist muscles and inhibition of antagonist muscles. For simplification commissural pathways between the right and left vestibular nuclei and pathways to the medial recti are omitted. Compared to the labyrinthine input to the vestibular nuclei, cervical input normally is minor and its interruption results in minimal functional loss.

ABNORMAL LABYRINTHINE FUNCTION

Much of our knowledge about labyrinthine function was accumulated at the turn of the century from clinical and experimental observations in humans and animals with unilateral and bilateral lesions of the peripheral labyrinth.[11, 24, 29, 49] At that time, a controversy existed concerning whether the symptoms associated with loss of labyrinthine function were due to irritation or paralysis of the affected labyrinth. The subsequent discovery of the continuous flow of action potentials in the unstimulated vestibular nerve led to the present concept that symptoms are usually caused by an imbalance of the normal resting state activity—by a unilateral decrease in activity; occasionally, such as during an acute attack of unilateral Meniere's syndrome, the symptoms result from an increase in activity.

The magnitude of symptoms and signs following labyrinthine lesions depends on 1) the extent of the lesion, 2) whether the lesion is unilateral or bilateral and 3) the rapidity with which the functional loss occurs. In most experimental animals simultaneous removal of both labyrinths does not produce severe abnormalities although vestibular reflex activity is lost and ocular and postural stability is impaired. Similarly, patients who have slowly lost vestibular function bilaterally (for example, secondary to streptomycin treatment) may not complain of any symptoms referrable to the vestibular loss. If closely questioned, however, they report visual blurring or oscillopsia with head movements and instability when

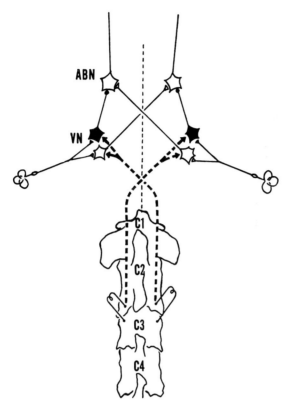

Figure 13. Diagram of cervicovestibular pathways. VN, vestibular nucleus, ABN, abducens nucleus, inhibitory interneurons in black. (From Hikosaka, O. and Maeda, M.: *Cervical effects on abducens motoneurons and their interaction with vestibulo-ocular reflex.* Exp. Brain Res. 18:512, 1973, with permission.)

walking at night (due to loss of vestibulo-ocular and vestibulospinal reflex activity).

In contrast, animals and humans develop severe symptoms and signs following unilateral labyrinthectomy. Lower mammals are initially unable to walk and develop head torsion toward the healthy side and decreased ipsilateral muscle tone. Nystagmus is prominent with the slow component directed toward the damaged side and the fast component toward the intact side. These signs abate with time but may remain for months after the operation.[16, 49]

A sudden unilateral loss of labyrinthine function in humans is a dramatic event. The patient complains of severe dizziness and nausea and is pale and perspiring and usually vomits repeatedly. He prefers to lie quietly but can walk if forced to (deviating toward the side of the lesion). Neck torsion and changes in extremity tone rarely occur. A brisk spontaneous nystagmus interferes with vision. These symptoms and signs are temporary and the process of compensation starts almost immediately. Within one week of the labyrinthine lesion a young patient can walk without difficulty and, with fixation, can inhibit the spontaneous nystagmus. Within one month most patients return to work with little, if any, residual symptoms. If a patient slowly loses vestibular function on one side over a period

17

of months or years (e.g. with a vestibular schwannoma) symptoms and signs may be absent.

APPROACH TO EVALUATION OF VESTIBULAR FUNCTION

Tests for vestibular function, as for function of other sensory systems, may be placed in two general categories: 1) those relying on a subjective response by the patient and 2) those relying on objective measurements of reflex activity. Although simple in concept, quantification of the sensation of movement derived from excitation of the vestibular receptors has been a difficult task for the clinician. With rotatory stimulation it is often impossible for the patient to differentiate those sensations that are strictly vestibular from tactile and proprioceptive sensations. Since vestibular sensations are more ambiguous than those produced by, for example, auditory or visual stimuli, the patient often has difficulty in sensing when the stimulus begins and ends and what its magnitude and direction of motion are. Even more important, the subjective awareness of vestibular stimulation depends on one's general state of alertness and degree of cooperation. Due to these difficulties with tests of subjective sensation, clinicians have increasingly turned their attention to objective tests to identify and quantify the components of vestibular reflex activity.

The vestibulo-ocular reflexes in particular have been extensively evaluated. The neurons in this reflex arc connect the labyrinthine receptor organs with the 12 extra-ocular muscles of the eyes, so that it should be possible to correlate vestibular lesions with impairment of function of the extra-ocular muscles through measurement of eye movements. Although experimental investigations of the vestibulo-ocular reflexes were initiated in the first quarter of this century, the contribution of each receptor organ and neural connection to the production of eye movements is still not completely known. The afferent signals from different vestibular receptors to each of the eye muscles overlap and the central neural pathways lie so close to each other that it is difficult to identify the receptor or pathway responsible for the deterioration of vestibular function. Nevertheless, the application of new methods of stimulation and quantification of reflexes has advanced to the level where substanial improvements in the diagnosis of vestibular disease are taking place. Through the combined work of basic and clinical investigators, a large number of observations are being made and integrated into an organized, logical picture of vestibular pathophysiology.

REFERENCES

1. ADES, H. W., AND ENGSTROM, H.: Form and innervation of the vestibular epithelia. In *Symposium on the Role of the Vestibular Organs in the Exploration of Space*. U.S. Naval School of Aviat. Med., Pensacola, Florida, 1965. NASA SP-77.

2. BAIRD, I. L.: Some aspects of the comparative anatomy and evolution of the inner ear in submammalian vertebrates. In Riss, W. (ed.): *Brain, Behavior and Evolution*. S. Karger, Basel, 1974.

3. BAKER, R. G., PRECHT, W., AND LLÍNAS, R.: *Cerebellar modullatory action on the vestibulotrochlear pathway in the cat*. Exp. Brain Res. 15:364, 1973.

4. BARD, P.: Postural coordination and locomotion and their central control. In Bard. P. (ed.): *Medical Physiology*, ed. 11. C. V. Mosby, Philadelphia, 1961.

5. BARLOW, J. S.: *Inertial navigation as a basis for animal navigation*. J. Theoret. Biol. 6:76, 1964.

6. BAUKNIGHT, R. S., STRELIOFF, D., AND HONRUBIA, V.: *Effective stimulus for the Xenopuslaevis lateral-line hair-cell system*. Laryngoscope 86:1836, 1976.

7. VON BÉKÉSY, G.: Experimental models of cochlea with and without nerve supply. In Rasmussen, G. L., Windle, W. F. (eds): *Neural Mechanisms of the Auditory and Vestibular System*. Charles C Thomas, Springfield, 1960.

8. VON BÉKÉSY, G.: *Pressure and shearing forces as stimuli of labyrinthine epithelium*. Arch. Otolaryngol. 84:122, 1966.

9. BIZZI, E., KALIL, R. E., AND TAGLIASCO, V.: *Eye-head coordination in monkeys: Evidence for centrally patterned organization*. Science 173:452, 1971.

10. BREUER, J.: *Über die Funktion der Bogengänge des Ohrlabyrinthes*. Wien. Med. Jahrb. 4:72, 1874.

11. BREUER, J.: *Über die Funktion der Otolithen-Apparate*. Pflügers Arch. Ges. Physiol. 48:195, 1891.

12. BRODÉL, M.: *Three Unpublished Drawings of the Anatomy of the Human Ear*. W. B. Saunders Co., Philadelphia, 1946.

13. BUDELMAN, B. U.: *Structure and function of the angular acceleration receptor systems in the statocysts of cephalopods*. Symp. Zool. Soc. London 38:309, 1977.

14. BUDELMAN, B. U., AND THIES, G.: *Secondary sensory cells in the gravity receptor system of the statocyst of Octopus vulgaris*. Cell. Tiss. Res. 182:93, 1977.

15. CAJAL, S.: *Histologie due Système nerveaux de l'homme et des Vertébrés*. Maloine, Paris, vols. 1 and 2, 1909.

16. CAMIS, M.: *La Fisiologia dell'Apparato Vestibolare*. Bologna, Zanichelli, 1928. Translated by R. S. Creed: *The Physiology of the Vestibular Apparatus*. Oxford, Clarendon, 1930.

17. COLLEWIJN, H.: *Oculomotor reactions in cuttlefish Sepia officinalis*. J. Exp. Biol. 52:369, 1970.

18. CORBIN, K. B., AND HINSE, J. C.: *Intramedullary course of the dorsal root fibers of each of the first four cervical nerves*. J. Comp. Neurol. 63:119, 1935.

19. CRUM-BROWN, A.: *On the sense of rotation and the anatomy and physiology of the semicircular canals of the internal ear*. J. Anat. Physiol. 8:327, 1874.

20. DAVIS, H.: *A model for transducer action in the cochlea*. Cold Spring Harbor Symp. Quant. Biol. 30:181, 1965.

21. DIJKGRAAF, S.: *Nystagmus and related phenomena in Sepia officinalis*. Experientia 19:29, 1963.

22. DIJKGRAAF, S.: *The functioning and significance of the lateral-line organs*. Biol. Rev. 38:51, 1962.

23. DOW, R. S.: *The effects of unilateral and bilateral labyrinthectomy in monkey, baboon and chimpanzee*. Am. J. Physiol. 121:392, 1938.

24. EWALD, J.: *Physiolgische Untersuchungen über das Endorgan des Nervus Octavus*. Bergmann, Wiesbaden, 1892.

25. FERNÁNDEZ, C., AND GOLDBERG, J. M.: *Physiology of peripheral neurons innervating otolith organs of the squirrel monkey. II. Directional selectivity and force-response relations*. J. Neurophysiol. 39:985, 1976.

26. FLOCK, Å.: Sensory transduction in hair cells. In Lowenstein, W. R. (ed.): *Handbook of Sensory Physiology, Principles of Receptor Physiology*, vol. 1. Springer-Verlag, New York, 1971.

27. FLOCK, Å., JORGENSEN, M., AND RUSSELL, I.: The physiology of individual hair cells and their synapses. In Miller, A. (ed.): *Basic Mechanisms in Hearing*. Academic Press, New York, 1973.

28. FLOCK, Å.: Transduction mechanism in the lateral line canal organ receptors. *Cold Spring Harbor Symp. Quant. Biol.* 30:133, 1965.

29. FLOURENS, P.: *Recherches Expérimentales sur les Propriétés et les Fonctions du Système Nerveux dans les Animaux Vertébrés*. Crevot, Paris, 1842.

30. FULTON, J. F., LIDDELL, E. G. T., AND RIOCH, D. McK.: *The influence of unilateral destruction of the vestibular nuclei upon posture and knee jerk*. Brain 53:327, 1930.

31. GACEK, R.: Efferent component of the vestibular nerve. In Rasmussen, G., and Windle, W. (eds.): *Neural Mechanisms of the Auditory and Vestibular Systems*. Charles C Thomas, Springfield, 1960.

32. GOLDBERG, J. M., AND FERNÁNDEZ, C.: *Physiology of peripheral neurons innervating semicircular canals of the squirrel monkey. I. Resting discharge and response to constant angular accelerations*. J. Neurophysiol. 34:635, 1971.

33. GRAY, O.: *A brief survey of the phylogenesis of the labyrinth*. J. Laryngol. 69:151, 1955.

34. HARRIS, G. G., FRISHKOPF, F. S., AND FLOCK, Å.: *Receptor potentials from hair cells of the lateral line*. Science 167:76, 1970.

19

35. HIKOSAKA, O., AND MAEDA, M.: *Cervical effects on abducens motoneurons and their interaction with vestibulo-ocular reflex.* Exp. Brain Res. 18:512, 1973.

36. HOAGLAND, H.: *Impulses from sensory nerves of catfish.* Proc. Nat. Acad. Sci., Washington, 18:701, 1932.

37. HONRUBIA, V., STRELIOFF, D., AND SITKO, S. T.: *Physiological basis of cochlear transduction and sensitivity.* Ann. Otol. Rhinol. Laryngol. 85:697, 1976.

38. ITO, M.: The vestibulo-cerebellar relationships: vestibulo-ocular reflex arc and flocculus. In Naunton, R. F. (ed.): *The Vestibular System.* Academic Press, New York and London, 1975.

39. KAPPERS, C. U. A., HUBER, G. C., AND CROSBY, E. D.: *The Comparative Anatomy of the Nervous System of Vertebrates, Including Man.* MacMillan, New York, 1936.

40. KIANG, N. Y. S., ET AL.: *Discharge Patterns of Single Fibers in the Cat's Auditory Nerve.* Res. Monograph 35, M.I.T. Press, Cambridge, 1965.

41. KRIGE, W. G. F.: *Functional Neuroanatomy,* ed. 2. Blakiston Co., New York, 1953.

42. LOEB, J.: *Forced Movements, Tropisms and Animal Conduct.* J. B. Lippincott Co., Philadelphia and London, 1918.

43. LORENTE DE NÓ, R.: *Anatomy of the eighth nerve. The central projection of the nerve endings of the internal ear.* Laryngoscope 43:1, 1933.

44. LORENTE DE NÓ, R., AND BERENS, C.: Nystagmus. In Piersol, G. M. and Bortz, E. L., (eds.): *Cyclopedia of Medicine, Surgery and Specialties,* vol. 9. F. A. Davis Company, Philadelphia, 1959.

45. LORENTE DE NÓ, R.: *Vestibulo-ocular reflex arc.* Arch. Neurol. Psych. 30:245, 1933.

46. LOWENSTEIN, O., AND WERSALL, J.: *A functional interpretation of the electron microscopic structure of the sensory hairs in the cristae of the elasmobranch Raja clavata in terms of directional sensitivity.* Nature 184:1807, 1959.

47. LOWENSTEIN, O. E.: Comparative morphology and physiology. In Kornhuber, H. H. (ed.): *Handbook of Sensory Physiology,* vol. VI, part 2. Springer-Verlag, New York, 1974.

48. MACH, E.: *Grundlinien der Lehre von den Bewegungsempfindungen.* Engelmann, Leipzig, 1875 (Translation: Bonset, Amsterdam, 1967).

49. MAGNUS, R.: *Körperstellung.* Springer-Verlag, Berlin, 1924.

50. MAGNUS, R.: *On the cooperation and interference of reflexes from other sense organs with those of the labyrinths.* Laryngoscope 36:701, 1926.

51. MAGNUS, R.: *Some results of studies in the physiology of posture. I.* Lancet 2:531, 1926.

52. MAGNUS, R.: *Some results of studies in the physiology of posture. II.* Lancet 2:585, 1926.

53. MARKL, H.: The perception of gravity and of angular acceleration in invertebrates. In Kornhuber, H. H. (ed.): *Handbook of Sensory Physiology,* vol. VI, part 2. Springer-Verlag, New York, 1974.

54. MAXWELL, S. S.: *Labyrinth and Equilibrium.* Lippincott, Philadelphia and London, 1923.

55. MELVILL-JONES, G.: Organization of neural control in the vestibulo-ocular reflex arc. In Bach-Y-Rita, P., Collins, C. C., and Hyde, J. E. (eds.): *The Control of Eye Movements.* Academic Press, New York, 1971.

56. MILES, F. A.: *Single unit firing patterns in the vestibular nuclei related to voluntary eye movements and passive body rotation in conscious monkeys.* Brain Res. 71:215, 1974.

57. MILES, F. A., AND FULLER, J. H.: *Visual tracking and the primate flocculus.* Science 189:1000, 1975.

58. McCOUCH, G. P., DEERING, I. D., AND LING, T. H.: *Location of receptors for tonic neck reflexes.* J. Neurophysiol. 14:191, 1951.

59. MEHLER, W. R.: Comparative anatomy of the vestibular nuclear complex in submammalian vertebrates. In Brodal, A. and Pompeiano, O. (eds.): *Basic Aspects of Central Vestibular Mechanisms.* Elsevier Publishing Co., New York, 1972.

60. MONEY, K. E., ET AL.: *Physical properties of fluids and structures of vestibular apparatus of the pigeon.* Am. J. Physiol. 220:140, 1971.

61. PURKINJÉ, J. E.: *Beiträge zur näheren Kenntnis des Schwindels aus heautognostischen Daten.* Med. Jahrb. (Wien.) 6:79, 1820.

62. RASMUSSEN, G.: *The olivary peduncle and other fiber projections of the superior olivary complex.* J. Comp. Neurol. 84:141, 1946.

63. ROBINSON, D. A.: *Adaptive gain control of vestibulo-ocular reflex by the cerebellum.* J. Neurophysiol. 39:954, 1976.

64. SCHÖNE, H.: Gravity receptors and gravity orientation in Crustacea. In Gordon, S., and Cohen, M. (eds.): *Gravity and Organism.* University of Chicago Press, Chicago, 1971.

65. SMITH, C. A.: *The Nervous System,* vol. 3. Raven Press, New York, 1975.

66. STRELIOFF, D., HAAS, G., AND HONRUBIA, V.: *Sound-induced electrical impedance changes in the guinea pig cochlea.* J. Acoust. Soc. Am. 51:617, 1972.

67. TAKEMORI, S., AND COHEN, B.: *Loss of visual suppression of vestibular nystagmus after flocculus lesions.* Brain Res. 72:213, 1974.

68. TAKEMORI, S.: *Visual suppression test.* Ann. Otol. Rhinol. Laryngol. 86:80, 1977.

69. DE VRIES, H.: *The mechanics of labyrinth otoliths.* Acta Otolaryngol. 38:262, 1950.

70. WERSÄLL, J.: Electron micrographic studies of vestibular hair cell innervation. In Rasmussen, G. L. and Windle, W. F. (eds.): *Neural Mechanisms of the Auditory and Vestibular System.* Charles C Thomas, Springfield, 1960.

71. WERSÄLL, D. J., AND BAGGER-SJÖBÄCK, D.: Morphology of the vestibular sense organs. In Kornhuber, H. H. (ed.): *Handbook of Sensory Physiology,* vol. VI, part 2. Springer-Verlag, New York, 1974.

72. WEVER, E., AND BRAY, C.: *The nature of acoustic response: The relation between sound intensity and the magnitude of responses in the cochlea.* J. Exper. Psychol. 19:129, 1936.

73. WOLFF, H. G.: *Efferente Aktivität in den Statonerven einiger Landpulmonaten (Gastropoda).* Z. Vergl. Physiol. 70:401, 1970.

74. WOLFF, H. G.: *Einige Ergebnisse zur Ultrastruktur der Statocysten von Limax maximus, Limax flavus und Arion empiricorum (Pulmonata).* Z. Zellforsch. 100:251, 1969.

CHAPTER 2

The Peripheral Vestibular System

THE EAR

The ear is a compound organ sensitive to sound and the forces associated with linear and angular acceleration. It is divided into three anatomic parts: the external, middle and inner ear. Except for the auricle and soft tissue portion of the external auditory canal the ear is enclosed within the temporal bone of the skull.

Temporal Bone

The temporal bone contributes to the base and lateral wall of the skull and forms part of the middle and posterior fossae.[3] It is divided into four parts: the squamous, mastoid, petrous and tympanic (Fig. 14). The tympanic portion, the smallest, forms the anterior, inferior, and part of the posterior wall of the external auditory canal. The petrous portion or pyramid contains the sense organs of the inner ear. The seventh and eighth cranial nerves enter the petrous portion through the internal auditory canal; the facial nerve exits via the stylomastoid foramen of the mastoid portion (Fig. 15). The internal carotid artery and internal jugular vein enter the skull through the temporal bone, their bony canals forming part of the antero-inferior wall of the middle ear.

The cross section of the temporal bone in Figure 16 illustrates the relationship between the three parts of the ear. Although the external and middle ear are auditory organs with no direct bearing on vestibular function, a knowledge of their structure and development, particularly that of the middle ear, is important for understanding diseases involving the inner ear.[55] For example, infection arising in the middle ear can spread directly through its medial wall into the inner ear or it can enter the intracranial cavity by breaking through the roof of the epitympanic recess. Passageways interconnect the epitympanic recess and air cells throughout the temporal bone so that infection beginning in the middle ear can spread to the vessels and nerves passing through the temporal bone.

Tympanic Membrane

The ear drum or tympanic membrane forms a partition between the external and middle ear.[3] The tympanic membrane has a thickness of 0.1 mm and a diameter of 8.5 to 10 mm. It consists of three layers: an inner mucosal layer, a middle fibrous layer and an external epidermal layer. It is attached to the tympanic ring in the external canal at a distance of 2 to 5 mm from the opposite (medial) wall of the

23

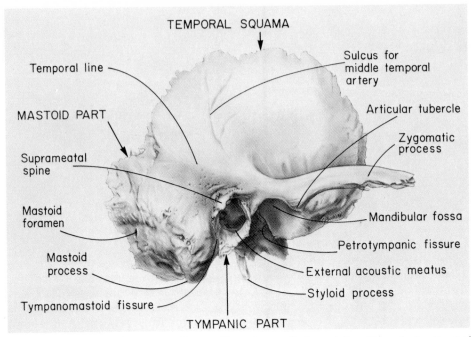

TEMPORAL SQUAMA

Temporal line

Sulcus for middle temporal artery

MASTOID PART

Articular tubercle

Zygomatic process

Suprameatal spine

Mastoid foramen

Mandibular fossa

Petrotympanic fissure

Mastoid process

External acoustic meatus

Styloid process

Tympanomastoid fissure

TYMPANIC PART

Figure 14. Lateral view of temporal bone. (From Anson, B. J., and Donaldson, J. A.: *Surgical Anatomy of the temporal Bone and Ear.* W. B. Saunders Co., Philadelphia, 1973, with permission.)

middle ear. From the external canal the tympanic membrane appears as a thin semitransparent disc that normally has a glistening pearly-gray color (see Fig. 49a, Chapter 4). It is concave on its external surface as if under traction from the manubrium of the malleus. The mallear stria (the manubrium shining through the tympanic membrane) passes from slightly inferior and posterior of the center (umbo) toward the superior margin of the tympanic membrane. Near the superior margin the mallear prominence is formed by the lateral process of the malleus. From the mallear prominence two folds stretch to the tympanic sulcus of the temporal bone enclosing the triangular area of the pars flaccida or Shrapnell's membrane.

Middle Ear

Functional Anatomy

The middle ear or tympanic cavity is a flat cleft with a volume of approximately 2.0 cc containing an assembly of tiny bones whose main role is to provide an interface for transmitting to the inner ear the changes in atmospheric pressure produced by sound waves.[11, 95] The long (5.8 mm) process of the malleus, the manubrium, is attached like the radius of a circle to the inner side of the tympanic membrane in a supero-anterior direction. Superiorly, the head of the malleus is bound to the incus, forming the incudomalleal articulation, a type of diarthric joint. The so-called long process of the incus (7 mm), directed down and anteriorly, is connected to the stapes, the smallest of the three middle ear ossicles. The footplate of the stapes articulates with the walls of the vestibule at the oval window to which it is attached by a ring of ligaments. The dimensions of the window are 1.2 by 3 mm with a total area that is one seventeenth that of the

24

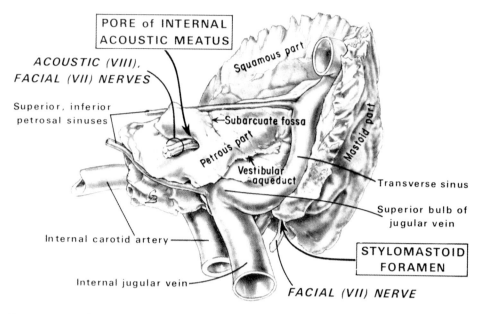

Figure 15. Medial view of temporal bone. (From Anson, B. J., and Donaldson, J. A.: *Surgical Anatomy of the Temporal Bone and Ear*. W. B. Saunders Co., Philadelphia, 1973, with permission.)

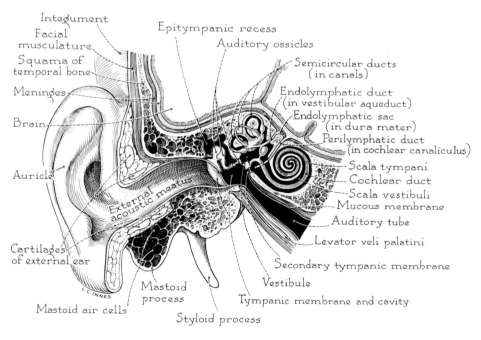

Figure 16. Cross section of the ear. (From Anson, B. J., and Donaldson, J. A.: *Surgical Anatomy of the Temporal Bone and Ear*. W. B. Saunders Co., Philadelphia, 1973, with permission.)

25

tympanic membrane. Sound-induced displacements of the tympanic membrane and its attached manubrium are transmitted through the medial arm of the assembly of middle ear bones acting as a lever to the inner ear; in this fashion the middle ear functions as a mechanical transformer. Additional amplification is produced as the force applied over the surface of the tympanic membrane is funneled into the smaller area of the oval window. The middle ear compensates for the loss of energy that would occur if sound were directly transmitted from air to the fluids of the inner ear. Without the middle ear structures approximately 99.9 percent of the sound energy would be lost during this transmission.[95]

The ossicles are suspended by several ligaments and are dynamically controlled by the action of two muscles. The tensor tympani, innervated by a branch of the trigeminal nerve, is connected by a tendon into the upper part of the manubrium. Coursing in a lateral direction from the anterior part of the medial wall of the tympanic cavity, this muscle draws the manubrium medially, tensing the tympanic membrane. The stapedius muscle, innervated by the facial nerve, is attached to the posterior wall of the tympanic cavity and is directed anteriorly to anchor in the upper part of the stapes. Its contraction hinders the transmission of sound to the inner ear.

Boundaries

For descriptive purposes the tympanic cavity can be thought of as being bounded by six walls facing one another in pairs. The *lateral* wall in large part is made up of the cone-shaped tympanic membrane. The *medial* or labyrinthine wall is an irregular surface because of structures bulging from the inner ear: the promontory of the basal turn of the cochlea and the prominences of the facial canal and horizontal semicircular canal. Beneath the cochlear prominence is the membrane of the cochlea or round window which seals the scala tympani of the cochlea and its fluid from the middle ear. It provides an outlet for equilibrium of pressure in the inner ear whenever sound displaces the stapes. Without this compliance sound energy could not displace the basilar membrane of the cochlea since the endolymph fluid is incompressible. The vestibular or oval window is located just above the cochlear prominence where it is closed by the base of the stapes and the annular ligament.

The *anterior* wall of the tympanic cavity is marked by three important structures: the eustachian tube orifice, the wall of the carotid canal and the opening of the channel for insertion of the tensor tympani muscle. The eustachian tube connects the middle ear cavity with the nasopharynx, providing ventilation of the tympanic cavity spaces. The tubal orifice at the nasopharynx is normally closed but during deglutition it opens due to the contraction of palate muscles which attach to the cartilage and elastic ligaments in the opening. The most important of the muscles, the tensor veli palate, is innervated by the trigeminal nerve. In the embryo, the eustachian tube is an extension of the pharyngeal pouch between the first (mandibular) and second (hyoid) branchial arches. As the pouch of entodermal origin presses towards the temporal bone the mesenchymal tissue that fills the middle ear cavity of the fetus recedes.[4, 5] The epithelium of the pouch covers the tympanic cavity and mastoid forming an endless variety of small cavities in a process known as pneumatization. This process takes place during the third to seventh month of fetal life. Two main cavities result: the epitympanic recess in the upper part of the tympanic cavity and the mastoid antrum located posteriorly to the tympanic cavity. The antrum is lined with mucus membrane continuous with that of both the tympanic and epitympanic cavities. It communicates with the epitympanum by an aperture, the aditus ad antrum, in the posterior side of the epitympanic recess. The antrum is a relatively large, irregular, bean-shaped cavity about 1 cm long. Many mastoid air cells open into this cavity located behind and below the antrum within the mastoid process of the temporal bone. Besides the antrum the *posterior* wall of the tympanic cavity contains an aperture transmitting the tendon of the stapedius muscle, a foramen by which the chorda tympani nerve enters the tympanic cavity and a fossa where the posterior ligament of the incus is attached.

The *roof* of the tympanic cavity is formed by the tegmen tympani, a thin plate of bone separating the epitympanic recess of the tympanic cavity from the middle cranial fossa. The *floor* is composed of the jugular bulb upon which are located irregular pneumatized cells.

Facial Nerve

The facial nerve arises at the inferior border of the pons and proceeds to the internal auditory canal on the superior surface of the cochlear nerve. Within the temporal bone four portions of the facial nerve can be classified: 1) the canal (meatal) segment (7 to 8 mm), 2) the labyrinthine segment (3 to 4 mm), 3) the tympanic (horizontal) segment (12 to 13 mm) and 4) the mastoid (vertical) segment (15 to 20 mm) (Fig. 17). The canal segment runs in close company with the vestibular and cochlear division of the eighth nerve while in its remaining segments the facial nerve lies separately within a bony canal, the facial or fallopian canal. The labyrinthine segment runs at nearly a right angle to the petrous pyramid

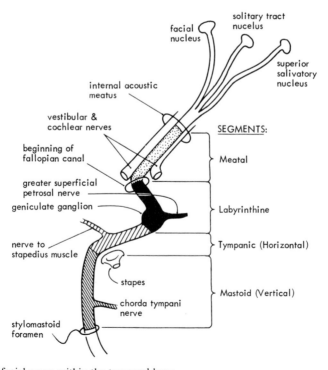

Figure 17. The facial nerve within the temporal bone.

27

superior to the cochlea and vestibule to reach the geniculate ganglion. At the geniculate ganglion the nerve takes a sharp turn posteriorly marking the beginning of the tympanic segment. The tympanic segment passes along the medial wall of the tympanic cavity superior to the oval window and inferior to the horizontal semicircular canal. At the sinus tympani the nerve bends inferiorly, marking the beginning of the mastoid segment.

Three major branches of the facial nerve lie within the temporal bone: 1) the greater superficial petrosal nerve arising from the geniculate ganglion, 2) the nerve to the stapedius muscle arising from the mastoid segment as it crosses the middle ear and 3) the chorda tympani leaving the facial nerve approximately 5 mm above the stylomastoid foramen.[19] The greater superficial petrosal nerve is composed of 1) parasympathetic efferent fibers originating in the superior salivatory nucleus for innervation of the lacrimal glands and seromucinous glands of the nasal cavity and 2) afferent cutaneous sensory fibers from parts of the external canal, tympanic membrane and middle ear destined for the nucleus of the solitary tract. The nerve to the stapedius muscle and the main facial nerve trunk are motor nerves originating from the facial nucleus in the caudal pons. The chorda tympani, like the greater superficial petrosal, is a mixed nerve containing 1) parasympathetic efferent fibers from the superior salivatory nucleus destined for the sublingual glands and 2) afferent taste fibers from the anterior two-thirds of the tongue ending in the nucleus of the solitary tract.

Knowledge of the structure and function of each division of the facial nerve allows the clinician to localize disease affecting the nerve within the temporal bone. Lesions in the internal auditory canal commonly involve both the seventh and eighth cranial nerves. Lesions of the labyrinthine segment of the facial nerve above the geniculate ganglion impair ipsilateral 1) lacrimation, 2) stapedius reflex activity, 3) taste on the anterior two-thirds of the tongue and 4) facial muscular strength. A lesion of the tympanic segment central to the nerve of the stapedius muscle affects only 2, 3 and 4 of the above and a lesion of the mastoid segment before the origin of the chorda tympani affects only 3 and 4. Finally, a lesion at the stylomastoid foramen causes only ipsilateral facial muscle weakness or paralysis.

Inner Ear

Bony Labyrinth

Within the petrous portion of the temporal bone a series of hollow channels, the bony labyrinth, contains the auditory and vestibular sensory organs (see Fig. 16). The bony labyrinth consists of an anterior cochlear part and a posterior vestibular part.[3] The vestibule is a central chamber (about 4 mm in diameter) marked by the recesses of the utricle and saccule. The superior and posterolateral walls contain openings for the three semicircular canals and anteriorly the vestibule is continuous with the scala vestibuli of the snail-shaped cochlea.

Medial to the bony labyrinth is the internal auditory canal, a cul-de-sac housing the seventh and eighth cranial nerves and internal auditory artery. The aperture on the cranial side is located at approximately the center of the posterior face of the pyramid of the temporal bone (see Fig. 15). Two other important orifices are in this vicinity. Halfway between the canal and the sigmoid sinus, the slit-like aperture of the vestibular aqueduct contains the endolymphatic sac, a structure important in the exchange of endolymph. The second opening is that of the cochlear aqueduct at the same level as the auditory canal but on the inferior side of the pyramid. The labyrinthine opening of this channel is located in the scala tympani, providing a connection between the subarachnoid and the perilymphatic spaces.

Membranous Labyrinth

The membranous labyrinth is enclosed within the channels of the bony labyrinth (Fig. 18). A space containing perilymphatic fluid, a supportive network of connective tissue and blood vessels lies between the periostium of the bony labyrinth and the membranous labyrinth; the spaces within the membranous labyrinth contain endolymphatic fluid. The endolymphatic system develops in the embryo as an invagination of the germinal ectodermal layer.[4] Starting as a simple fold it soon becomes a closed cavity, the otocyst, isolated from the original ectoderm. By the end of the seventh week the endolymphatic duct system is lodged in mesenchymal tissue and by the fourteenth week it attains the size that it will have in the adult ear. By successive infolding of the wall of the otocyst, three main areas are formed: the endolymphatic duct and sac, the utricle and semicircular canals and, lastly, the saccule and cochlear duct. The membranous cochlea holds the organ of Corti for the transduction of sound energy. The utricle, saccule and semicircular canals (the receptor organs for the sense of position and motion) constitute the membranous labyrinth proper. Finally, the endolymphatic duct provides a channel for the exchange of chemicals and to balance the pressure between the endolymphatic and subarachnoid spaces.

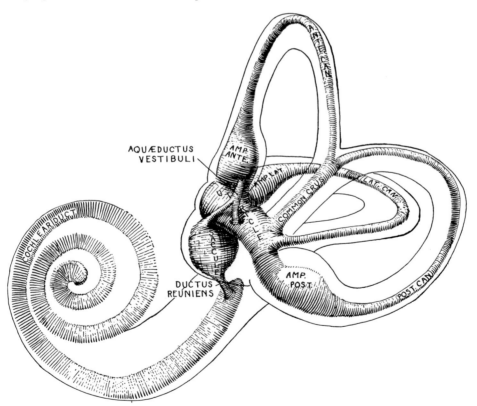

Figure 18.   The membranous labyrinth. (From Krieg, W. J. S.: *Functional Neuroanatomy*, ed. 2. Blakiston Co., New York, 1953, with permission.)

THE VESTIBULAR LABYRINTH

Structure of the Vestibular End Organs

Semicircular Canals

The semicircular canals are three membranous tubes with a cross-sectional diameter of 0.4 mm, each forming about two-thirds of a circle with a diameter of 6.5 mm.[42] They are aligned to form a coordinate system (Figs. 18 and 19b).[12] The horizontal semicircular canal with two openings on the lateral wall of the utricule makes a 30 degree angle with the horizontal plane. The other two canals are in a vertical position orthogonal to each other. The anterior one is directed medial and lateral over the roof of the utricle, and the posterior, behind the utricle, is directed down and lateral. The two vertical canals share a common opening on the posterior side of the utricle.

At the anterior opening of the horizontal and anterior canal and the inferior opening of the posterior canal, each tube enlarges to form the ampulla (see Fig. 18). A crest-like septum, the crista, crosses each ampulla in a perpendicular direction to the longitudinal axis of the canal (see Fig. 19a). It rests on the bone of the canal, and consists of sensory epithelium resting on a mound of connective tissue, where blood vessels and nerve fibers reach the sensory receptor area. Hair cells

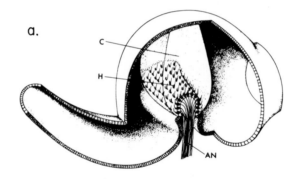

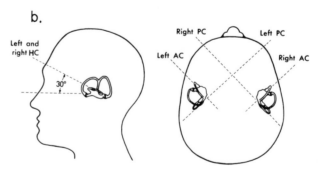

Figure 19. (a) The semicircular canal crista and (b) planes of individual semicircular canals. C, cupula, H, hair cells, AN, afferent nerve, HC, horizontal semicircular canal, AC, anterior semicircular canal, and PC, posterior semicircular canal. (From Barber, H. O., and Stockwell, C. W.: *Manual of Electronystagmography*. The C. V. Mosby Co., St. Louis, 1976, with permission.)

are located on the surface of the crista with their cilia protruding into the cupula, a gelatinous mass of the same composition as the otolithic membrane. The cupula extends from the surface of the crista to the ceiling of the ampulla, forming what appears to be a watertight seal.[42] A higher proportion of type I hair cells are located in the center of the crista than in the periphery (see Chapter 1 for definition of hair cell types). The margins of the crista contain zones of transitional epithelium, consisting of cells rich with infoldings believed to have secretory function (the so-called dark cells).[46] The hair cells cannot be regenerated after birth, so when they are damaged, function is lost permanently.[24]

The hair cells within each crista are all oriented with their kinocilium in the same direction. However, in the vertical canals the kinocilia are directed toward the canal side of the ampulla while in the horizontal canal the kinocilia are directed toward the utricular side.[94] The different morphologic polarization is the reason for the difference in directional sensitivity between the horizontal and vertical canals.[61] The afferent nerve fibers of the horizontal canals are stimulated by endolymph movement in the utricular or ampullopetal direction while those of the vertical canals are stimulated by ampullofugal endolymph flow.

Otoliths

The membranous labyrinth forms two globular cavities within the vestibule, the utricle and saccule. The saccule lies on the medial wall of the vestibule in a spherical recess inferior to the utricle with which it is in contact but without direct connection. It communicates with the endolymphatic duct (and thus the utricular duct) by the saccular duct and with the cochlea by the ductus reuniens (see Fig. 18). The sensory area of the saccule, the macule, is a differentiated patch of

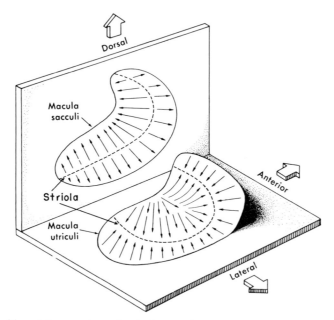

Figure 20. Position of the saccular and utricular macules. Arrows indicate the direction of hair cell polarization on each side of the striola. (From Barber, H. O., and Stockwell, C. W.: *Manual of Electronystagmography.* The C. V. Mosby Co., St. Louis, 1976, with permission.)

membrane in the medial wall, hood-shaped and predominantly in a vertical position (Fig. 20). The utricular cavity (superior to the saccule) is oval in shape, connecting to the membranous semicircular canals via five openings. The macule of the utricle is located next to the anterior opening of the horizontal semicircular canal and lies mostly in a horizontal position in a recess on the anterior part of the utricle (see Fig. 20).

The surfaces of the utricular and saccular macules are covered by the otolithic membrane, a structure consisting of a mesh of fibers embedded in a gel composed of acid mucopolysaccharides.[43, 53] This membrane contains a superficial calcareous deposit, the otoconia. The otoconia consist of small calcium carbonate crystals, ranging from 0.5 to 30 microns in diameter, and having a density more than twice that of water.[21] As discussed in Chapter 1, the stereocilia of the macular hair cells protrude into the otolithic membrane. The striola, a distinctive curved zone running through the center, divides each macule into two areas (see Fig. 20). The hair cells on each side of the striola are oriented so that their kinocilia are in opposite direction. In the utricle the kinocilia face the striola and in the saccule they face away from it (see Fig. 20). As a consequence, displacement of the macule's otolithic membrane in one direction (as illustrated in Fig. 1) has an opposite physiologic influence on the set of hair cells on each side of the striola. Furthermore, because of the curvature of the striola, hair cells are oriented at different angles, making the macule multi-directionally sensitive. A higher proportion of type I hair cells are located near the striola than in the rest of the macule.[54, 88]

Labyrithine Fluids

Two separate fluid compartments exist within the inner ear: the perilymph and the endolymph. The compartments do not communicate and each has a different chemical composition.

Dynamics of Fluid Formation

The mechanism of formation of the inner ear fluids is still not well established. The perilymph is in part a filtration of cerebrospinal fluid (CSF) and in part a filtration from blood vessels in the ear.[23, 83] CSF directly communicates with the perilymphatic space through the cochlear aqueduct, a narrow channel 3 to 4 mm long with its inner ear opening at the base of the scala tympani. In most instances this channel is filled by a loose net of fibrous tissue continuous with the arachnoid. The size of the bony canal varies from individual to individual. Necropsy studies in some patients who died of subarachnoid hemorrhage or meningitis reveal free passage of leukocytes and red blood cells into the inner ear, while in others the cells are blocked from passing through the aqueduct.[41, 74] Blood cells have also been found passing into the internal auditory canal and through the porous canaliculi that contain the vestibular and cochlear nerves, suggesting another route for CSF-perilymph communication.[41] Probably the most important source of perilymph, however, is filtration from blood vessels within the perilymph space, since blocking the cochlear aqueduct apparently does not affect inner ear morphology or function.[45, 82, 92]

The most likely site for production of endolymph is the secretory cells in the stria vascularis of the cochlea and the dark cells of the vestibular labyrinth.[46] Resorption of endolymph is generally agreed to take place in the endolymphatic sac. Dye and pigment experimentally injected into the cochlea of animals accumulate in the endolymphatic sac; electron microscopic studies of the lining membrane of the sac reveal active pinocytotic activity.[1, 38, 62, 78] Destruction of the epithelium lining the sac or occlusion of the duct results in an increase of endolymphatic volume in experimental animals.[47, 48, 92] The first change is an expansion of cochlear and saccular membranes which may completely fill the perilymphatic spaces. The anatomic changes resulting from this experiment are comparable to those found in the temporal bones of patients with Meniere's syndrome (either idiopathic or secondary to known inflammatory disease).

Fluid Chemistry

The chemical composition of the fluids filling the inner ear is similar to that of the extracellular and intracellular fluid throughout the body. The endolymphatic system contains intracellular-like fluids with a high potassium and low sodium concentration, while the perilymphatic fluid resembles the extracellular fluid having a low potassium and high sodium concentration.[15, 71, 83, 90] Figure 21 illustrates the relationship between electrolytes and protein concentration of the different fluid compartments.[84] The high protein content in the endolymphatic sac as compared to the endolymphatic space is consistent with the sac's role in the resorption of endolymph. The difference in protein concentration between perilymph and CSF argues against a free communication between these two fluid compartments and in favor of an active process of perilymph production. The electrolyte composition of the endolymph is critical for normal functioning of the sensory organs bathed in fluid. Ruptures of the membranous labyrinth in experimental animals cause destruction of the sensory and neural structures at the site of the endolymph-perilymph fistula.[81]

Recently it has become possible to sample the fluid in the vestibule by introducing a micropipette through a tiny fistula in the footplate of the stapes.[83, 85, 86] Normally the fluid obtained has the chemical composition of perilymph given in Fig-

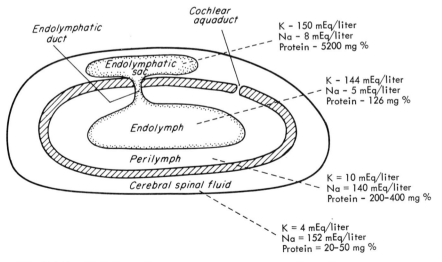

Figure 21. Relationship between electrolyte and protein concentration of fluid compartments within the ear. (From Schuknecht, H. F.: *Pathology of the Ear*. Harvard University Press, Massachusetts, 1974, with permission.)

33

ure 21. In 29 patients with vestibular schwannomas the protein content of the perilymph was consistently elevated with an average value of 1800 mg percent. [86] Elevation of perilymph protein can occur when the protein content of CSF is normal or only slightly elevated. The electrolyte composition of perilymph remains normal in such patients. In patients with Meniere's syndrome the markedly dilated saccule or herniated cochlear duct are usually in contact with the footplate so that endolymph rather than perilymph is obtained from tapping the vestibule. The chemical composition of perilymph obtained from other regions of the labyrinth at the time of surgery is normal in patients with Meniere's syndrome. [83, 86]

Blood Supply

The artery that irrigates the membranous labyrinth and its neural structures is a branch of an intracranial vessel and does not communicate with arteries in the otic capsule and the tympanic cavity. [31, 40, 66, 67] This vessel usually originates from the antero-inferior cerebellar artery, but exceptionally it arises directly from the basilar artery or some of its branches. As it enters the temporal bone it forms branches that irrigate the ganglion cells, nerves, dura and arachnoidal membranes in the internal auditory canal. [7, 31, 66] Shortly after entering the inner ear the labyrinthine artery divides into two main branches: the common cochlear artery and the anterior vestibular artery (Fig. 22a). Because the arteries course independently within the canal, it is possible that alterations in one branch result in changes only in the part of the inner ear to which it provides the blood supply. The common cochlear artery forms two branches: the posterior vestibular artery and the main cochlear artery. The latter enters the central canal of the modiolus where it generates the radiating arterioles, forming a plexus within the cochlea irrigating the spiral ganglion, the structures in the basilar membrane, and the stria vascularis. The posterior vestibular artery, a branch from the common cochlear artery, is the source of blood supply to the inferior part of the saccule and the ampulla of the posterior semicircular canal. The other primary branch of the labyrinthine artery, the anterior vestibular branch, provides irrigation to the utricle and ampulla of the anterior and horizontal semicircular canals as well as some blood to a small portion of the saccule.

The anterior vestibular vein drains the utricle and the ampullae of the anterior and horizontal canals; the posterior vestibular vein drains the saccule, ampulla of the posterior canal and the basal end of the cochlea (Fig. 22b). [9, 89] The confluence of these veins and the vein of the round window becomes the vestibulocochlear vein. Blood from the cochlea is primarily carried by the common modiolar vein and when joined by the vestibulocochlear vein becomes the vein at the cochlear aqueduct. This large venous channel enters a bony canal near the cochlear aqueduct to empty into the inferior petrosal sinus. The semicircular canals are drained by veins that pass toward the utricle and form the vein of the vestibular aqueduct which accompanies the endolymphatic duct and drains into the lateral venous sinus.

Interruption of the blood supply in the internal auditory artery or any of its branches seriously impairs the function of the inner ear since the labyrinthine arteries do not anastomose with any other major arterial branch. [49, 72, 73] Within 15 seconds of blood flow interruption the auditory nerve fibers become inexcitable and the receptor and resting potentials in the ear abruptly diminish. [49] If the interruption lasts for a prolonged period of time the changes are irreversible: loss of

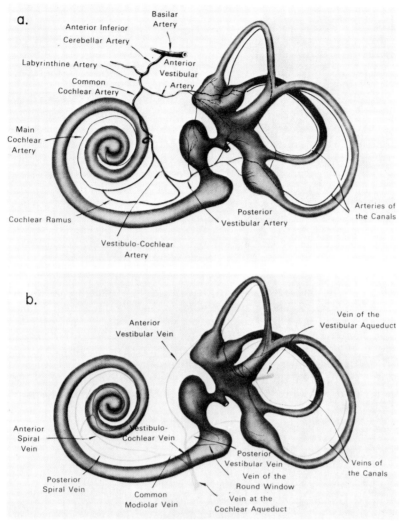

Figure 22. Arterial (a) and venous (b) labyrinthine circulation. (From Schuknecht, H. F.: *Pathology of the Ear.* Harvard University Press, Massachusetts, 1974, with permission.)

function is followed by degenerative changes wherein ganglion cells and sensory cells undergo autolysis and new bone growth fills the ear cavity.[72]

Innervation

The internal auditory canal is a tubular excavation in the petrous portion of the temporal bone about 15 mm in length and 6 mm in width.[2] The medial end of the tube opens into the cerebellopontine angle cistern; the lateral end is closed by a thin bony plate, the lamina cribosa. Through tiny perforations in the lamina cribosa the afferent and efferent vestibular and cochlear nerve fiber endings pass into the labyrinthine cavity to contact the sensory organs. The lamina cribosa is divided into an upper and lower section by the crista falciformis; each of these halves is in turn divided by vertical bony cristae into an anterior and posterior section. The auditory nerve consisting of approximately 30,000 fibers occupies the anteroinferior part of the internal auditory canal and the vestibular nerve containing approximately 20,000 fibers occupies the posterior half.[37, 46] The facial nerve is located in the remaining anterosuperior quadrant.

The afferent bipolar ganglion cells of the vestibular nerve (Scarpa's ganglion) are arranged in two cell masses in a vertical column within the internal auditory canal: the superior group forming the superior division of the vestibular nerve and the inferior forming the inferior division (see Fig. 7).[33, 56, 57, 79] The superior division innervates the cristae of the anterior and horizontal canals, the macule of the utricle and the anterosuperior part of the saccular macule. It exits the internal auditory canal through the posterosuperior fossa of the lamina cribosa. The inferior division innervates the crista of the posterior canal and the main portion of the macule of the saccule and exits the internal auditory canal through the posteroinferior area of the lamina.

Detailed study of the superior division of the vestibular nerve in animals reveals a highly organized arrangement of the nerve fibers originating from the different receptors and from the two types of hair cells within each receptor.[33, 69, 79] Large nerve fibers arise primarily from ganglion cells in the rostral part of the ganglion and small nerve fibers arise from the caudal portion of the ganglion. Within the ampullary nerves the large fibers assume a central position to end predominantly in the large chalice endings of the type I hair cells at the crest of the cristae. The surrounding smaller fibers end on the type II hair cells, more numerous at the slopes of the cristae. These selective peripheral origins of the large and small nerve fibers and the different central connections that will be discussed later suggest a different functional role for the type I and type II vestibular hair cells.

Physiology of the Vestibular End Organs

Semicircular Canals

BACKGROUND. The functional role of the semicircular canals was first linked to their gross anatomic features by Flourens in 1842.[32] While studying the auditory labyrinth in pigeons, he noted that opening a semicircular canal resulted in characteristic head movements in the plane of that canal. Several subsequent investigators proposed that movement of endolymphatic fluid within the canal was responsible for excitation of the cristae.[16, 20, 63] It was not until the studies of Ewald in 1892,[26] however, that a clear relationship was established between the planes of the semicircular canals, the direction of endolymph flow and the direction of induced eye and head movements. Exposing the membranous labyrinth of the semicircular canals of pigeons, Ewald applied positive and negative pressure to each canal membrane to cause ampullopetal and ampullofugal endolymph flow. Three important observations that later became known as Ewald's laws were: 1) the eye and head movements always occurred in the plane of the canal being stimulated and in the direction of endolymph flow, 2) ampullopetal endolymph flow in the horizontal canal caused a greater response (i.e. induced movements) than ampullofugal endolymph flow, and 3) in the vertical canals ampullofugal endolymph flow caused a greater response than ampullopetal endolymph flow.

Steinhausen and later Dohlman visualized the movement of the cupula during endolymph flow.[22, 91] By injecting India ink into the semicircular canals of fish, these investigators demonstrated that the cupula formed a seal with the ampullary wall and moved with the endolymph. Steinhausen, noticing the similarity between the cupular movement and that of a pendulum in a viscous medium, proposed a model for the description of cupular kinematics that became known as the pendulum model. Verification of this model awaited detailed study of the relationship between angular head acceleration and the flow of action potentials in an isolated ampullary nerve. These studies were first conducted in elasmobranches by Lowenstein and Sand,[58, 60] later in frogs,[14, 51, 69, 75] pigeons,[52] mammals,[13, 25, 80] and most recently in primates by Goldberg and Fernández.[30, 36, 37]

MECHANISM OF STIMULATION. The pendulum model is the most useful didactic model for describing the physiologic properties of the semicircular canals and, as will be shown later, for describing the semicircular canal-induced reflexes, especially the vestibulo-oculomotor reflexes.[39, 93, 97]

The cupula acts as the coupler between the force due to angular acceleration of the head and the hair cells (the transducer of mechanical to biological energy), leading to the production of action potentials in the vestibular afferent fibers. Because of the configuration and dimensions of the canals, the endolymph can move in only one direction along the cylindrical cavity. According to Newton's third principle, when an angular acceleration [and hence a force $M\ddot{\theta}_h(t)$] is applied to the head, displacement of the cupula-endolymph system acting as a solid mass is opposed by three restraining forces: (a) an elastic force [$K\theta_c(t)$] due to the cupula's springlike properties (which is proportional to the magnitude of its displacement), (b) the force due to the cupula-endolymph viscosity [$C\dot{\theta}_c(t)$] (whose magnitude is proportional to the velocity of its displacement), and (c) an inertial force [$M\ddot{\theta}_c(t)$] due to the fluid's mass (proportional to the acceleration of the fluid-cupula complex). Cupular displacement can be described by the following equation which is referred to as the equation of the pendulum model of semicircular canal function:

$$M\ddot{\theta}_c(t) + C\dot{\theta}_c(t) + K\theta_c(t) = M\ddot{\theta}_h(t) \qquad 1$$

where θ_c is the angular displacement of the cupula-endolymph system with respect to the wall of the canals, $\dot{\theta}_c$ and $\ddot{\theta}_c$ are the first (velocity) and second (acceleration) time derivatives of the cupular displacement and $\ddot{\theta}_h$ is the angular acceleration of the head. M is the moment of inertia, C the moment of viscous friction and K the moment of elasticity.

For natural to-and-fro head movements the magnitude of the elastic and inertial forces is negligible and the following simplified equation describes the kinematics of the cupula system.

$$C\dot{\theta}_c(t) \approx M\ddot{\theta}_h(t) \qquad 2$$

The force applied to the cupula-endolymph system during angular head acceleration is opposed mostly by the viscous drag of the cupula. Integrating Equation 2 we have:

$$\theta_c(t) \approx \frac{M}{C}\dot{\theta}_h(t) \qquad 3$$

Thus the displacement of the cupula system during natural head movements is proportional to the velocity of head motion rather than head acceleration. The magnitude of the proportionality constant (M/C) relating angular deviation of the cupula in degrees to the velocity of the head in degrees per second has been estimated by different authors to range between 10^{-1} and 10^{-4}.[65, 68] Most likely, during fast head movements with velocities as great as 800 deg/sec, the deviation of the cupula does not exceed one degree of deflection.[70]

Figure 23 illustrates the relationship between the time course of head acceleration, head velocity and cupular displacement as predicted by the pendulum model for three different types of angular rotation commonly used in clinical testing. The sinusoidal rotation in Figure 23a most closely resembles natural head movements since movement in one direction is followed by movement in the opposite direction. Most natural head movements can be broken down into a series of sine waves with different frequencies and amplitudes. According to Equation 3, the cupular displacement $\theta_c(t)$ is given by $\omega A \cos \omega t$ (the differential of head displacement $A \sin \omega t$) where ω is the radian frequency ($2\pi f$) of head rotation and A

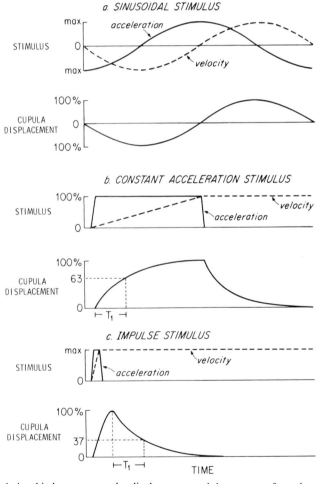

Figure 23. Relationship between cupular displacement and three types of angular acceleration of the head as predicted by the pendulum model.

38

is the angular head displacement. The head velocity at a given time t is proportional to the value of the cosine function at that instant in the cycle of motion. Since this value oscillates between $+1$ and -1, the head velocity ranges between $+\omega A$ and $-\omega A$. These relationships are felt to apply for sinusoidal rotations between 0.025 and 4.0 Hz and therefore cover the range of most natural to-and-fro head movements.[39]

The description of cupular displacement during constant angular acceleration (Fig. 23b) is more complex but can also be derived from Equation 1. At the beginning of head acceleration, endolymph movement lags behind the displacement of the head and thereby that of the walls of the semicircular canals. After a few seconds, however, a balance is established between the applied and restraining forces, and the endolymph moves simultaneously with the walls of the labyrinth. At this time the position of the ring of fluid within the canal and therefore the position of the cupula $\theta_c(t)$ differ from the initial conditions, having been displaced by a certain amount in the direction of the force. The magnitude of the displacement can easily be calculated. Once the endolymph is stationary the cupula velocity $\dot{\theta}_c(t)$ and its acceleration $\ddot{\theta}_c(t)$ in relation to the walls are zero, and consequently the terms for viscous and inertial restraining forces vanish in Equation 1, which now reduces to:

$$K\theta_c(t) = M\ddot{\theta}_h(t)$$

$$\text{or} \qquad \theta_c(t) = \frac{M}{K}\ddot{\theta}_h(t) \qquad\qquad 4$$

That is, the final displacement of the cupula depends on a proportionality constant and on the magnitude of the constant angular acceleration.

The relationships embodied in Equations 3 and 4 are two of the fundamental concepts of cupular function. To restate them: the maximum deviation of the cupula increases proportionally to the magnitude of head velocity during sinusoidal head rotations and to the magnitude of head acceleration during rotation with constant angular acceleration.

Cupula displacement after a constant angular acceleration stimulus follows an exponential time course (Fig. 23b) which can be determined by a more detailed mathematical treatment of Equation 1. Sixty-three percent of the total cupular deviation, regardless of its final value, always takes place after a fixed delay determined by what is known as the slow time constant (T_1) of the system (estimated to be about 4 seconds). The subsequent deviation of the cupula increases at the same rate (63 percent of the remainder every 4 seconds) so that 95 percent of the final deviation will take place after approximately 12 seconds. The magnitude of the time constant depends on the viscous and elastic coefficients: $T_1 = C/K$. That is, the time the cupula takes to reach a maximum deviation is directly proportional to the viscosity of the endolymph and inversely proportional to the elasticity of the cupula.

According the pendulum model, not only is the initial deviation of the cupula related to the constant acceleration stimulus, but after the stimulus is terminated the cupula returns to the resting position with the same exponential time course. It was precisely the observation by Steinhausen[91] of the slow exponential-like return of the cupula to the resting position after it had been deviated that led to the formulation of the pendulum model.

The cupular displacement following a brief impulse of angular acceleration is given in Figure 23c. This type of angular acceleration, although the least natural, is of great value in clinical vestibular testing. An impulse of acceleration is generated by changing the velocity of the head ($\Delta\dot{\theta}_h$) with the maximum acceleration possible. The maximum deviation of the cupula takes place almost immediately and is proportional to the magnitude of the instantaneous change in head velocity $\theta_c(t) \approx \Delta\dot{\theta}_h$. Of particular note, the cupular deviation thereafter decays exponentially with the same time course as that following the constant acceleration stimulus. That is, it takes one time constant to return 63 percent of the maximum deviation.

CHARACTERISTICS OF PRIMARY AFFERENT NEURONS. As described in Chapter 1 the primary vestibular afferent fibers maintain a constant baseline firing rate of action potentials. Recordings from the primary afferent fibers of the cristae in mammalian and nonmammalian species reveal that physiologic stimulation producing endolymph flow toward the ampulla in the horizontal semicircular canal increases the baseline firing rate. Conversely, endolymph flow away from the ampulla decreases the baseline firing rate. In the vertical canals the reverse occurs, ampullopetal endolymph flow decreases the baseline firing rate and ampullofugal flow increases the firing rate. Considering these observations and the previous anatomic descriptions, it is apparent that endolymph displacement that deviates the hairs of the sensory cells toward the kinocilium results in increased firing of the afferent nerve while displacement away from the kinocilium results in decreased firing of the afferent nerve.

Detailed measurements of afferent nerve activity from the cristae of squirrel monkeys reveal that the firing rate associated with physiologic rotatory stimuli follows the prediction of the pendulum model.[30] That is, the magnitude of change in frequency of action potentials is proportional to the theoretic deviation of the cupula. For example, during sinusoidal head rotation the firing rate follows the time course of cupular displacement shown in Figure 23a. A sinusoidal change in firing frequency is superimposed on a rather high resting discharge (70 to 90 spikes per second). The peak firing rate occurs at the time of the peak angular head velocity. For a small magnitude of sinusoidal rotation the modulation is almost symmetrical about the baseline firing rate. For higher stimulus magnitudes the responses become increasingly asymmetrical. For the largest stimuli the excitatory responses can increase up to 350 to 400 spikes per second in proportion to the stimulus magnitude while the growth of inhibitory response is limited to the disappearance of spontaneous activity. This asymmetry in afferent nerve response to large-magnitude stimuli explains Ewald's second and third laws since the "pneumatic hammer" that he used to apply pressure to the canals produced a massive stimulus.[26]

Quantitative study of the primary afferent nerve firing rate associated with different types of rotatory stimuli demonstrates some deviation from the prediction of the pendulum model.[36] Such deviation is relevant to understanding the vestibular reflexes that will be discussed later. When the cristae are subjected to prolonged constant acceleration a substantial proportion of nerve fibers undergo a slow decline in firing rate (adaptation) rather than maintaining a steady state as predicted in Figure 23b. Because of adaptation, the firing rate does not return to baseline after the cessation of acceleration, but rather drops to a lower level before slowly returning to the resting level.[13,36] Similar overshooting of the baseline occurs following stimulation with an impulse of acceleration. Instead of the monotonic response predicted by the pendulum model (Fig. 23c) the afferent nerve firing pattern exhibits a biphasic reaction with a prolonged secondary phase that slowly returns to baseline. As will be shown later the vestibulo-ocular reflex also reflects this deviation from the predicted pattern (see Fig. 62).[6, 22, 39, 64, 96]

Recordings from single primary afferent neurons innervating different parts of the cristae reveal that neurons demonstrating adaptation have an irregular spontaneous firing rate, and are sensitive to small magnitudes of stimulation and high frequencies of rotation. These neurons apparently innervate type I hair cells at the center of the cristae.[35, 37, 69]

Otoliths

BACKGROUND. Over a century ago, Mach,[63] Crum-Brown[20] and Breuer[16] each concluded that linear and angular acceleration had to be mediated by different end organs, and Breuer in particular postulated the mechanism by which the otoliths sense linear acceleration.[17] As in the case of the semicircular canals, a gross anatomic feature of the macules, the dense calcified otolithic membrane, suggested the mechanisms by which they sense the direction of gravitational force. The afferent neuronal activity from the macules associated with precise static and dynamic linear acceleration forces has only recently been investigated in primates.[27, 28, 29] These studies confirm that the utricular and saccular macules are responsive to static tilt and dynamic linear acceleration, resolving earlier controversy as to whether the saccular macule functions as an auditory or vestibular organ. The pattern of afferent nerve response is complex with various neurons exhibiting different resting activity, frequency response, and adaptation properties.

MECHANISMS OF STIMULATION. During head displacement, the calcified otolithic membrane is affected by the combined forces of applied linear acceleration and gravity and tends to move over the macule which is mounted in the wall of the membranous labyrinth (see Fig. 1). The otolith is restrained in its motion by elastic, viscous and inertial forces analogous to the forces associated with cupular movement. de Vries[21] measured the displacement of the large saccular otoliths of several fish and obtained estimates of the forces restraining the otoliths to the macules. He proposed a model analogous to the pendulum model that described the dynamics of otolith displacement as those of a low-pass filter. Displacements due to a sinusoidal linear acceleration would be greatest for low frequencies, including static head tilts. For greater frequencies the otolith displacement would decrease by one half each time the frequency is doubled.

CHARACTERISTICS OF PRIMARY AFFERENT NEURONS. The nerve fibers innervating the macules are activated by changes in position of the head in space.[59] Each neuron has a characteristic functional polarization vector that defines the axis of greatest sensitivity. It is as though the terminal fibers of each afferent neuron were stimulated only by hair cells with kinocilia oriented in a given direction in space, forming one functional neuronal unit. The combined polarization vectors of neurons from both macules cover all possible positions of the head in three-dimensional space. The majority of polarization vectors, however, are near the horizontal plane for the utricular macule and the sagittal plane for the saccular macule.[27, 28, 29] Diagrams of the functional polarization vectors determined by electrophysiologic analysis in the squirrel monkey are remarkably similar to the morphologic maps that plot the polarization of hair cells within each macule (see Fig. 20). None of the neuronal units records a response to compressive forces, confirming previous findings in lateral line systems that displacement of hairs is the only adequate stimulus for the hair cell.[10, 28]

With the subject in the normal upright position gravity does not stimulate most of the neuronal units of the utricular macule (since it is orthogonal to most polarization vectors). The average resting discharge of macular units in this position is approximately 65 spikes per second.[27] The macule is roughly divided into a medial and lateral section by the striola. Since in the utricular macule hair cell polarization (the direction of the kinocilia) is toward the striola, ipsilateral tilt results in an increase in the baseline firing of the units medial to the striola and a decreased firing of the units lateral to the striola. Because of the curvature of the striola many utricular macule units are also sensitive to forward and backward tilt.

In contrast, the saccular macule is in a sagittal plane when a subject is in the upright position and most of its functional polarization vectors are parallel to the gravity vector. Most neuronal units, therefore, are either excited or inhibited by the effect of 1 g acceleration. The saccular macule exhibits less curvature and most of its units have a preferred dorsoventral orientation. Saccular units at rest discharge at a rate essentially the same as the utricular units.[27] As in the case of the cristae, their spontaneous firing rate subdivides two main classes of neuronal units in both macules: regular and irregular.[29] The irregular units adapt rapidly when stimulated with constant linear acceleration, are more sensitive to small changes in linear acceleration and have a wider frequency response than the regularly firing units. During stimulation with static tilts the regular units maintain a constant ratio between the applied force and the response. During stimulation with sinusoidal linear acceleration (back and forth linear displacement) their sensitivity is constant up to 0.1 Hz but steadily declines at higher frequencies. These regular units therefore conform to the expectations of the de Vries model of otolith function.

The irregular units, on the other hand, appear to respond not only to otolith displacement but also to the velocity of the displacement. Following a change in head position, they undergo an immediate increase in firing followed by a decline. This difference between the presumed displacement of the otolithic membrane and the afferent unit response may be related to the mechanical linkage between the hair cell cilia and the membrane.[53] The irregular units might innervate type I hair cells whose cilia are not rigidly embedded in the otolithic membrane but rather are enclosed in fluid-filled chambers in the membrane. The cilia could sense the velocity of displacement of the otoliths by viscous coupling through the fluid. If so, the observed variation in unit response may reflect different types of coupling between different hair cells and the otolithic membrane. Another possibility is that the hair cell coupling is the same but synaptic connections on type I (calyciform) and II (button) hair cells have different transmission properties.

Just how different afferent units produce different vestibular reflexes is poorly understood. Could the larger fibers innervating type I hair cells in both the macules and cristae be mainly responsible for vestibulo-ocular reflexes? Do the regular units serve to maintain postural muscle tone? Only that fraction of the hair cells in each macule with their polarization vector in the plane of motion respond to one direction of tilt. In the crista, on the contrary, during angular acceleration in the horizontal plane all the hair cells are stimulated since they are uniformly oriented. If all the fibers were to contribute equally in vestibular reflexes, a vastly different number of receptor units in the macules and cristae would be involved in producing compensatory eye movements for linear and angular acceleration. No one yet knows just how these variables regulate the normal or abnormal reflex activity that originates in the macules and cristae.

REFERENCES

1. ALTMANN, F., AND WALTNER, J.: *Further investigations on the physiology of labyrinthine fluids.* Ann. Otol. Rhinol. Laryngol. 59:657, 1950.

2. ANIJAD, A. H., SCHEER, A. A., AND ROSENTHAL, J.: *Human internal auditory canal.* Arch. Otolaryngol. 89:709, 1969.

3. ANSON, B. J., AND DONALDSON, J. A.: Surgical Anatomy of the Temporal Bone and Ear. W. B. Saunders Co., Philadelphia, 1973.

4. ANSON, B. J.: Developmental anatomy of the ear. In Paparella, M. F., and Shumrick, D. A. (eds.): *Otolaryngology, I.* W. B. Saunders Co., Philadelphia, 1973.

5. ANSON, B. J., AND BAST, T. H.: *Development of the otic capsule of the human ear.* Quarterly Bulletin, Northwestern Univ. Med. School, 32:157, 1958.

6. ASCHAN, G., AND BERGSTEDT, M.: *The genesis of secondary nystagmus induced by vestibular stimuli.* Acta. Soc. Med. Upsaliensis 60:113, 1955.

7. AXELSSON, A.: The blood supply of the inner ear of mammals. In Keidel, W. D., and Neff, W. D. (eds.): *Handbook of Sensory Physiology-Auditory System,* vol. V, part 1. Springer-Verlag, New York, 1974.

8. BARBER, H. O., AND STOCKWELL, C. W.: *Manual of Electronystagmography.* The C. V. Mosby Co., St. Louis, 1976.

9. BAST, T., AND ANSON, B.: *The Temporal Bone and the Ear.* Charles C Thomas, Springfield, 1949.

10. BAUKNIGHT, R. S., STRELIOFF, D., AND HONRUBIA, V.: *Effective stimulus for the Xenopus laevis lateral-line hair-cell system.* Laryngoscope 86:1836, 1976.

11. VON BÉKÉSY, G., AND ROSENBLITH, W.: The mechanical properties of the ear. In Stevens, S. S. (ed.): *Handbook of Experimental Psychology.* John Wiley and Son, Inc., New York, 1951.

12. BLANKS, R. H. I., CURTHOYS, I. S., AND MARKHAM, C. H.: *Planar relationships of semicircular canals in the cat.* Am. J. Physiol. 223:55, 1972.

13. BLANKS, R. H. I., ESTES, M. S., AND MARKHAM, C. H.: *Physiologic characteristics of vestibular first-order canal neurons in the cat. II. Response to constant angular acceleration.* J. Neurophysiol. 38:1250, 1975.

14. BLANKS, R. H. I., AND PRECHT, W.: *Functional characteristics of primary vestibular afferents in the frog.* Exp. Brain Res. 25:369, 1976.

15. BOSHER, S. K., AND WARREN, R. L.: *Observations on the electrochemistry of the cochlear endolymph of the rat: a quantitative study of its electrical potential and ionic composition as determined by means of flame spectrophotometry.* Proc. Roy. Soc. B. 171:227, 1968.

16. BREUER, J.: *Über die Funktion der Bogengänge des Ohrlabyrinthes.* Wien. Med. Jahrb. 4:72, 1874.

17. BREUER, J.: *Über die Funktion der Otolithen-Apparate.* Pflügers Arch. ges. Physiol. 48:195, 1891.

18. CAJAL, S.: *Histologie due système nerveaux de l'homme et des vertébrés,* vol. 1. Maloine, Paris, 1909.

19. CARPENTER, M. B.: *Core Text of Neuroanatomy.* Williams & Wilkins, Baltimore, 1972.

20. CRUM-BROWN, A.: *On the sense of rotation and the anatomy and physiology of the semicircular canals of the internal ear.* J. Anat. Physiol. 8:327, 1874.

21. DE VRIES, H.: *The mechanics of the labyrinth otoliths.* Acta Otolaryngol. 38:262, 1950.

22. DOHLMAN, G. F.: *Some practical and theoretical points of labyrinthology.* Proc. Roy. Soc. Med. 28:1371, 1935.

23. DOHLMAN, G. F.: *The mechanism of secretion and absorption of endolymph in the vestibular apparatus.* Acta Otolaryngol. 59:275, 1965.

24. ENGSTROM, H., ADES, H. W., AND ANDERSSON, A.: *Structural Pattern on the Organ of Corti.* Williams & Wilkins, Baltimore, 1966.

25. ESTES, M. S., BLANKS, R. H. I., AND MARKHAM, C. H.: *Physiologic characteristics of vestibular first-order canal neurons in the cat. I. Response plane determination and resting discharge characteristics.* J. Neurophysiol. 38:1232, 1975.

26. EWALD, R.: *Physiologische Untersuchungen über das Endorgan des Nervus Octavus.* Bergmann, Wiesbaden, 1892.

27. FERNÁNDEZ, C., AND GOLDBERG, J. M.: *Physiology of peripheral neurons innervating otolith organs of the squirrel monkey. I. Response to static tilts and to long-duration centrifugal force.* J. Neurophysiol. 39:970, 1976.

28. FERNÁNDEZ, C., AND GOLDBERG, J. M.: *Physiology of peripheral neurons innervating otolith organs of the squirrel monkey. II. Directional selectivity and force-response relations.* J. Neurophysiol. 39:985, 1976.

29. FERNÁNDEZ, C., AND GOLDBERG, J. M.: *Physiology of peripheral neurons innervating otolith organs of the squirrel monkey. III. Response dynamics.* J. Neurophysiol. 39:996, 1976.

30. FERNÁNDEZ, C., AND GOLDBERG, J. M.: *Physiology of peripheral neurons innervating semicircular canals of the squirrel monkey. II. Response to sinusoidal stimulation and dynamics of peripheral vestibular system.* J. Neurophysiol. 34:661, 1971.

31. FISCH, U.: *Transtemporal surgery of the internal auditory canal. Report of 92 cases, technique, indications and results.* Adv. Oto-Rhino-Laryngol. 17:203, 1970.

32. FLOURENS, P.: *Recherches Expérimentales sur les Propriétés et les Fonctions due Système Nerveux dans les Animaux Vertébrés.* Crevot, Paris, 1842.

33. GACEK, R. R.: *The innervation of the vestibular labyrinth.* Ann. Otol. Rhinol. Laryngol. 77:676, 1968.

34. GACEK, R., AND RASMUSSEN, G. L.: *Fiber analysis of the acoustic nerve of cat, monkey, and guinea pig.* Anat. Rec. 127:417, 1957.

35. GOLDBERG, J., AND FERNÁNDEZ, C.: *Conduction times and background discharge of vestibular afferents.* Brain Res. 122:545, 1977.

36. GOLDBERG, J., AND FERNÁNDEZ, C.: *Physiology of peripheral neurons innervating semicircular canals of the squirrel monkey. I. Resting discharge and response to constant angular accelerations.* J. Neurophysiol. 34:635, 1971.

37. GOLDBERG, J. M., AND FERNÁNDEZ, C.: *Physiology of peripheral neurons innervating semicircular canals of the squirrel monkey. III. Variations among units in their discharge properties.* J. Neurophysiol. 34:676, 1971.

38. GUILD, S.: *The circulation of endolymph.* Amer. J. Anat. 39:57, 1927.

39. HALLPIKE, C. S., AND HOOD, J. D.: *The speed of the slow component of angular nystagmus induced by angular acceleration of the head: its experimental determination and application to the physical theory of the cupular mechanism.* Roy. Soc. Lond. Proc. 141:216, 1953.

40. HANSEN, C.: *Vascular anatomy of the human temporal bone: I. Anastomoses between the membranous labyrinth and its bony capsule; II. Anastomoses inside the labyrinthine capsule; III. The vascularization of the vestibulo-cochlear nerve.* Arch. Ohr. Nas.-Kehlk.-Heilk. 200:83, 1971.

41. HOLDEN, H., AND SCHUKNECHT, H.: *Distribution pattern of blood in the inner ear following spontaneous subarachnoid hemorrhage.* J. Laryngol. 82:321, 1968.

42. IGARASHI, M.: Dimensional study of the vestibular end organ apparatus. In *Second Symposium on the Role of the Vestibular Organs in Space Exploration.* U.S. Government Printing Office, Washington, 1966.

43. IURATO, S.: *Submicroscopic Structure of the Inner Ear.* Pergamon Press, New York, 1967.

44. KELLER, E. L.: *Behavior of horizontal semicircular canal afferents in alert monkey during vestibular and optokinetic stimulation.* Exp. Brain Res. 24:459, 1976.

45. KIMURA, R., SCHUKNECHT, H., AND OTA, C.: *Blockage of the cochlear aqueduct.* Acta Otolaryngol. 77:1, 1974.

46. KIMURA, R. S.: *Distribution, structure and function of dark cells in the vestibular labyrinth.* Ann. Otol. Rhinol. Laryngol. 78:542, 1969.

47. KIMURA, R. S.: Experimental Production of Endolymphatic Hydrops. In Pulec, J. (ed.): *Meniere's Disease.* W. B. Saunders, Philadelphia, 1968.

48. KIMURA, R., AND SCHUKNECHT, H.: *Membranous hydrops in the inner ear of the guinea pig after obliteration of the endolymphatic sac.* Pract. Oto-Rhino-Laryngol. 27:343, 1965.

49. KONISHI, T., BUTLER, R. A., AND FERNÁNDEZ, C.: *Effect of anoxia on cochlear potentials.* J. Acoust. Soc. Amer. 33:349, 1961.

50. KRIEG, W. J. S.: *Functional Neuroanatomy.* (ed. 2). Blakiston Co., New York, 1953.

51. LEDOUX, A.: *Les canaux semi-circulaires Etude électrophysiologique. Contribution à l'effort d'uniformisation des épreuves vestibulaires. Essai d'interprétation de la sémiologie vestibulaire.* Acta Oto-Rhino-Laryngol. Belgica 12:109, 1958.

52. LIFSCHITZ, W. S.: *Responses from the first order neurons of the horizontal semicircular canal in the pigeon.* Brain Res. 63:43, 1973.

53. LIM, D. J.: *Ultrastructure of the otolithic membrane and the cupula.* Adv. Oto-Rhino-Laryngol. 19:35, 1973.

54. LINDEMAN, H. H.: *Studies on the morphology of the sensory regions of the vestibular apparatus.* Adv. Anat. Embryol. Cell Biol. 42:1, 1969.

55. LINDSAY, J. R.: *Petrous pyramid of the temporal bone: Pneumatization and roentgenologic appearance.* Arch. Otolaryngol. 31:231, 1940.

56. LORENTE DE NÓ, R.: *Anatomy of the eighth nerve. The central projection of the nerve endings of the internal ear.* Laryngoscope 43:1, 1933.

57. LORENTE DE NÓ, R.: *Etudes Sur L'Anatomie et la Physiologie due Labyrinthe de L'Oreille et due VIII Nerf.* Madrid Univ. Lab. Recherches Biologiques Travaux. 24:53, 1926.

58. LOWENSTEIN, O., AND SAND, A.: *The individual and integrated activity of the semicircular canals of the elasmobranch labyrinth.* J. Physiol. 99:89, 1940.

59. LOWENSTEIN, O., AND ROBERTS, T. D. M.: *Oscillographic analysis of the responses of the otolith organs of the thornback ray.* J. Physiol. 110:392, 1949.

60. LOWENSTEIN, O., AND SAND, A.: *The mechanism of the semicircular canal. A study of the responses of single-fiber preparations to angular accelerations and rotations at constant speed.* Proc. Roy. Soc. London, Ser. B. 129:256, 1940.

61. LOWENSTEIN, O., AND WERSÄLL, J.: *A functional interpretation of the electron-microscopic structure of the sensory hairs in the cristae of the elasmobranch raja clavata in terms of directional sensitivity.* Nature 184:1807, 1959.

62. LUNDQUIST, P.-G.: *The endolymphatic duct and sac in the guinea pig.* Acta Otolaryngol. 201 (Suppl.):1, 1965.

63. MACH, E.: *Grundlinien der Lehre von den Bewegungsempfindungen.* Engelmann, Leipzig, 1875; Bonset, Amsterdam, 1967 (translation).

64. MALCOLM, R., AND JONES, G. M.: *Quantitative study of vestibular adaptation on humans.* Proc. 4th Symp. on the Role of the Vestibular Organs in Space Explor., Pensacola, 1968.

65. MAYNE, R.: A systems concept of the vestibular organs. In Kornhuber, H. H. (ed.): *Handbook of Sensory Physiology,* vol. VI, part 2. Springer-Verlag, New York, 1974.

66. MAZZONI, A.: *Internal auditory artery supply to the petrous bone.* Ann. Otol. Rhinol. Laryngol. 81:13, 1972.

67. MAZZONI, A.: *Internal auditory canal, arterial relations at the porus acusticus.* Ann. Otol. Rhinol. Laryngol. 78:797, 1969.

68. MONEY, K. E., ET AL.: *Physical properties of fluids and structures of vestibular apparatus of the pigeon.* Am. J. Physiol. 220:140, 1971.

69. O'LEARY, D. P., DUNN, R., AND HONRUBIA, V.: *Functional and anatomical correlation of afferent responses from the isolated semicircular canal.* Nature 251:255, 1974.

70. OMAN, C. M., AND YOUNG, L. R.: *The physiological range of pressure differences and cupular deflection in the human semicircular canal.* Acta Otolaryngol. 14:324, 1972.

71. PAPARELLA, M.: *Biochemical Mechanisms in Hearing and Deafness.* Charles C Thomas, Springfield, 1970.

72. PERLMAN, H. B., KIMURA, R. S., AND FERNÁNDEZ, C.: *Experiments on temporary obstruction of the internal auditory artery.* Laryngoscope 69:591, 1959.

73. PERLMAN, H. B., AND KIMURA, R. S.: *Observations of the living blood vessels of the cochlea.* Ann. Otol. Rhinol. and Laryngol. 64:1176, 1955.

74. PERLMAN, H., LINDSAY, J.: *Relation of the internal ear spaces to the meninges.* Arch. Otolaryngol. 29:12, 1939.

75. PRECHT, W. LLINÁS, R., AND CLARKE, M.: *Physiological responses of frog vestibular fibers to horizontal angular rotation.* Exp. Brain Res. 13:378, 1971.

76. RASMUSSEN, A.: *Studies of the VIIIth cranial nerve of man.* Laryngoscope 50:67, 1940.

77. ROSS, D. A.: *Electrical studies on the frog's labyrinth.* J. Physiol. 86:117, 1934.

78. RUDERT, H.: *Experimentelle Untersuchungen zur resorption der Endolymphe im Innenohr des Meer-schweinchens.* Arch. Klin. exp. Ohr.-Nas.-Kehlk.-Heilk. 193:138, 1969.

79. SANDO, I., BLACK, F. O., AND HEMENWAY, W. G.: *Spatial distribution of vestibular nerve in internal auditory canal.* Ann. Otol. 81:305, 1972.

80. SCHNEIDER, L. W., AND ANDERSON, D. J.: *Transfer characteristics of first and second order lateral and vestibular neurons in gerbil.* Brain Res. 112:61, 1976.

81. SCHUKNECHT, H., AND EL SEIFI, A.: *Experimental observations on the fluid physiology of the inner ear.* Ann. Otol. Rhinol. Laryngol. 72:687, 1963.

82. SCHUKNECHT, H., AND KIMURA, R.: *Functional and histological findings after obliteration of the periotic duct and endolymphatic sac in sound conditioned cats.* Laryngoscope 63:1170, 1953.

83. SCHUKNECHT, H. F.: *Pathology of the Ear.* Harvard University Press, Massachusetts, 1974.

84. SILVERSTEIN, H.: *Biochemical studies of the inner ear fluids in the cat.* Ann. Otol. Rhinol. Laryngol. 75:48, 1966.

85. SILVERSTEIN, H., AND SCHUKNECHT, H.: *Biochemical studies of inner ear fluid in man.* Arch. Otolaryngol. 84:395, 1966.

86. SILVERSTEIN, H.: *Inner ear fluid proteins in acoustic neuroma, Meniere's disease and otosclerosis.* Ann. Otol. Rhinol. Laryngol. 80:27, 1971.

87. SMITH, C. A.: *Capillary areas of the membranous labyrinth.* Ann. Otol. Rhinol. Laryngol. 63:435, 1954.

88. SMITH, C. A., AND TANAKA, K.: Some aspects of the structure of the vestibular apparatus. In Naunton, R. F. (ed.): *The Vestibular System.* Academic Press, Inc., New York, 1975.

89. SMITH, C. A.: *The capillaries of the vestibular membranous labyrinth in the guinea pig.* Laryngoscope 63:87, 1953.

90. SMITH, C. A., LOWRY, O. H., AND WU, M. L.: *The electrolytes of the labyrinthine fluids.* Laryngoscope 64:141, 1954.

91. STEINHAUSEN, W.: *Über Sichtbarmachung und Funktionsprufung der Cupula terminalis in den Bogengangs-ampullen der Labyrinths.* Arch. Ges. Physiol. 217:747, 1927.

92. SUH, K. W., AND CODY, D. T. R.: *Obliteration of vestibular and cochlear aqueducts in animals.* Trans. A.A.O.O.O. 84:359, 1977.

93. VAN EGMOND, A. A. J., GROEN, J. J., AND JONGKEES, L. B. W.: *The mechanics of the semicircular canal.* J. Physiol. 110:1, 1949.

94. WERSÄLL, J., FLOCK, Å., AND LUNDQUIST, P.-G.: *Structural basis for directional sensitivity in cochlear and vestibular sensory receptors.* Cold Spring Harbor Symposia on Quantitative Biology. 30:115, 1965.

95. WEVER, E., AND LAWRENCE, M.: *Physiological Acoustics.* Princeton University Press, Princeton, 1954.

96. YOUNG, L. R., AND OMAN, C. M.: *Model for vestibular adaptation to horizontal rotation.* Aerospace Med. 40:1076, 1969.

97. YOUNG, L. R.: *The current status of vestibular system models.* Automatica 5:369, 1969.

CHAPTER 3

The Central Vestibular System

VESTIBULAR NUCLEI

Anatomy

The central process of the primary vestibular neurons enter the brain stem at the inner aspect of the restiform body and divide into an ascending and descending branch (Fig. 24).[21, 24, 70, 117] The ascending branch ends either in the rostral end of the vestibular nuclei or in the cerebellum while the descending branch ends in the caudal vestibular nuclei. Primary afferent endings in the vestibular nuclei extend from the caudal third of the rhomboid fossa to a point above the region of the knee of the facial nerve. The vestibular nuclei consist of a group of neurons located on the floor of the fourth ventricle bounded laterally by the restiform body, ventrally by the nucleus and spinal tract of the trigeminal nerve and medially by the pontine reticular formation. Four distinct anatomic groups of neurons have traditionally been considered to constitute the vestibular nuclei, although not all of the neurons in these nuclei receive primary afferent vestibular nerve fibers (Fig. 24).[24, 117] The largest contingent of afferent fibers to the vestibular nuclei originate in the cerebellum.[24] The main vestibular nuclei are: the superior, also known as the angular or Bechterew's nucleus, the lateral or Deiter's nucleus, the medial or triangular nucleus of Schwalbe and the descending or inferior or spinal vestibular nucleus. In addition, the vestibular nuclear complex includes several small groups of cells that are closely associated topographically with the main nuclei but have distinct morphologic characteristics and anatomic connections. As in the case of the main nuclei some regions of these smaller nuclei do not receive primary vestibular fibers.

Superior Vestibular Nucleus

The superior vestibular nucleus extends from the caudal pole of the trigeminal motor nucleus to a level slightly caudal to the nucleus of the abducens nerve. It mainly contains medium sized neurons with some large multipolar cells at the center.[166] The bulk of afferent projections to the superior vestibular nucleus comes from the cristae of the semicircular canals where the fibers innervating type I hair cells terminate preferentially on the larger neurons in the center of the nucleus (Fig. 24).[24, 70] Another group of afferent fibers originates in the cerebellum. Those

47

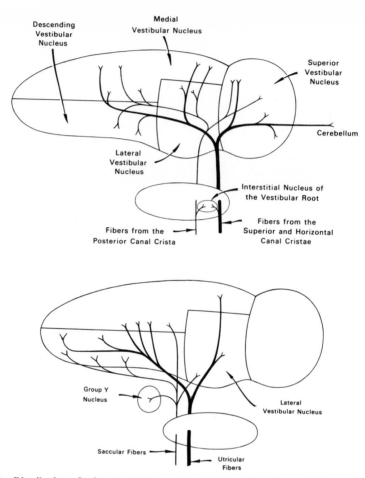

Figure 24. Distribution of primary vestibular afferent fibers within the vestibular nucleus. See text for details. (Adapted from Gacek, R.: Laryngoscope 81:1559, 1971 and Schuknecht, H. F.: *Pathology of the Ear,* 1974.)

from the floccule end in the central region and those from the fastigial nucleus, nodule and uvula end in the peripheral region. A group of fibers from the contralateral descending nucleus connect the two sides. Axons from the neurons in the superior nucleus run in the medial longitudinal fascicle (MLF) to innervate the motor nuclei of the extrinsic eye muscles. The dendrites of the neurons in the periphery of the nucleus extend into the adjacent reticular formation and into the principal trigeminal nucleus. Because of the pattern of afferent and efferent connections, the superior vestibular nucleus is a major relay center for ocular reflexes mediated by the semicircular canals.

Lateral Vestibular Nucleus (Deiter's Nucleus)

Beginning at the level of the superior nucleus and ending at the level of the abducens nucleus, the lateral nucleus is distinguished by the presence of giant cells (30 to 45 μ m) that are relatively more numerous in the dorsocaudal than in the rostroventral part.[24, 166] No sharp anatomic distinction divides these two parts of the nucleus; only the rostroventral part receives primary vestibular afferents (mostly from the utricular macule) (Fig. 24). the dorsocaudal part receives afferent fibers from the vermis and fastigial nucleus of the cerebellum (see Fig. 44). Afferent components from other sources (spinal and commissural fibers) are few in comparison with those from the cerebellum and vestibular nerve. The lateral nucleus sends most of its efferent fibers to the spinal cord as the ipsilateral vestibulospinal tract (see Fig. 43). This projection is somatotopically organized in that fibers to the cervicothoracic cord originate from the rostroventral part of the nucleus while fibers to the lumbosacral cord originate from the dorsocaudal part.[151] The lateral nucleus also sends efferent fibers to the MLF bilaterally that connect with the various oculomotor nuclei. Based on its fiber connections the lateral vestibular nucleus is an important station for the control of vestibulospinal reflexes, particularly those involving the forelimbs.

Medial Vestibular Nucleus

The medial vestibular nucleus is located beneath the floor of the fourth ventricle caudal to the superior and medial to the descending nucleus. It consists of cells of many different sizes and shapes relatively close together, embedded in a fine meshwork of fibers that course in almost all directions.[24, 166] Anatomic separation from the superior nucleus is not well defined. Neurons in the upper part of the nucleus receive afferent fibers from the cristae of the semicircular canals as well as from the fastigial nucleus and floccule of the cerebellum. The ventral and caudal parts receive their main afferents from the cerebellum (the contralateral fastigial nucleus and the ipsilateral nodule). Utriculomacular afferents project to the lateral region (Fig. 24). Other afferent contributions include some fibers from the reticular formation, but these are few in comparison to the vestibular and cerebellar connections.

Efferent connections from the medial nuclei run in the descending MLF to the cervical and thoracic spinal levels by way of the medial vestibulospinal tract (see Fig. 43). From the rostral area (receiving afferent input from the cristae) efferent fibers pass to the ascending MLF bilaterally to reach the nuclei of the oculomotor nerves. Other efferents are distributed to the vestibular cerebellum, the reticular formation, and the contralateral vestibular nuclei. Because of its projections in the MLF to extraocular muscles and the cervical cord, the medial vestibular nucleus appears to be an important center for coordinating eye, head and neck movements.

Descending Vestibular Nucleus

The descending or inferior vestibular nucleus is difficult to differentiate anatomically from the adjacent medial vestibular nucleus. It consists of small and medium sized cells with occasional giant cells.[24, 166] Primary afferent fibers arrive from the utricular and saccular macules (utricular—medial, saccular—lateral) with a small contribution to the rostral tip from the cristae (Fig. 24).[70] Cerebellar afferents from the floccule, nodule and uvula are scattered throughout the nucleus intermingling with the vestibular afferents. Projections from other sources including spinal afferents are minimal. Most of the efferent fibers from the descending nucleus pass to the cerebellum and to the reticular formation. Numerous commissural fibers supply the contralateral descending, medial and lateral nuclei. The descending nucleus apparently integrates vestibular signals from the two sides with signals from the cerebellum and reticular formation.

Interstitial Nucleus of the Vestibular Nerve

Of the small groups of cells associated with the vestibular nuclei the interstitial nucleus is most clearly defined.[24] It consists of small strands of elongated cells interspersed between the root fibers of the vestibular nerve (Fig. 24). The interstitial nucleus receives afferent collaterals from the cristae of all three semicircular canals but none from the macules of the utricule or saccule. Efferent projections from the interstitial nucleus enter the MLF and are important in mediating canal-ocular reflexes.

Physiology

Introduction

Vestibular signals originating in the two labyrinths first interact with signals from other somatosensory systems in the vestibular nuclei. Only a fraction of the neurons receive direct vestibular connections and, with the exception of the interstitial nucleus of the vestibular nerve, the neurons that receive primary vestibular afferent fibers also receive afferents from the cerebellum, the reticular formation, the spinal cord and the contralateral vestibular nuclei.[24, 70, 117] Consequently, efferent signals from the vestibular nuclei reflect the interaction of these various afferent systems. For example, visual signals relayed through the cerebellar floccule to neurons in the superior and medial nuclei modulate the activity of the vestibulo-ocular reflexes.[102, 136, 137] The cerebellum influences the vestibulospinal reflexes by means of connections between the vermis and the lateral and descending vestibular nuclei.[150, 179] Through connections with the reticular substance, vestibular neuron outflow interacts with descending corticobulboreticular and reticulospinal signals.[118, 125]

Two different groups of secondary vestibular neurons have been identified from measurements of the electrical activity within the vestibular nuclei following stimulation of the vestibular nerve with a single brief electric pulse.[152, 153] After a short latency a characteristic field potential is recorded in the areas of the brain stem receiving the vestibular input (Fig. 25). This field potential consists of three components: an initial positive-negative deflection from action currents in the primary vestibular fibers, a negative wave (N_1) with a latency of about 1 msec generated by monosynaptic-activated secondary vestibular neurons and fibers and a delayed negative deflection (N_2) with a latency of about 2.5 msec generated by multisynaptic-activated neurons and fibers (Fig. 25a). By carefully placing micro-electrodes in the vicinity of or inside secondary vestibular neurons and tailoring the electric stimuli it has been demonstrated that some neurons produce action potentials at the time of the extracellular N_1 wave (Fig. 25b), suggesting that they receive monosynaptic input. Other neurons produce delayed action potentials (Fig. 25c), suggesting multisynaptic activation. Approximately 75 percent of neurons sampled in the vestibular nuclei are activated by vestibular nerve stimulation and approximately half of these are monosynaptically activated.[153, 171] All monosynaptic connections are ipsilateral and excitatory. Neurons receiving multisynaptic input, on the other hand, are frequently activated by contralateral vestibular nerve stimulation.

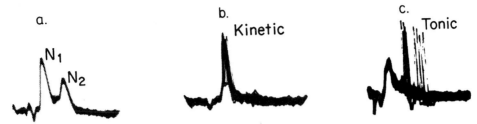

Figure 25. a. Field potential recorded in the medial vestibular nucleus after electric stimulation of the ipsilateral vestibular nerve. N_1 is generated by monosynaptic activated secondary vestibular neurons and N_2 by multisynaptic activated neurons. b. Response of a kinetic vestibular neuron, N_1 field potential is not seen because of superposition of spikes. c. Response of tonic vestibular neuron demonstrating spikes timed with N_2 field potential. Each recording is composed of about 20 superimposed traces. (Adapted from Precht, W., and Shimazu, H.: *Functional connections of tonic and kinetic vestibular neurons with primary vestibular afferents.* J. Neurophysiol. 28:1014, 1965.)

Semicircular Canal Connections

The anatomically determined specificity of canal projections to the vestibular nuclei has been verified electrophysiologically. The areas where the canal afferents terminate are identified by recording the activity in different vestibular nuclei following electric stimulation of afferent nerves from the cristae or physiologic stimulation of the semicircular canals with angular acceleration. Semicircular canal afferents are found primarily in the rostral nuclei, i.e. the superior nucleus and the rostral part of the medial vestibular nucleus. Most neurons in these areas respond to angular acceleration with the same pattern of firing as do vestibular nerve fibers.[133] That is, their firing rate primarily reflects the magnitude of cupular deflection, as exemplified in Figure 23. Not all neurons respond similarly, however. Type I neurons are excited, type II inhibited by ipsilateral rotation of the head (Fig. 26).

Among the type I neurons there are two subtypes: kinetic and tonic. Kinetic neurons are characterized by a lack of spontaneous activity and long latencies from the onset of physiologic stimulation to the onset of firing.[153,171,172] Once threshold is reached, however, these neurons exhibit great sensitivity, rapidly increasing their firing frequency in proportion to increases in the stimulus magnitude. Tonic neurons, on the other hand, have substantial spontaneous activity and shorter latencies and slowly increase their firing frequency with a stimulus of increasing magnitude. Kinetic neurons receive a monosynaptic input from vestibular nerve fibers while tonic neurons receive a multisynaptic input. Paradoxically kinetic type I neurons which have monosynaptic connections with spontaneously active primary vestibular fibers do not show resting activity.

Type II neurons receive their major input via commissural connections either from neurons in the reticular substance that act as interneurons or directly from contralateral type I neurons (Fig. 26).[172] Contralateral labyrinth stimulation excites type II neurons and they, in turn, inhibit ipsilateral type I tonic neurons. It follows that during head rotation the activity of ipsilateral type I tonic neurons is enhanced by excitation from the ipsilateral labyrinth and by decreased inhibition from neighboring type II neurons (whose input from the contralateral type I neurons has simultaneously decreased). Type I neurons (tonic and kinetic) are also affected by another inhibitory pathway mediated by neurons within the reticular substance (Fig. 26). This inhibitory pathway is monosynaptically activated

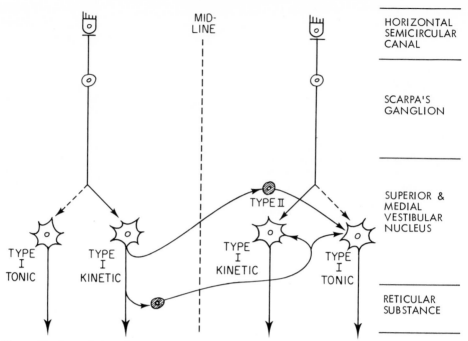

Figure 26. Interrelation of type I (tonic and kinetic) and type II secondary vestibular neurons. The broken line indicates multisynaptic activation, round dark neurons are inhibitory interneurons. (Adapted from Precht, W., and Shimazu, H.: *Functional connections of tonic and kinetic vestibular neurons with primary vestibular afferents.* J. Neurophysiol. 28:1014, 1965.)

by electric stimulation in the contralateral vestibular nuclei and is interrupted by shallow incisions of the midline of the floor of the fourth ventricle.[152, 172]

Mechanism of Compensation after Labyrinthectomy

Knowledge of the different types of secondary vestibular neurons and their interconnecting pathways is important for understanding the sequence of recovery following a unilateral loss of labyrinthine function.[154] Immediately after a labyrinthectomy the ipsilateral type I neurons lose their spontaneous activity and become unresponsive to ipsilateral angular rotation. At the same time contralateral healthy type II neurons lose their input and cease to exert inhibitory activity on neighboring type I neurons. Vestibular reflexes reflect the absence of ipsilateral excitatory activity and of contralateral inhibition. An imbalance in the tone of body and eye musculature results and the clinical signs of labyrinthectomy are produced: nystagmus, past pointing and imbalance. A few days after a labyrinthectomy in cats, the silent type I neurons on the damaged side recover their spontaneous activity and respond to physiologic stimulation of the contralateral labyrinth.[154] As a result of their connections with ipsilateral type II neurons these reactivated type I units are inhibited when the type I neurons on the healthy side are excited and excited by lack of inhibition when the contralateral type I neurons are inhibited. While the responses of the type I neurons on the damaged side are not as intense as those on the normal side they are qualitatively similar. The recovery of activity in the ipsilateral type I neurons after a labyrinthectomy parallels the time course of the relief of clinical symptoms and signs.

The genesis of the renewed tonic input to ipsilateral type I neurons several days after a labyrinthectomy is unknown.[152] The source is not an increase in tonic input from the healthy side since afferent activity in Scarpa's ganglion cells and in type I neurons in the normal side remains unchanged.[154] If a second labyrinthectomy is performed after complete compensation for the first occurs, the animal again develops signs of acute unilateral vestibular loss with nystagmus directed toward the previously operated ear (Bechterew's compensatory nystagmus)[16], as if the first labyrinthectomy had not taken place. Compensation after the second labyrinthectomy is slightly faster than the first but still requires several days. The most likely sources of tonic input to the type I neurons after labyrinthectomy are the cerebellum and reticular formation. Both areas have known anatomic connections with secondary vestibular neurons, and electric stimulation of parts of the cerebellum and reticular formation results in excitation of type I secondary vestibular neurons.[152]

Otolith Connections

Localization of secondary vestibular neurons responding to tilt or electric stimulation of the macular nerves corresponds to the anatomically determined distribution of primary vestibular fibers from the utricle and saccule; they are mainly found in the lateral, descending and caudal part of the medial vestibular nuclei.[1,54,152,201] Within the lateral nucleus a large percentage of rostroventral neurons are monosynaptically activated by electric pulse stimulation of the ipsilateral vestibular nerve.[201] On the other hand, neurons in the dorsocaudal part of the lateral nucleus are multisynaptically activated by ipsilateral vestibular nerve stimulation, a finding consistent with the fact that this area does not receive primary vestibular afferent fibers. Secondary vestibular neurons responsive to head tilt exhibit a variety of response patterns because of the variety of signals they receive from the macular afferent units.[67,149] Most second order neurons respond to tilt by only one axis. Some are phasic only showing a transient increase in firing during tilt while others develop a new tonic level of firing with the maintenance of a new position.

Semicircular Canal—Otolith Interaction

The activity of many secondary vestibular neurons reflects a convergence of input from different labyrinthine receptors.[54,126] Neurons sampled in the superior and medial nuclei often respond to stimulation of the macules as well as the horizontal and vertical canals. Most type I secondary neurons of the horizontal canal also receive excitatory stimulation from the ipsilateral utricular macule. The convergence of information at the level of the vestibular nucleus may partly explain the interaction of reflexes mediated by the canals and otoliths discussed in later sections.

VESTIBULO-OCULAR REFLEXES

Experimental Methods

Experiments employing a variety of research methods have documented that precisely organized projections connect the vestibular end organs to motoneurons innervating the extrinsic eye muscles. The experimental data include: 1) anatomic studies in normal animals using Golgi-stained preparations, cell and axon labeling techniques and demonstration of walleriann and retrograde cellular changes following sectioning of nerve fibers; 2) electrophysiologic studies monitoring action potentials in eye muscles, oculomotor nerves and neurons, secondary vestibular neurons and interconnecting pathways within the brain stem following stimulation of the vestibular end organs and vestibular nerves; 3) precise recordings of eye movements induced by physiologic and electric stimulation of vestibular pathways (the individual peripheral receptors, afferent nerves and the brain stem nuclei); and 4) studies of the alteration in eye movements resulting from focal lesions within the vestibulo-ocular pathways.

Organization of Eye Movement Control

Figure 27 summarizes the overall organization of eye movement control as perceived by Lorente de Nó in 1932.[116, 119] The only change from his original diagram is the addition of afferent impulses from proprioceptors in the neck relayed by the vestibular nuclei. Several important features of the control of eye movements deserve emphasis before proceeding to a more specific discussion of the vestibulo-ocular connections. Three main afferent influences control eye movements: visual, vestibular and neck proprioceptive. The visual signals are relayed through multiple centers including the lateral geniculate ganglion (l.g.g.), the superior colliculus (s.col.) and the visual cortex (C_1), all of which influence eye movements through nuclei in the reticular formation (ret.f.) of the midbrain, pons and medulla. Visually controlled (C_1) or voluntarily controlled (C_3) optomotor pathways from the cerebral cortex do not directly reach the oculomotor nuclei (Oc.n.) but rather end in the correlation nuclei of the reticular formation. These same correlation nuclei receive collaterals from secondary vestibular neurons (V.p.) which are influenced by signals from the vestibular and neck proprioceptive receptors. The vestibular nuclei also send a direct pathway to the oculomotor neurons. By drawing representative neurons in each center, Lorente de Nó emphasized the diversity of potential interaction between these neuronal centers.

Organization of the Vestibulo-Ocular Reflex Arcs

As illustrated in Figure 27 vestibulo-ocular connections run in two separate pathways: one a direct pathway from the secondary vestibular neurons to the oculomotor neurons and the other an indirect pathway relayed through the reticular substance of the brain stem. The so-called elementary vestibulo-ocular reflex is transmitted over a three-neuron arc consisting of neurons in Scarpa's ganglion, the vestibular nuclei and the oculomotor nuclei.[116, 185] Many of the direct connections from the vestibular nuclei to the oculomotor neurons are part of a large fiber bundle, the medial longitudinal fascicle (MLF), lying along the floor of the fourth ventricle. This fiber bundle extends from the cervical cord to the reticular substance of the midbrain and thalamus, providing an interconnecting pathway between the vestibular and abducens nuclei in the middle brain stem and the oculomotor complex in the rostral brain stem.[26] In addition to sending axons into the third and fourth nuclei the MLF also sends collaterals into the reticular substance of the midbrain and thalamus. The indirect pathway between the vestibular and oculomotor nuclei is multisynaptic involving both short and long axonal interconnections within the reticular substance.

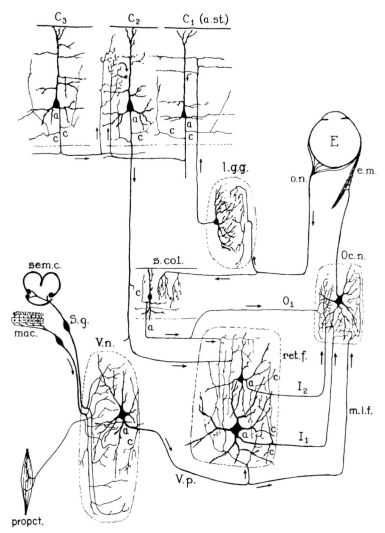

Figure 27. Organization of eye movement control as perceived by Lorente de Nó. See text for details. (Adapted from Lorente de Nó, R., and Berens, C.: Nystagmus. In Piersol, G. M., and Bortz, E. L. (eds.): *Cyclopedia of Medicine, Surgery and Specialties,* vol. 9. F. A. Davis Co., Philadelphia, 1959.)

The respective contribution of the reticular and MLF pathways to the production of vestibular-induced eye movements is not precisely known. Stimulation of either fiber bundle can produce eye movements, but precise vestibulo-ocular control requires the combination of activity in both pathways. Vestibulo-ocular reflexes are reduced but not abolished by sectioning the axons in the MLF or by lesions in the pontine reticular formation.[56, 116] Anesthetics and tranquilizers abolish the fast components of nystagmus but the slow tonic deviation of the vestibulo-ocular reflex is relatively preserved.[181] The polysynaptic pathways that generate fast components (see Nystagmus Fast Component Generation) are more sensitive to the drug effect than the oligosynaptic pathways that generate the slow component. The MLF and reticular pathways appear to complement each other, the former providing a quick communication channel and the latter acting as a modulator. By way of reverberating circuits the reticular formation maintains a level of spontaneous activity or tonus and integrates information from several neural centers. It creates the necessary delays for summation of signals from the visual, proprioceptive, and vestibular systems to produce accurate compensatory eye movements. It acts, therefore, as a fine tuner of vestibular-induced eye movements.[119, 163]

Semicircular Canal—Ocular Reflexes

Detailed information about the connections that link vestibular receptors and different eye muscles was initially obtained by recording the eye muscle response following either physiologic or electric stimulation of each receptor.[33, 81, 92, 116, 118, 182, 185] By measuring the muscle contraction or relaxation the excitatory or inhibitory nature of each connection was established. Table 1 summarizes the primary excitatory and inhibitory connections of each semicircular canal with the muscles of both eyes. Note that each semicircular canal is connected to the eye muscles in such a way that stimulation of the canal nerve results in eye movement in the plane of that canal. For example, stimulation of the left posterior canal nerve causes excitation of the ipsilateral superior oblique and the contralateral inferior rectus muscles while inhibiting the ipsilateral inferior oblique and the contralateral superior rectus. An oblique downward movement in the plane of the left posterior canal is the end result. As suggested in Chapter 1 (see Classification of Vestibular Reflexes), tonic activity arriving at each eye muscle from all the labyrinthine organs provides an important background upon which these more specific reflexes act.[116]

As suggested earlier, stimulation of the vestibular nerve with a brief electric pulse results in monosynaptic activation of ipsilateral secondary vestibular neurons. Intracellular recording in the oculomotor nuclei reveals that oculomotor neurons are disynaptically activated after vestibular nerve stimulation.[7, 81, 122, 173] Within 1 to 2 msec following a shock to the vestibular nerve, excitatory post-synaptic potentials are recorded in oculomotor neurons of agonist muscles, inhibitory postsynaptic potentials in antagonist oculomotor neurons. By system-

Table 1. Connections of the semicircular canals with muscles of the eyes

Semicircular Canal	Excitation	Inhibition
Horizontal	*I — MR C — LR	C — MR I — LR
Posterior	I — SO C — IR	I — IO C — SR
Anterior	I — SR C — IO	I — IR C — SO

* I = Ipsilateral; C = contralateral; MR = medial rectus; LR = lateral rectus; SO = superior oblique; IO = inferior oblique; SR = superior rectus; IR = inferior rectus.

56

atically recording in different vestibular and oculomotor nuclei after selective stimulation of each semicircular canal it has been possible to trace most of the disynaptic excitatory and inhibitory pathways connecting the semicircular canals with the extraocular muscles.[28, 71, 92, 174, 189, 196] These pathways are diagrammed in Figure 28. The pathways from the horizontal canals to the horizontal extraocular muscles deserve particular attention since they are the focus of most clinical vestibular testing. The excitatory secondary vestibular neurons lie in the medial vestibular nucleus while the inhibitory secondary neurons reside in the superior nucleus. Excitatory connections with the ipsilateral medial rectus are made through the ipsilateral MLF and inhibitory connections with the contralateral medial rectus run in the reticular substance beneath the MLF. Input to the lateral rectus muscles (excitatory and inhibitory) runs directly to the contralateral and ipsilateral abducens nuclei respectively.

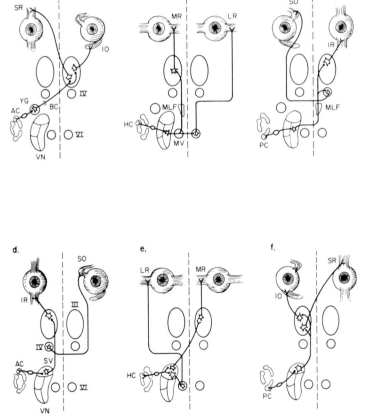

Figure 28. Excitatory (a, b, c) and inhibitory (d, e, f) pathways between the individual semicircular canals and eye muscles. SR, superior rectus, IO, inferior oblique, MR, medial rectus, LR, lateral rectus, SO, superior oblique, IR, inferior rectus, AC, anterior canal, HC, horizontal canal, PC, posterior canal, VN, vestibular nuclei, YG, satellite vestibular nucleus, SV, superior vestibular nucleus, MV, medial vestibular nucleus, BC, brachium conjunctivum, VI, abducens nucleus, IV, trochlear nucleus, III, oculomotor complex. (Adapted from Ito, M.: The vestibulo-cerebellar relationships: vestibulo-ocular reflex arc and flocculus. In Naunton, R. F. (ed.): *The Vestibular System*. Academic Press, New York, 1975.)

Otolith—Ocular Reflexes

The pathways from the macules to the extraocular muscles are less clearly defined than those from the semicircular canals. The latency of eye muscle activation after stimulation of the utricular and saccular nerves is similar to that recorded after semicircular canal nerve stimulation; disynaptic pathways also exist from the macules to the extraocular muscles.[6, 169, 185] Because of the varied orientation of hair cells within the macules, simultaneous stimulation of all the nerve fibers coming from the macule produces a nonphysiologic excitation and the induced eye movements fail to represent the naturally occurring ones. Selective stimulation of different parts of the utricle and saccule results in mostly vertical and vertical-rotatory eye movements.[62, 92, 183] As one would expect, stimulation on each side of the striola produces oppositely directed rotatory and vertical components. Each of the vertical eye muscles appears to be connected to specific areas of the macules so that groups of hair cells whose kinocilia are oriented in opposite directions excite agonist and antagonist muscles.

Summary

Several basic principles underlie the connections between the labyrinthine end organs and eye muscles. First, a receptor organ is connected to a group of motoneurons whose activity produces an eye muscle contraction that compensates for a specific head movement with the objective of maintaining gaze stability. Second, blind spots do not exist in the receptive field of the inner ear organs because the organs in each ear form a complementary set of acceleration sensors capable of reacting to the individual components of linear and angular acceleration associated with head movement in any direction in three-dimensional space. Third, each receptor organ simultaneously activates an excitatory and an inhibitory pathway to agonist and antagonist muscles and thus produce conjugate ocular responses. Because of the bilateral symmetry of the labyrinthine organs, physiologic stimuli activate a push-pull system of control as illustrated in Figure 11. Fourth, alternate pathways complement the elementary disynaptic connections. These pathways consist of chains of interneurons that form reverberating circuits by means of which different reflexes interact and "fine tune" the more specific end organ reflexes.

Characteristics of Eye Movements Induced by Stimulation of Semicircular Canals

Compensatory Eye Movements

The characteristics of semicircular canal-induced eye movements vary among different animal species. In phylogenetically lower animals, such as the rabbit, sinusoidal angular head rotation of small amplitude within the frequency range of natural head movements (0.1 to 1.0 Hz) results in compensatory sinusoidal eye movements 180 degrees out of phase with the head (as illustrated in Fig. 4a and b). The use of sinusoidal angular rotation simplifies the study of the phase relationships between the eyes and the head.[3, 75, 84, 130, 164] Figure 29 illustrates how in the rabbit the vestibular signal produced by a sinusoidally changing head position (a) is converted to an equal and opposite signal in the oculomotor neurons controlling eye position (g). The effective stimulus to the cristae is the force associated with the angular head acceleration (b) but, as was discussed earlier, the cupular deflec-

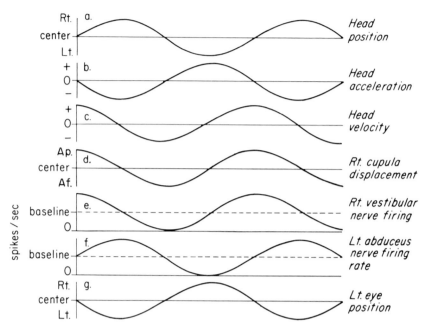

Figure 29. Mechanism by which sinusoidal changing head position (a) is converted to an equal and opposite eye position (g). Ap, ampullopetal, Af, ampullofugal. See text for details.

tion (d) and vestibular nerve firing rate (e) reflect the temporal course of head velocity (c) rather than head acceleration. For eye movements at this frequency (0.1 Hz) the external rectus muscle contraction and the frequency of action potentials in the abducens nerve are in phase with eye position.[160, 164, 174, 176] A puzzling question arises, therefore: where has the one-fourth cycle phase shift between the firing rates of the vestibular and abducens nerves (between e and f) taken place?

The phase shift could result from a delay in the transmission of impulses from one nuclear complex to the next. Such a delay would have to be 2.5 seconds during rotation at a frequency of 0.1 Hz and even greater for lower frequencies. This is an extraordinarily long latency when one considers that the distance between the vestibular and abducens nuclei is a few millimeters. A second more reasonable possibility is that neurons in the brain stem act as mathematical integrators transforming the velocity signal coded in the firing rate of the vestibular nerve fibers (which is the first time derivative of motion) into its integral displacement signal. Such an integration could occur through the interaction of circuits of neurons in the reticular substance in the medulla and pons with the vestibular nuclei and oculomotor neurons although the precise cellular mechanism is unknown.[161] Initial electrophysiologic studies in anesthetized animals suggested that the integration occurred in vestibulo-ocular reflex pathways central to the vestibular nuclei since secondary vestibular neurons were found to fire in phase with the vestibular nerve.[133, 134] Subsequent studies in alert animals, however, showed that although some neurons in the vestibular nuclei fired in phase with the vestibular nerve, others fired in phase with the oculomotor neurons.[66, 101, 136, 193] Apparently the primary afferent signals were integrated in the reticular formation and then returned to neurons in the vestibular nuclei before being passed on to the oculomotor neurons (by the pathways outlined in Fig. 28). These integrated sig-

59

nals were not found in secondary vestibular neurons in earlier studies because the anesthetics inhibited the polysynaptic pathways responsible for the integration.

In summary the vestibulo-ocular reflex involves the activity of many nuclei and a countless number of neurons whose group behavior may differ from that of the isolated units. This complexity must be kept in mind when attempting to evaluate the effects of lesions on vestibulo-ocular reflex activity. It is often impossible to interpret the results of vestibular tests in terms of deficits in a single neural pathway.

Nystagmus

DESCRIPTION. If the stimulus to the semicircular canals is of large magnitude—one that cannot be compensated for by the motion of the eye in the orbit—the slow vestibular induced eye deviation is interrupted with a quick movement in the opposite direction (Fig. 4c and d). This combination of rhythmic slow and fast movements in opposite direction is called nystagmus. Although the eye movement during the slow component takes place in different locations in the orbit, gaze stabilization is still possible because the eye velocity during the slow component is approximately equal and opposite to that of the head.[3, 131] Because of the resetting fast components, the trajectory of the eye motion during the slow components effectively compensates for the head rotation as if the eye had unlimited freedom of motion.

NEURONAL MECHANISMS FOR THE PRODUCTION OF NYSTAGMUS. The relationship between the firing rate of oculomotor neurons and the movements of the eyes during each phase of nystagmus has been studied extensively. Figure 30 shows the membrane potential changes of an abducens motoneuron associated with nystagmus in both directions. During the production of an agonist slow

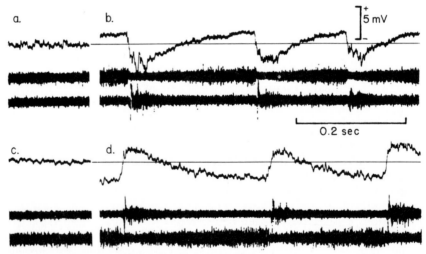

Figure 30. Intracellular recording of membrane potential changes in a left abducens motoneuron (upper traces) and firing rate of the left (middle traces) and right (lower traces) abducens nerve before (a and c) and during nystagmus induced by stimulation of the right (b) and left (d) vestibular nerve. Horizontal lines indicate the membrane potential levels (-41 mv in b and -43 mv in d). (From Maeda, M., Shimazu, H., and Shinoda, Y.: *Nature of synaptic events in cat abducens motoneurons at slow and quick phase of vestibular nystagmus.* J. Neurophysiol. 35:279, 1972, with permission.)

component (Fig. 30b) the membrane potential is slowly depolarized by excitatory postsynaptic potentials arriving via the vestibulo-ocular pathways discussed in the previous sections.[7,122,173] Toward the end of the slow component, the membrane potential rapidly becomes hyperpolarized and the motoneuron abruptly terminates its discharge. This hyperpolarization is produced by inhibitory activity from a group of neurons different from those producing the slow component. The firing rate of the ipsilateral abducens nerve shown in the middle trace of Figure 30 reflects the build up of excitatory and inhibitory activity recorded intracellularly. The opposite membrane potential changes and abducens nerve firing rate occur when the neuron is participating antagonistically in the production of the slow component of nystagmus (Fig. 30d).

Figure 31 illustrates the firing rate of a single right abducens nerve fiber during sinusoidal angular rotation at three different magnitudes. The concurrent nystagmus of the left eye is shown above each firing record. With slow components to the right the right abducens nerve is innervating an agonist muscle and a steady increase in nerve firing occurs that is roughly proportional to the eye displacement. Just before initiation of the fast component in the opposite direction (to the left) the firing of the right abducens nerve suddenly decreases and, in many instances, stops completely. During the subsequent slow component the nerve fiber remains silent until the eye reaches a position in the orbit that is above threshold for this particular abducens neuron. With slow components to the left, an abrupt increase in firing rate occurs just before the onset of the fast component followed by a slow decrease during the slow components. While the change in nerve firing rate during the slow component bears a close relationship to the change in eye

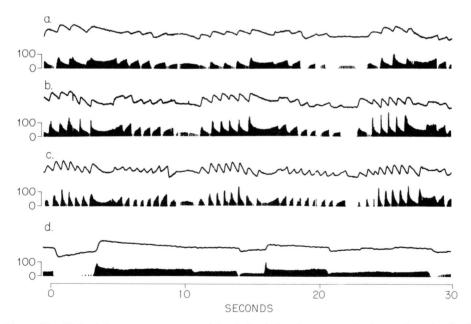

Figure 31. Right abducens motoneuron activity during induced nystagmus in the cat. In each pair of traces, the top trace represents the EOG recording of eye movement and the bottom trace the motoneuron firing frequency. In a, b and c, the animal was rotated at the frequency of 0.1 Hz at peak velocities of 30, 60 and 120 deg/sec respectively. Spontaneous eye movements (saccades) are shown in d.

position, during the fast component a much larger increase in action potentials occurs per unit of time.

Measurement of the relationship between motoneuron firing rates and eye movement induced by vestibular or visual stimuli has shown that the motoneurons behave the same regardless of the nature of the stimulus.[156, 160, 176] Almost all oculomotor neurons exhibit a threshold above which they increase their firing rate roughly in proportion to the change in eye position in the orbit. A small percentage of the change in firing rate (approximately 20 percent) is proportional to the velocity of the eye movement.[156, 160] It is as though the firing rate of the oculomotor neurons was designed to overcome the elastic and viscous forces (roughly in a ratio of 5 to 1) restraining the eye in the orbit. This relationship can best be appreciated by examining the rate of firing of an oculomotor neuron associated with a visually induced refixation saccade (Fig. 31d) where the goal is to move the eyes as rapidly as possible from one position in the orbit to another and to maintain the new position once it is reached. During the high velocity saccade the oculomotor neuron increases its firing rate to a high level to compensate for the viscous drag of the eye ligaments.[161] Once the new position is reached a much lower rate of discharge produces compensation for the elastic restraining force and maintains the new position. Although the reflex pathways for vestibular and visually induced eye movements involve different neuronal circuits, the motoneurons governing the extrinsic eye muscles fire in the same manner regardless of the original sensory input.[156]

FAST COMPONENT GENERATION. Groups of neurons in the parapontine reticular formation fire in short bursts of activity just before the onset of horizontal fast components and voluntary saccades.[80, 100, 177] Apparently fast eye movements, whether voluntary or involuntary, are generated by a common neuronal mechanism.[35, 118, 127, 178] The parapontine reticular formation is not a discrete anatomic structure but rather a region that has been designated because of its apparent functional specificity. Stimulation in the parapontine reticular formation produces ipsilateral slow and rapid eye movements depending on the stimulus variables.[100] The latency of induced eye movements suggests that 1 or 2 synapses lie between the pontine neurons and the oculomotor neurons. Anatomic pathways between this area of the reticular formation and the eye muscle motor nuclei were first reported by Lorente de Nó and subsequently confirmed by other investigators.[32, 118] Numerous documented anatomic pathways also interconnect the vestibular nuclei with the parapontine reticular formation.[83] Apparently neurons in the parapontine reticular formation monitor vestibulo-ocular signals and intermittently discharge to produce corrective fast components based on certain features of the vestibulo-ocular signal (see below).

PATTERN OF EYE MOTION. It had been intuitively assumed that during the slow phase of nystagmus the eyes deviated toward the periphery of the orbit and that the fast component was a resetting movement rotating the globe back to the center.[44] Recently it has been shown, however, that the fast component acts as an anticipatory movement taking the eyes toward the periphery.[86, 132, 180] During physiologic stimulation (such as angular rotation), the fast components of the initial beats of nystagmus attain a larger amplitude than the preceding slow components and the eyes deviate in the direction of the fast component (see Fig. 67a). The apparent advantage of this strategy is that the eyes are ready to focus on newly arriving targets in the field of rotation and fixation can be maintained during the subsequent slow component.

The initiation of fast components can be related to the eye position in the orbit and to a lesser degree on the eye velocity during the slow component.[106] The same highly organized pattern occurs whether the nystagmus is induced by vestibular or visual stimuli. A fast component is generated when the slow component returns the eyes to a certain position near the midline as though there were an orbital threshold position for the initiation of fast components. The exact threshold position varies with the velocity of the slow component of nystagmus but it is usually near the midposition.[86] Rotatory-induced nystagmus has a pattern so reproducible that any alterations provide clinically useful information (see Fig. 67).

EFFECT OF EXPERIMENTAL LESIONS. *Spontaneous Nystagmus.* Spontaneous vestibular nystagmus is produced in animals by lesions of the labyrinth, the vestibular nerve and the vestibular nuclei.[16,57,60,191] A key ingredient for the production of spontaneous nystagmus is an imbalance in the vestibulo-ocular pathways. Damage to one labyrinth results in spontaneous nystagmus whose slow component is directed toward the lesion side; the tonic input from the intact side is no longer balanced by input from the damaged side. This spontaneous nystagmus is indistinguishable from nystagmus produced by stimulation of the normal labyrinth. If a process simultaneously removes both labyrinths spontaneous nystagmus does not result, demonstrating that for production of nystagmus the relative balance of input is more important than the absolute magnitude of input.

Spontaneous nystagmus produced by sectioning of the vestibular nerve duplicates that resulting from labyrinthectomy. The slow component is directed toward the side of the lesion. The direction of spontaneous nystagmus associated with lesions of the vestibular nuclei, however, is less predictable, and depends on the location and extent of the lesion. Uemura and Cohen[191] produced spontaneous nystagmus in monkeys with small focal lesions in the vestibular nuclei. They found that the slow phase of nystagmus developed contralateral to lesions in the superior and rostral medial nuclei and ipsilateral to lesions in the lateral and caudal medial nuclei. The imbalance between inhibitory and excitatory secondary vestibular neurons undoubtedly determined the direction of spontaneous nystagmus.

Induced Nystagmus. Lesions involving the vestibulo-ocular pathways in animals may effect either the slow or fast component and occasionally both phases of induced nystagmus. Interruption of the connections linking the semicircular canals to the oculomotor neurons decreases the velocity of the slow components of induced nystagmus. Lesions involving the peripheral vestibular structures (end organ and nerve) affect the nystagmus in both eyes equally since the central pathways are symmetrically connected. A single remaining labyrinth senses angular rotation in both directions and produces conjugate nystagmus in both directions. The maximum slow component velocity of induced nystagmus is asymmetric, however, because of the asymmetry in afferent nerve firing rate produced by ampullopetal and ampullofugal endolymph flow (see Characteristics of Afferent Responses, Chapter 2). Central lesions lying anywhere from the vestibular nuclei to the oculomotor neurons often produce disconjugate nystagmus since the pathways to the eye muscles diverge beginning at the vestibular nuclei. A lesion of the MLF, for example, impairs slow and fast components made by the ipsilateral medial rectus muscle but leaves normal slow and fast components at the contralateral lateral rectus (see Fig. 67d).

The proposed role of the parapontine reticular formation in the production of rapid horizontal eye movements is largely based on the results of experimental lesions in several species of animals.[34] Animals with unilateral lesions of the parapontine reticular formation lose all types of rapid ipsilateral eye movement and the eyes move in the contralateral hemifield. Ipsilateral voluntary saccades and quick phases of vestibular and optokinetic nystagmus are affected equally. Stimuli that normally would produce nystagmus with ipsilateral fast components simply cause a strong tonic contralateral deviation of the eyes (see Fig. 67c). On the other hand, stimuli that produce contralateral fast components result in normal nystagmus. Lesions in the pretectal region have a similar effect on vertical rapid eye movements without affecting horizontal eye movements,[28,147] an effect consistent with the separate neural organization of horizontal and vertical saccades (see Organization of Visual-Ocular Control).

HABITUATION. The term habituation refers to a reduction in response with repeated stimulation. More specifically, with regard to nystagmus, it refers to a long lasting decrease in the velocity of the slow component after repeated stimulation of the semicircular canals. Habituation has been reported with both physiologic and electric stimulation of the semicircular canal nerves in animals and with caloric and rotatory stimulation of the canals in man.[43] Habituation is not a single phenomenon but represents the end effect of multiple factors, some known and others entirely unknown.

Adaptation. As discussed earlier, adaptation refers to the slow decline in the firing rate of afferent nerves associated with a long lasting constant stimulus to the cristae. After the stimulus stops the firing rate transiently decreases below its baseline value. Although adaptation could account for decreased slow component velocity of induced nystagmus on repeated stimulation several kinds of evidence indicate that it is not a major factor in the production of habituation. Adaptation is a transient phenomenon while habituation occurs when the interval between stimulation varies from a few minutes to as long as several days.[25,48,87] In fact, spacing the stimulation sessions days apart results in greater habituation than massing the sessions on a single day.[25,58] Once habituation is established it remains for several weeks.[25,27,87,135]

The two most convincing pieces of evidence showing that habituation is not a result of adaptation at the primary afferent neuron level are: 1) that double caloric irrigations do not cause habituation[39] and 2) unilateral caloric irrigation results in habituation of nystagmus in one direction regardless of the ear stimulated or the temperature of water used.[27,38,155] In the first instance afferent nerves from both horizontal semicircular canals are stimulated by a caloric irrigation of the same temperature and since the balance of input to the vestibular nuclei is unchanged nystagmus is not produced. If peripheral adaptation were a significant factor in producing habituation, subsequent unilateral caloric infusions should exhibit habituation. In the second instance warm caloric infusion in one ear results in habituation to subsequent cold infusions in the opposite ear, both of which result in nystagmus directed toward the ear receiving the warm infusion. Adaptation at the end organ level could not account for this transfer of habituation from one ear to the other.

Level of Arousal. Since the turn of the century numerous investigators have noted a relationship between the magnitude of induced nystagmus and the state of arousal of the animals or human subjects receiving vestibular stimulation.[42] A systemic study of the level of arousal as part of the habituation phenomenon, however, has only recently been undertaken. If a subject who has developed habituation with repeated stimulation is alerted with different types of stimuli (auditory, tactile) the suppressed nystagmus returns to near the prehabituation

64

level.[36, 37] Adrenalin or amphetamine given to animals who have developed habituation reinstates the suppressed nystagmus and impairs the development of subsequent habituation.[48] These alerting maneuvers affect the level of habituation whether the testing is performed in darkness or in the light, which permits visual-vestibular interaction.

Collins and his associates first began a systemic evaluation of the instructions given to human subjects aimed at controlling alertness during rotational and caloric testing and found that the velocity of the slow components of induced nystagmus depended on the type of mental activity.[36, 37, 42, 43] If the subject was instructed to relax and daydream the velocity was less than when he was instructed to perform continuous mental arithmetic (successive division). Although other techniques of mental alerting such as having the subject report on the turning sensation or estimate the time of auditory stimuli were also effective, mental arithmetic tasks were most effective in maintaining mental alertness. The mental task had to achieve a certain degree of complexity since simple forward counting was not effective in maintaining the nystagmus response.[42] Abolition of nystagmus does not occur with repeated stimulation in darkness if the subject is properly alerted but some reduction in nystagmus slow component velocity and changes in nystagmus pattern occur even if the subject is maximally alerted.[43]

Suppression with Visual Input. When caloric or rotatory testing is performed in the light permitting the subject to fixate the resulting nystagmus is markedly diminished compared to testing in the dark. This is the mechanism by which dancers and skaters effectively inhibit vestibular nystagmus during high velocity spins.[40, 52, 68, 146] They develop fixation suppression to such an extent that nystagmus is not produced by caloric or rotatory stimuli when fixation is permitted.[40] When dancers and skaters are tested in the dark, however, their vestibular induced nystagmus is indistinguishable from that of normal subjects.[41] The mechanism of visual-vestibular interaction is discussed in detail in a later section.

Normal subjects, given repeated unidirectional rotatory stimulation while fixating develop a directional imbalance of induced nystagmus that remains on subsequent testing either with fixation or in total darkness.[76, 77] Therefore, habituation is transferred from testing in the light with fixation to subsequent testing in total darkness. Barr and coworkers[14] recently demonstrated that the slow component velocity of rotatory induced nystagmus could be markedly diminished in the dark by instructing the subject to visualize an imaginary target moving with the rotatory chair. The nystagmus inhibition occurred despite mental alerting tasks. If the subject was instructed to imagine a target that was stationary relative to the moving chair the induced nystagmus was enhanced as though a synergistic optokinetic stimulus were added to the vestibular stimulus. The nervous system is apparently able to generate a "visual" frame of reference when vision is not available. These observations emphasize the importance of giving a clear set of instructions to subjects undergoing vestibular testing since without such instructions the subject might adopt his own strategy regarding an imaginary fixed or moving frame of reference.

Suppression with Other Sensory Input. Although visual signals are effectively removed when subjects are rotated in the dark, other sensory clues (tactile, auditory and proprioceptive) may provide information for establishing a frame of reference and potentially inhibiting or enhancing induced nystagmus.[104, 105] For example, a fixed sound source such as an air conditioner would provide a stationary frame of reference while tactile stimulation from the rotating chair might provide a moving frame of reference. If the subject is able to move his neck during vestibular stimulation he might diminish the vestibulo-ocular signals with competing cervico-ocular signals. The mechanism of cervicovestibular interaction is discussed in a later section.

The organism is constantly required to adjust to new sensory input by a process of rearranging sensory-perceptual and sensory-motor relations. This is essentially what the learning process represents—a rearrangement of priorities. With repeated vestibular stimulation a rearrangement of vestibulo-ocular relations occurs such that a more efficient oculomotor control is achieved. This may result through a rearrangement of other sensory input for ocular control or through "voluntary" control mechanisms.[43]

Characteristics of Eye Movements Induced by Otolith Stimulation

General Properties

Because the sensory cells of each macule are oriented in multiple directions, the firing rate of the macular afferent nerve reflects a complex pattern of excitation and inhibition of different units within the macule. By comparison, all the sensory cells of a semicircular canal crista are aligned in the same direction and are either excited or inhibited by a stimulus acting in the plane of the canal. The organization of the otolith-ocular reflexes is therefore more complex than that of canal-ocular reflexes. To simplify the discussion of otolith-ocular reflexes it is helpful to think of the otolith organs (utricle and saccule combined) as a unitary sensor capable of resolving all of the linear forces acting on the head into a single resultant vector force. This "unitary" three-dimensional otolith receptor is positioned at the center of the head with the x and z axes orthogonal to and the y axis parallel to the earth's vertical axis. The receptor computes the angle (θ) between the resultant vector force and the earth's vertical axis and sends this information to the CNS where a compensatory eye deviation is generated with the goal of maintaining the eyes normal to the earth's vertical axis. The perfect macular reflex would be one that rotates the eyes at an angle equal and opposite to θ. In the case of head tilt in the x-y plane as illustrated in Figure 32, the efficiency or gain of the reflex can be

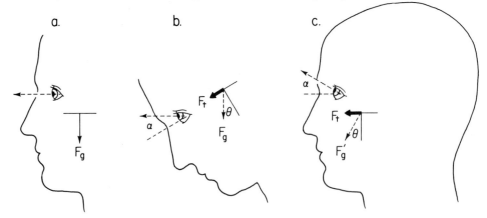

Figure 32. Compensatory eye movement induced by static head tilt (b) and by linear acceleration tangential to the "unitary" otolith receptor (c). α equals the angle of eye rotation and θ equals the angle between the resultant force of gravity and a line orthogonal to the receptor.

represented by the relation of the angle of eye deviation to the angle of head tilt θ (gain equals α/θ).

With these concepts in mind it is interesting to compare the eye movements produced by head tilt (Fig. 32b) with those produced by linear displacement of the head (Fig. 32c). During static head tilt, θ is equal to the angle of tilt and the resulting ocular rotation α compensates for the tilt, maintaining the eyes in the horizontal plane. The otolith signal also provides the brain with an awareness of the true earth vertical (the direction of the gravitational vector F_g). The situation is different when linear acceleration is applied parallel to the x axis (Fig. 32c). If a linear force F_t is chosen that is exactly equal to the F_t produced by static head tilt in Figure 32b, the eye rotation α will be the same as that associated with the head tilt. The eyes will not be aligned with the earth horizontal, however, but rather in a plane perpendicular to the direction of the resulting vector F_g'. Furthermore, the subject will erroneously interpret the direction of F_g' as that of the earth vertical.

Eye Movements Produced by Head Tilt

Compensatory eye movements produced by static head tilt in different animals are either rotational or torsional depending on the direction of tilt and the position of the orbits in the skull. In rabbits and fish lateral tilt causes a vertically directed rotational movement and forward-backward tilt causes a torsional eye movement (Fig. 2). In humans countertorsional movements are produced by lateral tilt (ocular counterrolling) while vertical rotation results from forward-backward tilt (Fig. 32). Eye movements associated with static tilt have been studied most extensively in the rabbit. Head tilt in the dark within a range of ± 45 degrees about the normal position causes a compensatory eye deviation with a gain of approximately 0.6.[4] That is, the angle of eye rotation (α) is approximately 60 percent of the angle of tilt (θ). In human subjects the ocular response to tilt is much less efficient. The maximum ocular torsion for a lateral tilt of 50 degrees is only 5 to 6 degrees (a gain of approximately 0.1).[138]

Eye Movements Produced by Linear Acceleration of the Head

Linear acceleration forces, acting upon the head and hence upon the otoliths, interact with the constantly active gravitational force. The resultant vector force F_g' forms an angle θ with the earth vertical. In the two-dimensional model illustrated in Figure 32 the magnitude of θ can be computed by dividing the value of the linear acceleration vector F_t (in units of m/sec²) by that of the gravitational acceleration F_g (9.8 m/sec²). This ratio defines the value of the tangent of the angle θ so that $\theta = \arctan \dfrac{F_t}{F_g}$. By comparing θ with the induced angular deviation of the eyes (α) the gain of the otolith-ocular reflex can be computed for different magnitudes of linear acceleration.

LINEAR TRACK ACCELERATION. Continuous linear acceleration in a vehicle along a straight track theoretically constitutes an ideal stimulus to test the function of the otolith-ocular reflex arc. The direction of the linear acceleration vector lies perpendicular to the earth vertical and the effective stimulus is the result of interaction of the force due to the vehicle acceleration with that of gravity.

Unfortunately from a clinical point of view the length of track required to produce measurable otolith-ocular reflexes is much greater than is practically feasible. Eye movements induced in experimental animals by constant linear acceleration take several seconds to reach a steady state of deviation.[4, 114] For example, with a constant acceleration of approximately one-tenth of the gravitational acceleration (0.90 m/sec^2), the eyes take 4 seconds to reach an angular deviation of only 3 degrees.[4] The gain of this compensatory eye movement is approximately 0.5 ($F_t/F_g \approx 0.1$; θ = arctan 0.1 = 5.7 degrees; α = 3 degrees; gain = α/θ = 3/5.7 = 0.53). Assuming a similar gain, a minimum of approximately 110 m/sec^2 are required to produce an angular eye deviation of 45 degrees. Considering the slowness of these reflexes, in order to produce this large eye deviation the subject would have to be displaced in a longitudinal track of approximately 1000 meters. Because of the obvious difficulties in generating such a stimulus other types of linear acceleration have been used clinically.

PARALLEL SWING. The parallel swing consists of a platform suspended from the ceiling by four stiff bars about 2 to 3 meters in length (Fig. 33). The moving parts are connected by ball bearings so that the platform can be displaced in only one direction. The natural period (T) in seconds of the swing is dependent on the length of arms (λ) in meters by $T = 2\pi \sqrt{\lambda/g}$. The oscillation amplitude and hence the acceleration depend on the initial deviation of the platform, which, once released, exhibits a damped oscillation of frequency $1/T$. The parallel swing has a vertical displacement as well as a horizontal displacement but the former is minor compared to the latter (less than 10 percent).

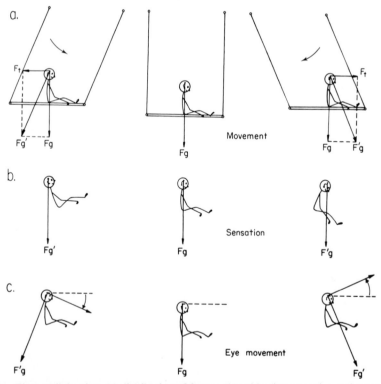

Figure 33. The parallel swing. (a) distribution of forces, (b) subjective sensation and (c) compensatory eye movements at different swing positions. Curved arrows indicate direction of acceleration. (Adapted from Jongkees, L. B. W.: Pathology of the vestibular sensation. In Kornhuber, H. H. (ed.): *Handbook of Sensory Physiology,* vol. VI, part 2. Springer-Verlag, New York, 1974.)

A human subject seated on the platform and displaced along an occipitofrontal axis in total darkness experiences the sensation of being tilted backward with acceleration forward and of being tilted forward with acceleration backward (Fig. 33).[96, 98] As discussed earlier, the subjective sensation of the earth vertical corresponds to the resultant force F_g' (Fig. 33b). The direction of the compensatory vertical eye deviation also depends on the direction of F_g'. When the sensation is that of the head being tilted backward the eyes deviate toward the feet and when the sensation is one of forward tilt, the eyes deviate upward. The eyes move to maintain the direction of gaze orthogonal to the direction of the apparent gravitational vector F_g' (Fig. 33c).

Only qualitative data exist concerning the efficiency in humans[98] of the compensatory eye movements induced by the parallel swing. The amplitude of the eye movements (α) is small compared to the angle θ between the resultant force F_g' and the earth vertical (gain usually less than 0.3). In the rabbit, where most quantitative studies have been performed, the gain of compensatory eye movements is frequently dependent.[4] The gain is highest (0.3 to 0.4) at low frequencies (0.05 to 0.1 Hz) and decreases to less than 0.1 for frequencies greater than 0.3 Hz, falling even more at higher frequencies.

NYSTAGMUS AND OTOLITH STIMULATION. Another method of stimulating the otolith organs is to rotate a subject around the cephalocaudal axis, like a barbeque rotation. Stimulation of the semicircular canals can be minimized by maintaining a constant angular velocity. The otolith organs are subjected to a periodically changing linear acceleration of ± 1 g. Barbeque rotation in animals and humans produces compensatory eye movements which at times have the characteristics of nystagmus.[47, 78]

The relationship between otolith stimulation and the production of nystagmus in humans has been studied in more detail by means of a linear track and horizontal sinusoidal linear acceleration acting in the frontal and transverse planes of the head.[141] Figure 34 illustrates horizontal nystagmus induced in a normal human subject by sinusoidal linear acceleration applied in the horizontal plane at a frequency of 0.2 Hz on a 40 foot linear track. The maximum velocity of the slow

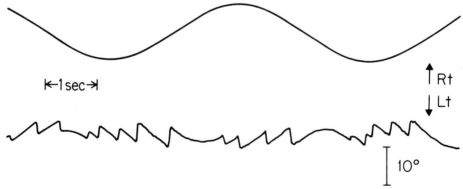

Figure 34. Horizontal nystagmus in a normal human subject induced by sinusoidal linear acceleration (0.2 Hz, 15 feet/sec maximum velocity) applied in the horizontal plane. Upper trace represents motion of subject, lower trace is EOG recording. (Adapted from Niven, J. I., Carroll Hixson, W., and Correia, M. J.: An experimental approach to the dynamics of the vestibular mechanisms. In *Symposium on the Role of the Vestibular Organs in the Exploration of Space*. U.S. Government Printing Office, Washington, 1965.)

components is comparable to that produced by sinusoidal angular acceleration at 0.2 Hz and 15 deg/sec peak velocity suggesting that a common mechanism produces nystagmus by macular and semicircular canal stimulation.

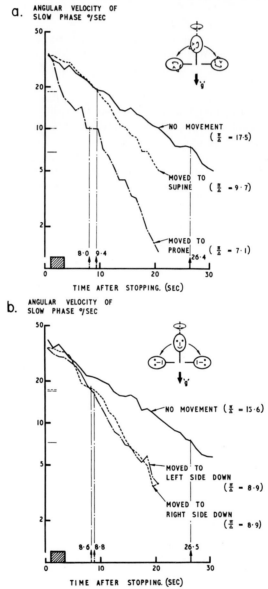

Figure 35. Effect of changing head position on responses to angular rotation in normal human subjects. After rotation about the vertical axis at a constant velocity of 60 deg/sec, the subject was suddenly stopped. The shaded block on the abscissa indicates the time period in which the subject was moved from the vertical to horizontal position. The mean duration of the after sensation in seconds is indicated by the arrows on the abscissa. π/Δ = mean time constant decay in seconds. Mean values are from 8 subjects. (From Benson, A. J., and Bodin, M. A.: *Effect of orientation to the gravitational vertical on nystagmus following rotation about a horizontal axis.* Acta Otolaryngol. 61:517, 1966, with permission.)

An important question is whether lesions selectively involving the otolith organs can produce nystagmus. Intuitively this seems improbable since the disease process would be likely to affect the entire macule, resulting in a random loss of stimulation from many different sensory units all with different polarization vectors (see Fig. 20). The situation is distinctly different with lesions involving a single semicircular canal where all sensory cells are aligned with their kinocilia in the same direction and consequently nystagmus is produced in the plane of the damaged canal. Animal experiments in which a single macular nerve is either stimulated or cut have produced conflicting results. Suzuki and coworkers[183] reported that in the cat strong stimulation of the utricular nerve with recurrent pulses resulted in rotatory nystagmus, the uppermost movement beating toward the stimulated side. Fluur and Siegborn[63] selectively sectioned the utricular nerve on one side in cats and found horizontal spontaneous nystagmus directed toward the normal ear. Other investigators have found other types of nystagmus or have been unable to produce nystagmus with selective utricular nerve stimulation or sectioning.[33] These varying results probably reflect the difficulty in selectively stimulating or producing a lesion in a single macular nerve without affecting the remainder of the labyrinth.

Interaction of Semicircular Canal and Otolith-Induced Eye Movements

The existence of otolith-ocular reflexes was documented at the turn of the century, but reliable clinical tests of these reflexes are still not available. Because of the technical difficulties involved in stimulating the otolith-ocular reflexes investigators have attempted to measure otolith function indirectly by observing changes that otolith stimulation induces in the more easily elicited semicircular canal-ocular reflexes.[18] For example, the nystagmus that develops in response to an impulse of angular acceleration can be compared at different angles of tilt in relation to the earth vertical (Fig. 35). The effect on the canal-induced nystagmus of a change in linear acceleration of ± 1 g can be evaluated with this method. The semicircular canal-induced nystagmus reaction reaches a peak slow component velocity almost immediately and then slowly decays over the next 30 to 60 seconds. As suggested earlier, the otolith-ocular reflexes are sluggish, so if one changes the subjects' head position immediately after the impulse, the initial peak slow component velocity is not affected but the velocity of the slow components decays more rapidly and the total duration of nystagmus is decreased. Other studies, confirming the effect of positional change of the head on caloric-induced nystagmus and spontaneous nystagmus,[31, 61, 97] demonstrate an interaction between the otolith and canal-mediated ocular reflexes; these methods have not been evaluated for their usefulness in clinical assessment of otolith function.

VESTIBULO-OCULAR REFLEX INTERACTION WITH OTHER SYSTEMS

Neck-Vestibular Interaction

Introduction

Ocular stability during most natural head movements results from a coordinated interaction of signals originating in vestibular, visual and neck receptors. The compensatory nature of neck-induced eye movements has been documented in animals. De Kleyn in 1924[102] showed that if one holds an animal's head stationary and displaces the body, a compensatory eye deviation occurs which tends to preserve the relationship between gaze and the body axis (Fig. 36a). Nonfoveated animals, such as the rabbit, exhibit clear compensatory eye deviations since they possess almost no spontaneous eye movements.[74] Cervico-ocular and vestibulo-ocular reflex interaction is more difficult to study in humans because of the dominance of voluntary and visually controlled eye movements. Very few investigators have quantitatively assessed eye, head and neck movement coordination in humans and the clinical significance of lesions involving the cervico-ocular reflex pathways is uncertain (see Cervical Vertigo, Chapter 7).

Anatomic and Physiologic Basis

Animal studies have shown that the cervico-ocular reflex originates from nerve endings in the ligaments and capsules of the upper cervical articulations.[46, 82, 128] The reflex can be induced by electrically stimulating the capsules of the upper cervical joints, the C_1 to C_3 dorsal roots and the high cervical spinal cord. The reflex is not induced by stimulating the superficial muscles or skin of the neck. Bilateral sectioning of the high cervicodorsal roots or the application of local anesthetic agents around the cervical articulations abolishes the cervico-ocular reflexes. Unilateral interruption of the neck-ocular reflex pathways produces nystagmus in rabbits, cats and monkeys when fixation is inhibited although no consistent relationship exists between the side of dorsal root involvement and the direction of nystagmus.[91, 95] As with the vestibulo-ocular reflexes, the eye muscles are either exited or inhibited by neck stimulation depending on whether the muscle is agonistic or antagonistic for the required compensatory movement.

Recent electrophysiologic experiments suggest that the cervico-ocular reflexes are mediated via the vestibular nuclei (primarily in the medial and descending nuclei).[82, 165] The precise projections of the neck afferents to each vestibular nucleus are only partially known, but it can be anticipated that since the neck-

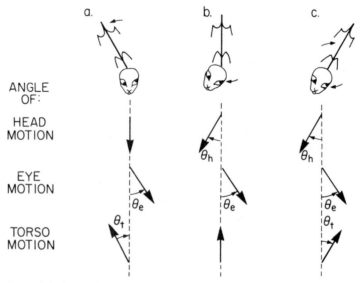

Figure 36. Synergistic interaction of cervico-ocular and vestibulo-ocular reflexes. See text for details.

induced eye movements compensate for displacement in the precise plane of body motion, the vestibular nuclei must contain a discrete topographic representation of cervical afferents in a manner similar to that of the vestibular afferents.

Electric stimulation of the high cervicodorsal roots in the cat produces evoked potentials in the contralateral vestibular nuclei[82] followed by excitation of the abducens nucleus ipsilateral to the neck stimulation and inhibition of the contralateral abducens nucleus (see Fig. 13). In addition, stimulation of the cervicodorsal roots enhances the amplitude of action potentials in the ipsilateral abducens nerve induced by contralateral vestibular nerve stimulation, and inhibits action potentials in the contralateral abducens nerve induced by ipsilateral vestibular nerve stimulation. Vestibulo-ocular and cervico-ocular reflex interaction, therefore, result from a convergence of neck and semicircular canal afferents on secondary vestibular neurons.

Characteristics of Neck-Induced Eye Movements

Figure 36 illustrates the synergistic interaction of neck and vestibulo-ocular reflexes. When the rabbit's head is turned to the right (clockwise about the cephalocaudal axis) the eyes turn counterclockwise in the orbit because the movement stimulates the horizontal semicircular canals and neck reflexes (Fig. 36b). The direction of the eye movement is the same as if the whole animal had been rotated, stimulating only the semicircular canals (Fig. 36c). The characteristics of the neck-ocular reflex alone are evaluated by rotating the body while the head is stationary (Fig. 36a). The same relationship between head and torso is produced as in Figure 36b and the eyes deviate in the same direction. In both instances the normal relationship between eyes and torso is maintained.

Since the time of Bárány, rotating the body with the head stationary and measuring the eye movements has been considered a potential functional test of the human neck-ocular reflex pathways.[10, 11] Several methodologic problems have been encountered, however. It is difficult to induce body motion and concurrently maintain the head completely stationary so as to avoid vestibular stimulation. As with vestibular-induced eye movements, care must be taken to inhibit fixation while monitoring the neck-induced eye movement. Even if these problems are overcome a body torsion of 50 to 60 degrees results in a compensatory eye deviation of only 4 to 5 degrees.[131, 187] The magnitude of the reflex response varies with the frequency of sinusoidal body rotation, being optimal between 0.1 and 1.0 Hz (when eye and body motion are in phase).[131] Compensatory sinusoidal eye movements induced by sinusoidal body rotation take on the appearance of nystagmus if the stimulus is large enough (Fig. 37). The direction of the slow phase of nystagmus is such that the eye is driven in phase with the motion of the trunk.

The neck-ocular reflexes exert a strong influence on both vestibular- and optokinetic-induced nystagmus. Tonic neck deviation in the rabbit produces an imbalance in the otherwise symmetrical nystagmus that results from rotating the animal sinusoidally with the head and body normally aligned. When the slow components of nystagmus are in the direction of the neck-induced tonic ocular deviation, the amplitude of the fast components and the velocity of the slow components are smaller than those of the nystagmus in the opposite direction. Figure 38 illustrates cervicovestibulo-ocular reflex interaction when a rabbit is sinusoidally rotated with the head maintained at three different positions with respect to the body. When the head is turned to the left (Fig. 38a) the mean eye position and slow components are displaced to the right and fast components to

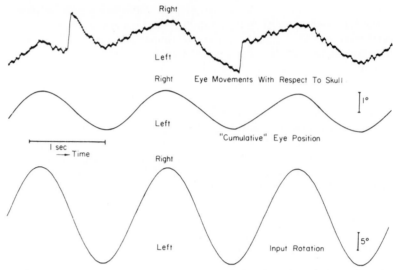

Figure 37. Compensatory eye movements (upper trace) induced by sinusoidal rotation of the trunk (lower trace) while the head is kept stationary (rotation frequency 0.6 Hz, amplitude ± 13.5 degrees). The "cumulative" eye position shows an angular travel of the eyeball of ± 1.0 degrees. The eye movements have a slow and fast component similar to vestibular nystagmus. (From Meiry, J. L.: Vestibular and proprioceptive stabilization of eye movements. In Bach-Y-Rita, P., Collins, C. C., and Hyde, J. E. (eds.): *The Control of Eye Movements.* Academic Press, New York, 1971, with permission.)

the left are inhibited. The reverse occurs when the head is tonically deviated to the right (Fig. 38c). Whether lesions of the neck-ocular reflex pathways or static neck deviations in humans change vestibular-induced nystagmus in a predictable fashion awaits further study.

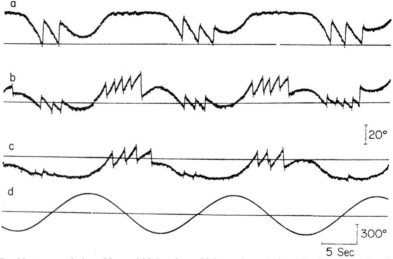

Figure 38. Nystagmus induced in a rabbit by sinusoidal angular rotation (d) with the head maintained at three orientations with respect to the torso. In a, b, and c the head is to the left, straight ahead and to the right, respectively. In a, the mean eye position is displaced to the right, and left beating nystagmus is inhibited. The reverse occurs in c.

74

Visual-Vestibular Interaction

Introduction

The relationship between the head and an object in the environment may change in several ways. The object may move relative to the head, the head may move relative to the object or the head and object may move simultaneously. The visual and vestibular signals interact synergistically to stabilize gaze during most natural head movements. As discussed in the previous section, if the neck is also turned, the neck-ocular reflex participates in the compensatory movement. The effect is better ocular stability than would be possible if each system worked alone. Occasionally vestibular and visual signals conflict and one signal must override the other in order to maintain gaze stability. In these instances the visually mediated ocular reflexes override the vestibulo-ocular reflex. For example, when the head and visual target are moving at the same velocity the vestibulo-ocular reflex is suppressed and gaze is maintained on the target (see Fig. 12).

Organization of Visual-Ocular Control

Two visually controlled ocular stabilizing systems produce versional eye movements, the saccadic and smooth pursuit.[53, 159, 197, 198, 204] The saccade system responds to an error in the direction of gaze with respect to the position of an object of interest by initiating a rapid eye movement (a saccade) to correct the "retinal position error," bringing the object to the fovea in the shortest possible time. The smooth pursuit system, responsible for maintaining gaze on a moving target, compares the eye velocity with that of the target velocity and produces a continuous match of the eye and target position. Optokinetic nystagmus is generally considered to be a form of smooth pursuit in which the eye tracking motion is periodically interrupted by corrective saccades in the opposite direction to relocate the gaze on new targets coming into the visual field.

SACCADES. *Basic Features.* Saccades are stereotyped in that their trajectory and velocity cannot be voluntarily altered.[20] If a subject attempts to slow his saccadic eye movements the size of the jumps is diminished but the velocity and duration is appropriate to the size. Saccades made in darkness or with eyes closed are slower than saccades of equal amplitude made in a lighted room which permits fixation.[17]

When following a target moving in small stepwise jumps (<10 degrees), the eyes normally accelerate rapidly, reaching maximum velocity midway to the target, then decelerate with minimal overshooting or undershooting.[8, 198] By contrast, when making large saccades (>25 degrees), the eyes reach peak velocity early in the trajectory, then undergo a prolonged deceleration. They consistently undershoot the target and require a second small saccade to reach the target. Overshooting of the target is uncommon in normal subjects. A characteristic delay period (reaction time) exists between the time of target jump and the induced saccade (approximately 200 msec in normal subjects). If the target moves twice in less than 200 msec, the eyes may jump to the site of the first target position followed by another delay period before jumping to the final target position. This fixed delay period suggests a sampled data system operating at a sampling period of approximately 200 msec. Several models of such a system have been proposed using modern control theory.[45, 158, 204]

Anatomic Pathways. The site of immediate supranuclear control of horizontal saccadic eye movements is the parapontine region and of vertical saccadic movements, the pretectal region.[88] Neurons in these centers generate the high rate of firing (pulse) needed to overcome the viscoelastic properties of the globe and accelerate it to the rapid saccadic velocities (see Fig. 31d). The parapontine region controls horizontal saccades through its connections with the ipsilateral sixth and contralateral third nerve nuclei (via the MLF), while the pretectal region fires into the nearby third nerve complex to generate vertical saccades. As suggested earlier, both voluntary and involuntary control of the saccade pulse generating centers exists. Stimulation of each frontal eye field produces horizontal saccades, whereas vertical saccades are only produced by simultaneous stimulation of identical locations in each hemisphere.[88] The nature of cerebellar and basal ganglia control of the brain stem saccade centers is poorly understood but both structures are important for generating accurate voluntary saccades. Involuntary saccades (fast components of vestibular and optokinetic nystagmus) are initiated via inputs to the saccade generating centers from the vestibular nuclei and optic pathways in the occipital lobe and tectal region of the brain stem. The mechanism by which a vestibular or visual signal producing a slow component initiates a fast component from the brain stem saccade centers is only partially understood (see Nystagmus, Fast Component Generation).

SMOOTH PURSUIT. *Basic Features.* The function of the smooth pursuit system is to stabilize a moving target on the fovea. Activated by responding to movement of a target across the retina, the smooth pursuit system produces an eye movement approximately equal in velocity to that of the target velocity.[53, 197] If the velocity of the target exceeds a critical maximum level (30 to 60 deg/sec in normal subjects) the eyes continually fall behind and must resort to frequent corrective saccades to bring the target to the fovea. A subject can pursue a target with constantly changing velocity only if the pattern of movement can be predicted (as with a sinusoidal pattern).[197]

Anatomic Pathways. The anatomic substrate for the smooth pursuit system is not fully known.[88] As with saccades the immediate supranuclear control is located in the pretectal and parapontine regions for vertical and horizontal pursuit, respectively. Visual signals relayed in the optic tracts to the occipital lobes and superior colliculi provide feedback control to allow the smooth pursuit system to maintain eye velocity near target velocity. Visual signals carried via the accessory optic tract to the inferior olives and midline cerebellum are important in generating the appropriate eye velocity.[137]

OPTOKINETIC NYSTAGMUS. *Basic Features.* Optokinetic nystagmus is induced by moving a striped pattern across a subject's visual field. When the subject attempts to follow the stripes he produces a large amplitude, low frequency nystagmus ("look" optokinetic nystagmus). If he is instructed to stare straight ahead at the striped surface and not follow the stripes, he produces a small amplitude high frequency nystagmus ("stare" optokinetic nystagmus).[85] In normal subjects the velocity of the slow components of induced nystagmus approaches the stripe velocity for velocities as high as 60 deg/sec.[85, 175] The slow component velocity of stare optokinetic nystagmus falls off faster for higher target velocities than that of look optokinetic nystagmus.

Anatomic Pathways. Many of the same brain stem centers that generate smooth pursuit and saccades also generate the slow and fast component of optokinetic nystagmus, but the pathways that control and interconnect these systems are poorly understood.

Comparison of Vestibular and Pursuit Eye Movements

The schematic diagrams of the smooth pursuit system and the vestibulo-ocular reflex in Figure 39 illustrate important similarities and differences between the two systems. In both instances the velocity of the reflex eye movement ($\dot{\theta}_e$) matches that of the stimulus velocity if the system is functioning perfectly. In the case of the smooth pursuit system the stimulus is the target velocity (or optokinetic drum velocity) ($\dot{\theta}_t$) while for the vestibulo-ocular reflex it is the head velocity ($\dot{\theta}_h$). The eye movement takes the form of either smooth pursuit or nystagmus. In the latter case, $\dot{\theta}_e$ equals the slow component velocity. The target velocity and head velocity must have opposite signs in order to produce $\dot{\theta}_e$ with the same sign. The smooth pursuit system functions as a closed loop system with negative feedback to compare eye and target velocity while the vestibulo-ocular reflex is an open loop system.

The concept of gain introduced in the section on otolith-ocular reflexes is useful for comparing the efficiency of the two systems. The gain simply compares the input and output of each system. For the smooth pursuit system, the gain equals $\dot{\theta}_e / \dot{\theta}_t$ and for the vestibulo-ocular reflex, the gain equals $\dot{\theta}_e / -\dot{\theta}_h$. Measurements of smooth pursuit and vestibulo-ocular reflex gain have been made in animals and humans under numerous different experimental conditions.

For both systems, the gain is dependent on the input velocity and frequency.[159] The smooth pursuit system is most efficient at low target velocities with a gain of approximately 0.95 when normal human subjects follow a sinusoidally moving target at 0.1 Hz and a maximum velocity of 30 deg/sec (unpublished observation). The gain rapidly falls off for target velocities greater than 60 deg/sec and frequencies greater than 1 Hz. The vestibulo-ocular reflex gain is approximately 0.4 when normal human subjects are sinusoidally rotated in the dark at 0.05 Hz and a maximum velocity of 30 deg/sec.[9] Unlike the pursuit system, however, the vestibulo-ocular reflex effectively responds to head movements with velocities greater than 100 deg/sec and frequencies from 1 to 4 Hz.[9, 103] The reader can test

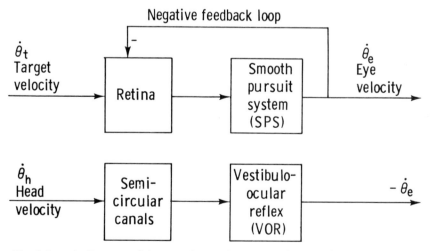

Figure 39. Schematic diagrams of the smooth pursuit system and the vestibulo-ocular reflex. The former is a closed loop negative feedback system and the latter is an open loop system.

this increased efficiency of the vestibulo-ocular reflex over the smooth pursuit system at high input velocities and frequencies by a simple maneuver. Rapidly move your hand back and forth with increasing velocity with your head stationary until your hand appears blurred. Then hold your hand stationary and rapidly move your head back and forth at the same high speed. Despite the rapid head movement the smallest detail of the palm remains clear.[133]

Anatomic and Physiologic Basis of Visual-Vestibular Interaction

Figure 40 diagrams the principal anatomic pathways for visual-vestibular interaction as proposed by Ito.[92] Retinal sensory information reaches the inferior olives by way of the accessory optic tract and the central tegmental tract.[92, 123] Neurons in the inferior olives activate Purkinje cells in the floccule, nodule and adjacent parts of the cerebellum. These areas of the cerebellum also receive primary vestibular afferent fibers and secondary vestibular fibers originating mostly in the medial and descending vestibular nuclei (not shown). Outflow from the cerebellar Purkinje cells terminates at secondary vestibular neurons and neurons in the adjacent reticular substance.[150]

Although Purkinje cell outflow to the vestibular nuclei is inhibitory (as with all Purkinje cell output), since it ends on both excitatory and inhibitory vestibular neurons it can enhance or inhibit the vestibulo-ocular reflex. Several types of experimental data confirm the floccular role in mediating visual-vestibular interaction.[93, 162, 164, 188, 199] Electric stimulation of the floccule inhibits nystagmus induced by physiologic and electric stimulation of the vestibular nerve.[59] The reflex contraction produced in agonist extraocular muscles by electric stimulation of an isolated canal nerve is inhibited by prior stimulation of the floccule, the accessory optic tract or the optic chiasm.[123] Finally, in animals with lesions of the floccule or

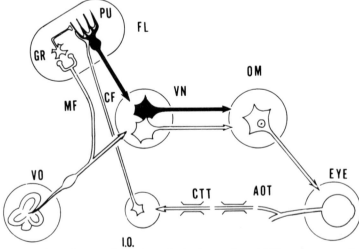

Figure 40. Anatomic pathways of visual-vestibular interaction. AOT, accessory optic tract, CTT, central tegmental tract, IO, inferior olive, VO, vestibular end organ, MF, mossy fiber, CF, climbing fiber, GR, granule cell, PU, Purkinje cell, Fl, flocculus, VN, vestibular nucleus, OM, ocular motoneuron. Inhibitory neurons are filled in black. (From Ito, M.: The vestibulo-cerebellar relationships: vestibulo-ocular reflex arc and flocculus. In Naunton, R. F. (ed.): *The Vestibular System.* Academic Press, New York, 1975, with permission.)

inferior olives, the vestibulo-ocular reflex cannot be modulated by visual stimulation.[93, 162, 188]

Quantitative Aspects of Visual-Vestibular Interaction

Figure 41 gives a simple linear interaction model for the smooth pursuit system and the vestibulo-ocular reflex. The two independent block diagrams in Figure 39 have been interrelated to produce a single output eye velocity ($\dot{\theta}_e$).[107, 167, 203] When the target is stationary, movement of the head results in an equivalent movement of the target in the opposite direction relative to the head. When both the target and head move the driving stimulus to the pursuit system is the angular velocity of the target relative to the head, that is, the difference between the target velocity relative to space ($\dot{\theta}_t$) and the head angular velocity relative to space ($\dot{\theta}_h$). This interaction between head movement and target movement is represented by the box labeled "stimulus interaction." The anatomic equivalent of the box labeled "visual-vestibular interaction" is assumed to be the visual-cerebellar-vestibular pathways discussed in the previous section. In the absence of head movements ($\dot{\theta}_h$ equals 0), the eye movement response is under the control of the closed loop smooth pursuit system, whereas, if the head is rotated in the dark, the pursuit system is inoperative and the eye movement response is under the control of the vestibulo-ocular reflex.

By application of principles derived from simple control theory it can be shown that the overall gain of the visual-vestibular system at low input velocities is given by the equation: $\dot{\theta}_e = 0.95\dot{\theta}_t - 0.97\dot{\theta}_h$. This equation assumes a gain of 0.4 for the vestibulo-ocular reflex alone and 0.95 for the smooth pursuit system alone (average normal values determined in our laboratory with sinusoidal stimulation at 0.05 Hz, maximum velocity 30 deg/sec). If a subject is rotated in a lighted room with a stationary background ($\dot{\theta}_t = 0$), the eye velocity $\dot{\theta}_e = -0.97\theta_h$. In other words, the eye movement is almost equal and opposite to the head movement. This value is more than twice the gain when the subject is rotated in the dark but only slightly greater than the gain of the pursuit system alone (if the head is still and background moves). If the head velocity and target velocity are the same ($\dot{\theta}_h = \dot{\theta}_t$), such as when a subject is rotated while fixating on his extended thumb, $\dot{\theta}_e = -0.02\theta_h$. In this case the eyes remain almost stationary and the vestibulo-ocular reflex is practically inhibited. The eye movements predicted by this linear interac-

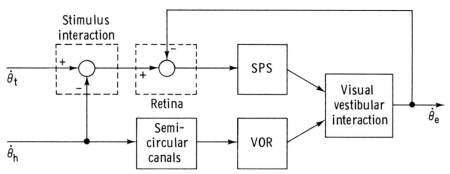

Figure 41. Interaction of the smooth pursuit system and the vestibulo-ocular reflex. See text for details. (Adapted from Lau, C. G. Y., et al.: *A linear model for visual and vestibular interaction.* Aviat. Space Environ. Med. In press.

tion model are remarkably close to those obtained with visual-vestibular interaction testing in normal human subjects and patients.[107]

This model demonstrates the overriding influence in normal subjects of the smooth pursuit system over the vestibulo-ocular reflex at the low frequencies of stimulation used in most clinical vestibular tests. It emphasizes that angular rotation of the head in the light allowing fixation on a stationary or moving background is primarily a test of the pursuit system.

VESTIBULOSPINAL REFLEXES

Comparison of Ocular and Spinal Vestibular Reflexes

It is helpful to consider the similarities and differences between the ocular and spinal vestibular reflexes as an introduction to the organization of vestibulospinal reflexes. If a rabbit is rotated at a constant speed on a turntable and suddenly stopped (producing an impulse of acceleration to the horizontal semicircular canal), a burst of ocular nystagmus results with the slow phase in the direction of the rotation prior to the deceleration (in the directon of endolymph flow). In addition, if the head is mobile it deviates slowly in the same direction as the slow phase eye deviation.[57, 60, 124] In some animals, if the stimulus is large enough quick return movements regularly interrupt the slow head deviation resulting in head oscillation ("head nystagmus"). The relationship between the magnitude of reflex head movement and nystagmus changes along the phylogenetic scale. For example, in pigeons the head movement predominates, in rabbits head movement and nystagmus are equally prominent while in primates nystagmus predominates.[89, 186] When present, head movement occurs in the plane of the stimulated canal; one can infer a highly organized pattern of connections between the individual semicircular canals and neck muscles similar to the connections between the individual canals and the eye muscles.

The rabbit on the turntable, if unrestrained and standing on four legs, tends to fall in the direction of the slow phase of eye and head deviation when the table is suddenly stopped. This falling tendency is counteracted by reflex activation of the antigravity muscles of the limbs on the side toward which the rabbit is falling, producing an increased extensor thrust in those limbs. At the same time the extensor tone of the contralateral limbs is diminished and the rabbit maintains his balance. These extremity muscle reflexes are mediated via the semicircular canals and are always appropriate to prevent falling regardless of the direction of the acceleration force.[124, 157]

The effector organs of the vestibulo-ocular reflexes are the extraocular muscles while those of the vestibulospinal reflexes are the "antigravity" muscles, the extensors of the neck, trunk and extremities. Figure 42 illustrates the organization of the vestibulospinal reflexes. Note the similarities between this figure and Figure 11 that illustrates the organization of the horizontal semicircular canal-ocular reflex. The same push-pull mechanism exists for controlling the balance between the extensor and flexor skeletal muscles as for the lateral and medial recti. A major difference between the organization of ocular and spinal reflexes is the increased complexity of the spinal muscle response compared to the eye movement produced by an agonist and antagonist muscle acting in the horizontal plane. Even a simple movement about an extremity joint in a two-dimensional plane

80

requires a complex pattern of contraction and relaxation in numerous muscles. Multiple agonist and antagonist muscles on both sides must receive appropriate signals to ensure a smooth coordinated movement. Unfortunately, a simple recording technique does not exist for quantifying this complex skeletal muscle response. These factors have hindered the mapping of connections between the labyrinthine receptors and the individual skeletal muscles.

Vestibulospinal Pathways

Secondary vestibular neurons influence spinal anterior horn cell activity by means of three major pathways: 1) the lateral vestibulospinal tract, 2) the medial vestibulospinal tract and 3) the reticulospinal tract. The first two arise directly from neurons in the vestibular nuclei while the third arises from neurons in the reticular formation that are influenced by vestibular stimulation (as well as several other kinds of input). The cerebellum is highly interrelated with each of these pathways.

Lateral Vestibulospinal Tract

It is generally agreed that the vast majority of fibers in the lateral vestibulospinal tract originate from neurons in the lateral vestibular nucleus (Fig. 43).[22] A somatotopic pattern of projections originates in the lateral vestibular nucleus such that neurons in the rostroventral region supply the cervical cord while neurons in the dorsocaudal region innervate the lumbosacral cord. Neurons in the intermediate region supply the thoracic cord. It should be recalled that primary vestibular afferent fibers terminate only in the rostroventral region of the lateral nucleus.

In the spinal cord the fibers run ipsilaterally in the ventral half of the lateral funicle and the lateral part of the ventral funicle (Fig. 43). The tract terminates throughout the length of the cord in the eighth lamina and the medial part of the seventh lamina, either directly on dendrites of anterior horn cells or on interneurons that project to anterior horn cells of the axial and proximal limb musculature.[143] Some of the cells of the eighth lamina send their axons to the contralateral cord, probably accounting for the bilateral effects that have been observed after stimulation in the lateral vestibular nucleus. Activation of vestibulospinal fibers

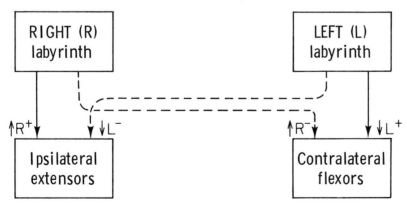

Figure 42. Organization of vestibulospinal tracts. See text for details.

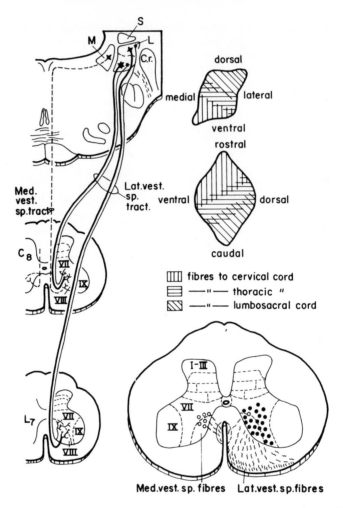

Figure 43. Lateral and medial vestibulospinal tracts. Topographical organization within the lateral vestibular nucleus (upper right) and endings within the spinal cord (lower right). (From Brodal, A.: Anatomical organization of cerebello-vestibulo-spinal pathways. In De Renck, A. V. S., and Knight, J. (eds.): *CIBA Foundtion Symposium: Myotatic, kinesthetic and vestibular mechansims.* Churchill Ltd., London, 1967, with permission.)

by electric stimulation in the lateral nucleus produces monosynaptic excitation of extensor motoneurons and disynaptic inhibition of flexor motoneurons.[55, 120] Both alpha and gamma motoneurons of extensor muscles receive monosynaptic excitatory postsynaptic potentials. Gamma motoneurons fire at lower magnitudes of stimulation, however, so that muscle spindles are activated before stronger stimulation evokes alpha discharge and muscle contraction.[72] The gamma system appears to function as a sensitizing device, ensuring smooth, continuous control, while the alpha system provides a rapid forceful contraction. Consistent with this interpretation is the fact that interrupting the gamma loop by cutting the dorsal roots only slightly reduces the tension that vestibular stimulation produces in the gastrocnemius muscle.[72]

82

Medial Vestibulospinal Tract

The fibers of the medial vestibulospinal tract originate from neurons in the medial vestibular nucleus and enter the spinal cord in the descending MLF (Fig. 43). The fibers travel in the ventral funicle as far as the midthoracic level. The majority end on interneurons in the seventh and eighth lamina of the cervical cord.[142] No monosynaptic connections appear to exist between the medial vestibulospinal tract and cervical anterior horn cells.[72, 200]

Functionally the medial vestibulospinal tract plays an important part in interaction of neck-vestibular-ocular reflexes. It has far fewer fibers than either the lateral vestibulospinal or reticulospinal tracts. Long latency excitatory and inhibitory postsynaptic potentials have been recorded intracellularly from both flexor and extensor cervical motoneurons after stimulation of the descending MLF.[72, 200]

Reticulospinal Tract

The reticulospinal tract originates from neurons in the bulbar reticular formation. The nuclei reticularis gigantocellularis and pontis caudalis provide most of the long fibers passing into the spinal cord although the majority of neurons in the caudal reticular formation also contribute fibers. Both crossed and uncrossed fibers transverse the length of the spinal cord, terminating in the seventh and eighth laminae of the gray matter.[21, 144]

Stimulation of the pontomedullary reticular formation in the regions where the long descending spinal projections originate results in inhibition of both extensor and flexor motoneurons throughout the spinal cord.[112, 113] If localized electric stimulation is applied to the more rostral or lateral regions of the reticular formation, facilitation is produced rather than inhibition.[190] This facilitatory influence must involve multisynaptic connections since the neurons in these regions have short axons and do not send fibers into the spinal cord. The inhibitory and facilitatory reticulospinal fibers do not form well defined tracts within the spinal cord although some separation of the inhibitory and facilitatory fibers occurs in the lateral funicle. As in the case of the lateral vestibulospinal tract, both alpha and gamma motoneurons are influenced by excitatory and inhibitory input from the reticulospinal tract.

The vestibular nuclei are one of many structures that send fibers to the reticular formation. Axonal branches and collaterals of cells in all four main vestibular nuclei are distributed to the pontomedullary reticular formation. Only a small number of primary vestibular fibers end in the reticular formation so that the main vestibular influence on reticulospinal outflow is mediated by way of the secondary vestibular neurons. A pattern exists within the vestiboreticular projections such that each nucleus projects to different areas of the reticular formation, but no detailed somatotopic organization has been identified.[24]

Cerebellar-Vestibular Interaction

The "spinal" cerebellum provides a major source of input to neurons whose axons form the lateral vestibulospinal and reticulospinal tracts. A somatotopic organization of projections to the lateral nucleus occurs in both the vermian cortex and fastigial nuclei (Fig. 44).[21, 150, 157] Direct projections connect the vermian cortex to the lateral vestibular nucleus and indirect projections pass through the

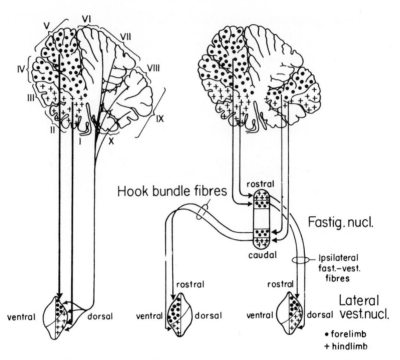

Figure 44. Topographical organization of cerebellar vermian, fastigial nucleus and lateral vestibular nucleus connections. (From Brodal, A.: Anatomy of the vestibular nuclei and their connections. In Kornhuber, H. H. (ed.): *Handbook of Sensory Physiology,* vol. VI, part 1. Springer-Verlag, New York, 1974, with permission.

fastigial nuclei. The caudal part of the fastigial nucleus gives rise to a bundle of fibers that cross the midline (Russell's hook bundle), curving around the brachium conjunctivum before running to the contralateral lateral vestibular nucleus and dorsolateral reticular formation. In addition, direct ipsilateral outflow passes from the fastigial nucleus to areas of the reticular formation that send long fibers to the spinal cord in the reticulospinal tract. The cerebellar-reticular pathways do not exhibit somatotopic organization.[150]

The cerebellar vermis and fastigial nuclei receive input from secondary vestibular neurons, the spinal cord and the pontomedullary reticular formation. The result is a close knit vestibular-reticular-cerebellar functional unit for the maintenance of equilibrium and locomotion.[150]

Vestibular Influence in the Control of Posture and Equilibrium

The elementary unit for the control of tone in the trunk and extremity skeletal muscles is the myotatic reflex (the deep tendon reflex). The myotatic reflexes of the antigravity muscles are under the combined excitatory and inhibitory influence of multiple supraspinal neural centers (Fig. 45).[12, 111] At least in the cat one finds two main facilitatory centers (the lateral vestibular nucleus and rostral reticular formation) and four inhibitory centers (the pericruciate cortex, basal ganglia, cerebellum and caudal reticular formation). The balance of input from these different centers determines the degree of tone in the antigravity muscles. If one removes the inhibitory influence of the frontal cortex and basal ganglia by section-ing the animal's midbrain, a characteristic state of contraction in the antigravity muscles results—so-called decerebrate rigidity. The extensor muscles increase their resistance to lengthening and the deep tendon reflexes become hyperactive. One may conclude that the vestibular system contributes largely to this increased extensor tone after witnessing the marked decrease upon bilateral destruction of the labyrinths.[5] Unilateral destruction of the labyrinth or the lateral vestibular nucleus results in an ipsilateral decrease in tone, indicating that the main excita-tory input to the anterior horn cells arrives from the ipsilateral lateral vestibulo-spinal tract.[69]

In a decerebrate animal with normal labyrinths the intensity of the extensor tone can be modulated in a specific way by changing the position of the head in space.[124, 170] The tone is maximal when the animal is in the supine position with the angle of the mouth 45 degrees above horizontal and minimal when the animal is prone with the angle of the mouth 45 degrees below the horizontal. Intermediate positions of rotation of the animal's body about the transverse or longitudinal axis result in intermediate degrees of extensor tone. If the head of the upright animal is tilted upward (without neck extension), extensor tone in the forelegs increases; downward tilting of the head causes decreased extensor tone and flexion of the forelegs. Lateral tilt produces extension of the extremities on the opposite side.

These tonic labyrinthine reflexes, mediated by way of the otoliths, seldom occur in intact animals or human subjects because of the inhibitory influence of the higher cortical and subcortical centers. They can be demonstrated in prema-ture infants, however, and in adults with lesions releasing the brain stem from the higher neural centers.[129]

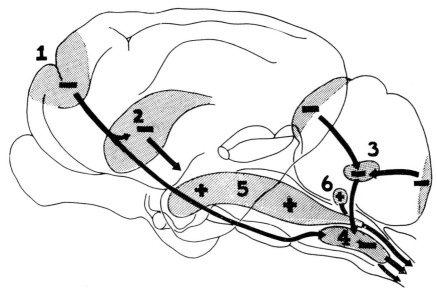

Figure 45. Facilitatory (+) and inhibitory (−) pathways influencing the myotatic spinal reflex in the cat. Inhibitory pathways are: 1) corticobulboreticular, 2) caudatospinal, 3) cerebelloreticular and 4) reticulospinal. Facilitatory pathways are: 5) reticulospinal and 6) vestibulospinal. (From Lindsley, D. B., Schreiner, L. H., and Magoun, H. W.: *An electromyographic study of spasticity.* J. Neurophysiol. 12:197, 1949, with permission.)

SUBJECTIVE VESTIBULAR SENSATION

Introduction

Unlike those sensory organs that respond to energy sources external to the body, the labyrinths respond to self generated forces within the head. During natural head movements these forces are not under voluntary control and therefore the vestibular responses are more automatic than those of the other sensory modalities. For example, one can remove vision simply by closing ones eyes whereas one cannot suppress vestibular stimuli during head movement.

The existence of a separate sense organ for the perception of motion was first appreciated over a hundred years ago through the imaginative experiments of Mach.[121] Recent progress in engineering has made it possible to quantify vestibular sensation in isolation from other sensory inputs (visual, proprioceptive). A sensory illusion experienced while travelling on a railroad train aroused Mach's interest in the study of vestibular sensation. He wrote:

> ". . . on the railroad, when riding a great curve, the horses and the trees often seem to deviate considerably from the vertical . . . This could be explained if one assumes that the direction of the vertical is perceived, and that the direction of the mass acceleration resulting from the interaction of the force of gravity and the centrifugal force, is always considered to be in the vertical direction."

Through a series of experiments Mach became aware that it was the acceleration (or change in velocity of movement) that was perceived. When rotating a subject inside a box about an earth vertical axis he found that

> ". . . every rotatory movement will be recognized immediately according to direction and approximate amount. But if the rotation is maintained uniformly for several seconds, the sensation of rotation will gradually cease entirely . . . As soon as the apparatus is stopped, one has the impression that one is executing, together with the box, a contrary rotation. If the rotating box is opened quickly, the entire visible space and its contents will rotate."

He made a similar observation regarding linear acceleration by producing vertical oscillations in a subject seated on a see-saw platform. The subject

> ". . . always stated that he is sinking shortly before arriving at the highest point of the oscillation . . . Likewise, the rise was always noticed shortly before, or at the lowest point (of displacement) itself, of course always with the eyes closed. Hence, one is very sensitive to oscillations of the amount of the gravity acceleration, and one does not perceive the position or the velocity in the vertical movements, but rather the accelerations."

Mach observed that the perception of motion in his different experiments could be altered by changing the position of the head in relation to the body, which suggested to him that the sensory organs were located in the head. His findings, along with the physiologic and histologic work of contemporaries such as Fluorens,[60] Crum-Brown[50] and Breuer,[19] led him to the conclusion that the semicircular canals and the otoliths were responsible for the perception of angular and linear acceleration, respectively.

Several important clinical observations support the existence of a specific vestibular sensation. Probably the most convincing is that patients without vestibular function (either on an acquired or congenital basis) do not experience a turning sensation when rotated in the dark if visual and tactile cues are eliminated.[79] Patients with complete spinal transections in the cervical region, on the other hand, perceive acceleration normally.[194] The sensation of movement is not dependent on vision or associated nystagmus since blind subjects and patients with complete oculomotor paralysis experience a spinning sensation comparable to that of normal subjects when their vestibular end organs are stimulated. Focal cortical lesions in the nondominant parietal lobe interfere with spatial orientation and the performance of three-dimensional construction tasks, and epileptic discharges from many different areas of the cortex can be associated with a subjective illusion of movement (usually spinning).[13, 49, 148] These observations imply a cerebrocortical representation for vestibular sensation.

Anatomy and Physiology of Vestibular Sensation

The first electrophysiologic identification of vestibulocortical projections was made in the cat by Watzl and Montcastle.[195] Following electric stimulation of the contralateral vestibular nerve, they recorded short latency monophasic potentials in the suprasylvian gyrus just anterior to the auditory area. In the rhesus monkey, Fredrickson and coworkers[64, 65] found the primary vestibular projection area of the vestibular nerve to be at the lower end of the intraparietal sulcus next to the face area of the postcentral gyrus (Fig. 46). Evoked potentials were elicited from other nearby cortical areas after contralateral vestibular nerve stimulation but these potentials had longer latencies, suggesting that they were secondary projection areas. In humans, electric stimulation of both the superior sylvian gyrus and the region of the inferior intraparietal sulcus produce a subjective sensation of rotation or bodily displacement.[148]

Large lesions in the vestibular nuclei of cats result in terminal degeneration of axons in the ventroposteriolateral nucleus (VPL) of the contralateral thalamus,

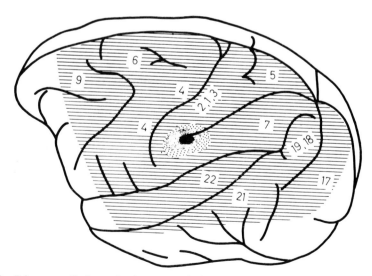

Figure 46. Primary vestibular projection area at the lower end of the intraparietal sulcus in the rhesus monkey. (From Fredrickson, J. M., et al.: *Vestibular nerve projection to the cerebral cortex of the rhesus monkey.* Exp. Brain Res. 2:318, 1966, with permission.)

suggesting direct connections between the vestibular nuclei and the thalamus.[110] Further support for the existence of such connections comes from the electrophysiologic findings of short latency potentials recorded in VPL after stimulation of the contralateral vestibular nerve, and antidromic activation of secondary vestibular neurons by electric stimulation in VPL.[109] Microelectrode recordings of potentials in and around VPL in the squirrel monkey demonstrate that the vestibular projections are scattered over large areas, thus evidence does not exist for a specific vestibular thalamic nucleus.[109] Of the VPL neurons activated by vestibular stinulation, only about one-fourth project to the sensorimotor cortex, some sending collaterals to both the precentral and postcentral gyri.[109]

From a functional point of view the vestibulothalamocortical projections appear to integrate labyrinthine and somatic proprioceptive signals and to provide one with a "conscious awareness" of body orientation. Beginning at the vestibular nuclei a stepwise integration of body orienting signals occurs, reaching its maximum at the level of the cortex.

Psychophysical Studies

Semicircular Canals

As Mach described,[121] a subject rotated about an earth vertical axis on a rotatory platform will perceive turning that is dependent on the magnitude of angular acceleration. The perceived "speed of turning" progressively increases with prolonged constant acceleration although the turning sensation increases at a lesser rate than the platform velocity. Below a minimum or threshold angular acceleration the subject does not perceive turning. Although considerable difference exists in reported values, the threshold to constant angular acceleration is in the range of 0.1 to 0.5 deg/sec^2.[29, 79] This is approximately an order of magnitude lower than the constant angular acceleration necessary to produce nystagmus.[90, 96]

Attempts to correlate the threshold and magnitude of subjective sensation with the magnitude of angular acceleration represent the earliest tests of vestibular function. Cupulometry developed by van Egmond and associates[192] is still a popular technique for assessing vestibular function on the basis of subjective sensation. With this test the subject is maintained at a constant velocity of angular rotation and then suddenly stopped. The durations of "after turning" sensation and induced nystagmus are measured for impulses of different amplitude (usually 15 to 60 deg/sec).

According to the pendulum model the duration of after sensation should be proportional to the amplitude of cupular deviation which in turn is proportional to the amplitude of the impulse of acceleration. The cupula returns to the resting position with an exponential time course. The duration of this return depends on the value of the so-called slow time constant (T_1) of the cupula (see Fig. 23). No matter how large the initial cupular deviation, it returns 63 percent of the way in T_1. Figure 47a plots the theoretic time course of cupular return after four different magnitudes of impulse deceleration (assuming $T_1 = 15$ seconds). On the ordinate, cupular deflection is represented by an arbitrary logarithmic scale. When the deflection is less than "threshold" (θs), the after sensation disappears. If the times at which the cupula crosses the threshold deviation (the theoretic duration of after sensation) are plotted against the log of the magnitude of angular impulse, a theoretic cupulogram is produced (Fig. 47b). The intercept of the line with the abscissa corresponds to the subjective sensation threshold; the slope of the line is equivalent to the time constant of cupular return shown in Figure 47a (15 seconds). Based on this theoretic foundation it was assumed that measuring the duration of after sensation in normal subjects and patients after impulses of different intensity would provide a quantitative measurement of cupular function.

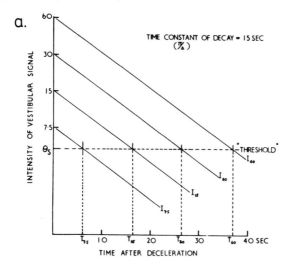

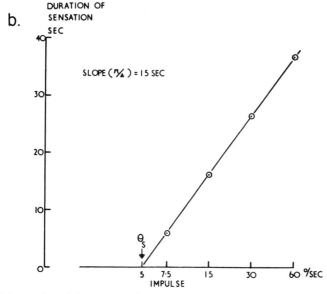

Figure 47. a) Magnitude and time course of cupular deflection produced by four impulses of angular acceleration (i.e. sudden stopping from a constant velocity of 7.5, 15, 30 and 60 degs/sec). Cupular deflection is represented by an arbitrary logarithmic ordinate scale. The after sensation disappears when the deflection is less than "threshold" intensity (θs). b) Theoretical cupulogram obtained by plotting the duration of after sensation from (a) ($T_{7.5}$ to T_{60}) against log intensity of the impulse. The intercept of the line with the abscissa corresponds to threshold, and the slope is the same as the time constant of decay of the cupula ($\pi/\Delta = 15$ seconds). (From Benson, A. J., and Bodin, M. A.: *Effect of orientation to the gravitational vertical on nystagmus following rotation about a horizontal axis.* Acta Otolaryngol. 61:517, 1966, with permission.)

The average sensation and nystagmus cupulogram from 50 normal subjects is shown in Figure 48.[96] In this normal population the average subjective threshold was 2.5 deg/sec and the average slope of the sensation cupulogram (T_1) was 7 seconds. A large scatter described the normal values, however, with the subjective threshold varying from 1 to 4 deg/sec and T_1 varying from 2 to 14 seconds. Surprisingly the average slope of the after sensation cupulogram is different from that of the after nystagmus cupulogram. Obviously there is only one cupular time constant T_1, even though these graphs suggest a different time constant for sensation and nystagmus.

This discrepancy means that either 1) the basic torsion pendulum model is inadequate to explain cupular dynamics or 2) the model is adequate but the nervous system in some way alters the stimulus-response relationship. The current consensus favors the second alternative.[79] The phenomena of peripheral adapta-

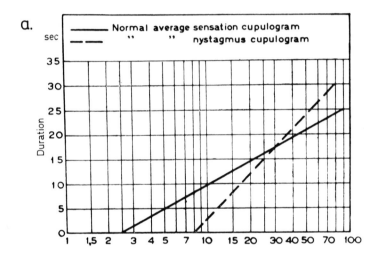

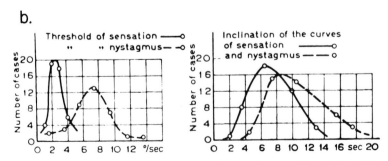

Figure 48. The average nystagmus—and sensation—cupulogram (a) and the distribution of threshold and slope measurements (b) in 50 normal subjects. (From Jongkees, L. B. W.: Pathology of vestibular sensation. In Kornhuber, H. H. (ed.): *Handbook of Sensory Physiology,* vol. VI, part 2. Springer-Verlag, New York, 1974, with permission.)

tion and central habituation and how they alter the response predicted by the pendulum model have already been discussed. The central pathways for subjective sensation and nystagmus are different even though both rely on the same basic input, that of cupular deviation.

Otolith Organs

A subject undergoing horizontal linear oscillation (for example on a parallel swing as in Fig. 33), reports experiencing two separate types of motion. One is a sensation of linear movement in the horizontal plane and the other is a sensation of tilt. Both sensations vary with the changing velocity (acceleration) of the platform.[96] Beginning with low amplitudes of oscillation the subject initially perceives motion without a specific direction. This is followed by perception of the direction of linear movement and finally at higher intensities of stimulation by a perception of tilting. Using dynamic stimuli, estimates of the minimal horizontal linear acceleration that normal subjects can perceive range from 5 to 15 cm/sec^2.[79] Interestingly these threshold values are similar to the values obtained by Mach for the perception of vertical linear acceleration (10 to 12 cm/sec^2).

The reason for the perception of tilt illustrated in Figure 33 is readily explained if one recalls the discussion related to Figure 1. When the swing is accelerating forward (upper left), F_t and F_g interact to produce a resulting force F_g' which is perceived as the true earth vertical. The same F_t could be produced by an actual backward tilt of the head, in which case F_g would be the true earth vertical. The otolith organs respond to F_t whether it results from linear acceleration or static head tilt and the nervous system perceives an angle of tilt proportional to F_t whether or not the body is acutally tilting.

The most complete data on threshold and accuracy of estimation of tilt have been obtained with static tilt experiments.[30, 73] The subject is strapped to a tilt platform in darkness and asked either to estimate the deviation of his head from the earth vertical or to adjust a luminous line on a dark field to a vertical position. Normal subjects respond with an accuracy of 2 to 4 degrees for tilt angles up to 40 degrees (accuracy falls off progressively for larger angles of tilt).[2, 15, 140] As expected from the discussion of F_t and F_g interaction, the subjective estimate of tilt depends on the gravitational force (F_g).[145] If the subject is asked to estimate the angle of tilt under different gravitational forces, the estimate will vary with F_g. For g values less than 1 the angle of tilt is underestimated while for g values greater than 1 the angle of tilt is overestimated. In experiments carried out at "zero g" in parabolic aircraft flights and in orbiting spacecraft, the subjects are unable to perceive tilt.

Motion Sickness

Motion sickness refers to the syndrome of dizziness, perspiration, nausea, vomiting, increased salivation, yawning and generalized malaise caused by excessive stimulation of the vestibular system.[94, 139] Although it is usually produced by prolonged stimulation of the labyrinthine end organs persistent visual stimulation with an optokinetic drum can also produce the syndrome.[51] Both linear and angular head acceleration induce motion sickness if applied for prolonged periods in susceptible subjects. Combinations of linear and angular acceleration or multiplanar angular accelerations are particularly effective. Rotation about the vertical axis along with either voluntary or involuntary nodding movements in the sagittal plane rapidly produce motion sickness in nearly everybody. This movement combines linear and angular acceleration (Coriolis effect).

Autonomic symptoms are usually the initial manifestation of motion sickness.[94] Sensitive sweat detectors can identify increased sweating as soon as 5 seconds after onset of motion and grossly detectable sweating is usually apparent before any noticeable nausea. Increased salivation and frequent swallowing movements occur. Gastric motility is reduced and digestion is impaired. Hyperventilation is almost always present and the resulting hypocapnea leads to changes in blood volume with pooling in the lower parts of the body, predisposing the subject to postural hypotension. Motion sickness effects the appetite so that even the sight or smell of food is distressing.

Some people are sensitive to development of motion sickness while others are highly resistant.[99] Most will adapt to prolonged vestibular stimulation but some never adapt (the chronically seasick ocean voyager). No completely reliable method exists for predicting who will develop motion sickness. Susceptible subjects often have a steeper sensation cupulogram than those who are resistant suggesting that the former have an increased sensitivity to vestibular stimulation.[99, 202] Thresholds for vestibular stimulation (rotatory or caloric) are usually normal in subjects susceptible to motion sickness, however, and they develop habituation at the same rate as subjects who are resistant.[99, 108] Patients whose labyrinths have been inactivated by congenital or acquired disease are resistant to motion sickness whether induced by vestibular or visual stimuli.[94]

REFERENCES

1. ADRIAN, E. D.: *Discharges from vestibular receptors in the cat.* J. Physiol. 101:389, 1943.

2. AUBERT, H.: *Eine scheinbare bedeutende Drehung von Objekten bei Neigung des Kopfes nach rechts oder links.* Virchows Arch. 20:381, 1861.

3. BAARSMA, E. A., AND COLLEWIJN, H.: *Vestibulo-ocular and optokinetic reactions to rotation and their interaction in the rabbit.* J. Physiol. 238:603, 1974.

4. BAARSMA, E. A., AND COLLEWIJN, H.: *Eye movements due to linear accelerations in the rabbit.* J. Physiol. 245:227, 1975.

5. BACH, L. M. N., AND MAGOUN, H. W.: *The vestibular nuclei as an excitatory mechanism for the cord.* J. Neurophysiol. 10:331, 1947.

6. BAKER, R., PRECHT, W., AND BERTHOZ, A.: *Synaptic connections to trochlear motoneurons determined by individual vestibular nerve branch stimulation in the cat.* Brain Res. 64:402, 1973.

7. BAKER, R., AND BERTHOZ, A.: *Organization of vestibular nystagmus in oblique oculomotor system.* J. Neurophysiol. 37:195, 1974.

8. BALOH, R. W., ET AL.: *Quantitative measurement of saccade amplitude, duration, and velocity.* Neurology 25:1065, 1975.

9. BALOH, R. W., SILLS, A. W., AND HONRUBIA, B.: *Impulsive and sinusoidal rotatory testing. A comparison with results of caloric testing.* Laryngoscope, In press.

10. BÁRÁNY, R.: *Augenbewegungen, durch thoraxbewegungen ausgelöst.* Zentvalkl. Physiol. 20:298, 1906.

11. BÁRÁNY, R.: *Üker einige Augen-und Halsmuskelreflexe bei Neugeborenen.* Acta Otolaryngol. 1:97, 1918.

12. BARD, P.: *Postural coordination and locomotion and their central control.* In Bard, P. (ed.): *Medical Physiology,* ed. 11. The C. V. Mosby Co., St. Louis, 1961.

13. BARLOW, J. S.: *Vestibular and non-dominant parietal lobe disorders.* Dis. Nerv. Syst. 31:624, 1970.

14. BARR, C. C., SCHULTHEIS, L. W., AND ROBINSON, D. A.: *Voluntary, non-visual control of the human vestibulo-ocular reflex.* Acta Otolaryngol. 81:365, 1976.

15. BAUERMEISTER, M.: *Effect of body tilt on apparent verticality, apparent body position, and their relation.* J. Exp. Psychol. 67:142, 1964.

16. BECHTEREW, W.: *Ergebnisse der Durchschneidung des N. acusticus, nebst Erörterung der Bedeutung der semicirculären Canäle für das Körpergleichgewicht.* Pfluegers Arch. Ges Physiol. 30:312, 1883.

17. BECKER, W., AND FUCHS, A. F.: *Further properties of the human saccadic system: Eye movements and correction saccades with and without visual fixation points.* Vision Res. 9:1247, 1969.

18. BENSON, A. J., AND BODIN, M. A.: *Effect of orientation to the gravitational vertical on nystagmus following rotation about a horizontal axis.* Acta Otolaryngol. 61:517, 1966.

19. BREUER, J.: *Über die Funktion der Bogengänge des Ohrlabyrinthes.* Wien. Med. Jahrb. 4:72, 1874.

20. BROCKHURST, R. J., AND LION, K. S.: *Analysis of ocular movements by means of an electrical method.* Arch. Ophthalmol. 46:311, 1951.

21. BRODAL, A.: *The Reticular Formation of the Brain Stem. Anatomical Aspects and Functional Correlations.* Oliver and Boyd, Edinburgh, 1957.

22. BRODAL, A., POMPEIANO, O., AND WALBERG, F.: *The Vestibular Nuclei and Their Connections, Anatomy and Functional Correlations.* The William Ramsay Henderson Trust, Oliver and Boyd, Edinburgh, 1962.

23. BRODAL, A.: Anatomical organization of cerebello-vestibulo-spinal pathways. In De Renck, A. V. S., and Knight, J. (eds.): *CIBA Foundation Symposium: Myotatic, kinesthetic and vestibular mechanisms.* Churchill Ltd., London, 1967.

24. BRODAL, A.: Anatomy of the vestibular nuclei and their connections. In Kornhuber, H. H. (ed.): *Handbook of Sensory Physiology,* vol. VI, part I. Springer-Verlag, New York, 1974.

25. BROWN, J. H.: *Acquisition and retention of nystagmic habituation in cats with distributed acceleration experience.* J. Comp. Physiol. Psychol. 60:340, 1965.

26. CAJAL, S.: *Histologie du système nerveaux de l'homme et des vertébrés,* vol. 1. Maloine, Paris, 1909.

27. CAPPS, M. J., AND COLLINS, W. E.: *Effects of bilateral caloric habituation on vestibular nystagmus in the cat.* Acta Otolaryngol. 59:511, 1965.

28. CARPENTER, M. B.: Central oculomotor pathways. In Bach-Y-Rita, P., Collins, C. C., and Hyde, J. E. (eds.): *The Control of Eye Movements.* Academic Press, New York, 1971.

29. CLARK, B.: *Thresholds for the perception of angular acceleration in man.* Aerospace Med. 38:443, 1967.

30. CLARK, B.: *The vestibular system.* Ann. Rev. Psychol. 21:273, 1970.

31. COATS, A. C., AND SMITH, S. Y.: *Body position and the intensity of caloric nystagmus.* Acta Otolaryngol. 63:515, 1967.

32. COHEN, B.: Vestibulo-ocular relations. In Bach-Y-Rita, P., Collins C. C., and Hyde, J. E. (eds.): *The Control of Eye Movements.* Academic Press, New York, 1971.

33. COHEN, B.: The vestibulo-ocular reflex arc. In Kornhuber, H. H. (ed.): *Handbook of Sensory Physiology. Vestibular System,* vol. VI, part 1. Springer-Verlag, New York, 1974.

34. COHEN, B., KOMATSUZAKI, A., AND BENDER, M. B.: *Electrooculographic syndrome in monkeys after pontine reticular formation lesions.* Arch. Neurol. 18:78, 1968.

35. COHEN, B., AND HENN, V.: *The origin of quick phases of nystagmus in the horizontal plane.* Bibl. Ophthalmol. 82:36, 1972.

36. COLLINS, W. E.: *Effects of mental set upon vestibular nystagmus.* J. Exp. Psychol. 63:191, 1962.

37. COLLINS, W. E.: *Manipulation of arousal and its effects upon human vestibular nystagmus induced by caloric irrigation and angular accelerations.* Aerospace Med. 34:124, 1963.

38. COLLINS, W. E.: *Nystagmus responses of the cat to rotation and to directionally equivalent and non-equivalent stimuli after unilateral caloric habituation.* Acta Otolaryngol. 58:247, 1964.

39. COLLINS, W. E.: *Effects of "double irrigations" on the caloric nystagmus of the cat.* Acta Otolaryngol. 59:45, 1965.

40. COLLINS, W. E.: *Vestibular responses from figure skaters.* Aerospace Med. 37:1098, 1966.

41. COLLINS, W. E.: *Special effects of brief periods of visual fixation on nystagmus and sensations of turning.* Aerospace Med. 39:257, 1968.

42. COLLINS, W. E.: Arousal and vestibular habituation. In Kornhuber, H. H. (ed.): *Handbook of Sensory Physiology. The Vestibular System,* vol. VI, part 2. Springer-Verlag, New York, 1974.

43. COLLINS, W. E.: Habituation of vestibular responses with and without visual stimulation. In Kornhuber, H. H. (ed.): *Handbook of Sensory Physiology. The Vestibular System,* vol. VI, part 2. Springer-Verlag, New York, 1974.

44. COLLINS, W E., ET AL.: *Some characteristics of optokinetic eye movement patterns: a comparative study*. Aerospace Med. 41:1251, 1970.

45. COOK, G., AND STARK, L.: *The human eye-movement mechanism: Experiments, modeling and model testing*. Arch. Ophthalmol. 79:428, 1968.

46. CORBIN, K. B., AND HINSEY, J. C.: *Intramedullary course of the dorsal root fibers of each of the first four cervical nerves*. J. Comp. Neurol. 63:119, 1935.

47. CORREIA, M. J. AND GUEDRY, F. E.: *Modification of vestibular responses as a function of rate of rotation about an earth-horizontal axis*. U.S. Navy Aerospace Med. Inst. NAMI-957, 1966.

48. CRAMPTON, G. H.: Habituation of ocular nystagmus of vestibular origin. In Bender, M. B. (ed.): *The Oculomotor System*. Harper and Row, New York, 1964.

49. CRITCHLEY, M.: *The Parietal Lobes*. Arnold, London, 1953.

50. CRUM-BROWN, A.: *On the sense of rotation and the anatomy and physiology of the semicircular canals of the internal ear*. J. Anat. Physiol. 8:327, 1874.

51. DICHGANS, J., AND BRANDT, T.: Visual-vestibular integration and motion perception. In Bizzi, E., and Dichgans, F. (eds.): *Cerebral Control of Eye Movements and Motion Perception*. S. Karger, Basel, 1972.

52. DIX, M. R., AND HOOD, J. D.: *Observations upon the nervous mechanism of vestibular habituation*. Acta Otolaryngol. 44:310, 1969.

53. DODGE, R.: *Five types of eye movements in the horizontal meridian plane of the field of regard*. Am. J. Physiol. 8:307, 1903.

54. DUENSING, F., AND SCHAEFER, K. P.: *Über die Konvergenz verschiedener labyrinthärer Afferenzen auf einzelne Neurone des Vestibulariskerngebietes*. Arch. Psychiat. 199:345, 1959.

55. ERULKAR, S. D., ET AL.: *Organization of the vestibular projection to the spinal cord of the cat*. J. Neurophysiol. 29:626, 1966.

56. EVINGER, L. C., FUCHS, A. F., AND BAKER, R.: *Bilateral lesions of the medial longitudinal fasciculus in monkeys: Effects on the horizontal and vertical components of voluntary and vestibular induced eye movements*. Exp. Brain Res. 28:1, 1977.

57. EWALD, R.: *Physiologische Untersuchungen über das Endorgan des Nervus Octavus*. Bergmann, Wiesbaden, 1892.

58. FEARING, F. S.: *The retention of the effects of repeated elicitation of the post-rotational nystagmus in pigeons. II. The retention of the effects of "distributed" stimulation*. J. Comp. Psychol. 31:47, 1941.

59. FERNÁNDEZ, C., AND FREDRICKSON, J. M.: *Experimental cerebellar lesions and their effect on vestibular function*. Acta Otolaryngol. Suppl. 192:52, 1964.

60. FLOURENS, P.: *Recherches Expérimentals sur les Propriétés et les Fonctions due Système Nerveux dans les Animaux Vertébrés*. Crevot, Paris, 1842.

61. FLUUR, E.: *Interaction between the utricles and the horizontal semicircular canals. IV. Tilting of human patients with acute unilateral vestibular neuritis*. Acta Otolaryngol. 76:349, 1973.

62. FLUUR, E., AND MELLSTRÖM, A.: *The otolith organs and their influence on oculomotor movements*. Exp. Neurol. 30:139, 1971.

63. FLUUR, E., AND SIEGBORN, J.: *Interaction between the utricles of the horizontal and semicircular canals. II. Unilateral selective section of the horizontal ampullar and the utricular nerve, followed by tilting around the longitudinal axis*. Acta Otolaryngol. 75:393, 1973.

64. FREDRICKSON, J. M., ET AL.: *Vestibular nerve projection to the cerebral cortex of the rhesus monkey*. Exp. Brain Res. 2:318, 1966.

65. FREDRICKSON, J. M., KORNHUBER, H. H., AND SCHWARZ, J. M.: Cortical projections of the vestibular nerve. In Kornhuber, H. H. (ed.): *Handbook of Sensory Physiology*, vol. VI., part 2. Springer-Verlag, New York, 1974.

66. FUCHS, A. F. AND KIMM, J.: *Unit activity in vestibular nucleus of the alert monkey during horizontal angular acceleration and eye movement*. J. Neurophysiol. 38:1140, 1975.

67. FUJITA, Y., ROSENBERG, J., AND SEGUNDO, J. R.: *Activity of cells in the lateral vestibular nucleus as a function of head position*. J. Physiol. 196:1, 1968.

68. FUKUDA, T., ET AL.: *Study on nystagmus during voluntary acts—observation of rotation in ballet*. J. Oto-Rhino-Laryngol. Soc. Jap. Suppl. 70:11, 1967.

69. FULTON, J. F., LIDDELL, E. G. T. AND RIOCH, D. M.: *The influence of unilateral destruction of the vestibular nuclei upon posture and the knee jerk*. Brain 53:327, 1930.

70. GACEK, R.: *The course and central termination of first order neurons supplying vestibular endorgans in the cat.* Acta Otolaryngol. Suppl. 254, 1969.

71. GACEK, R.: *Anatomical demonstration of the vestibulo-ocular projections in the cat.* Laryngoscope 81:1559, 1971.

72. GERNANDT, B. E.: Vestibulo-spinal mechanisms. In Kornhuber, H. H. (ed.): *Handbook of Sensory Physiology. The Vestibular System,* vol. VI, part 2. Springer-Verlag, New York, 1974.

73. GRAYBIEL, A.: Measurement of otolith function in man. In Kornhuber, H. H. (ed.): *Handbook of Sensory Physiology,* vol. VI, part 2. Springer-Verlag, New York, 1974.

74. GRESTY, M. A.: *A reexamination of "neck reflex" eye movements in the rabbit.* Acta Otolaryngol. 81:386, 1976.

75. GROEN. J. J.: *The semicircular canal systems of the organs of equilibrium II.* Physics in Med. Biol. 1:225, 1956-1957.

76. GUEDRY, F. E., AND GRAYBIEL, A.: *Compensatory nystagmus conditioned during adaptation to living in a rotating room.* J. Appl. Physiol. 17:398, 1962.

77. GUEDRY, F. W.: *Visual control of habituation to complex vestibular stimulation in man.* Acta Otolaryngol. 58:377, 1964.

78. GUEDRY, F. E.: *Influence of linear and angular accelerations on nystagmus.* NASA SP 115:185, 1966.

79. GUEDRY, F. E.: Psychophysics of vestibular sensation. In Kornhuber, H. H. (ed.): *Handbook of Sensory Physiology. The Vestibular System,* vol. VI, part 2. Springer-Verlag, New York, 1974.

80. HENN, V., AND COHEN, B.: Activity in eye motoneurons and brain stem units during eye movements. In Lennerstrand, G., and Bach-Y-Rita, P. (eds.): *Basic Mechanisms of Ocular Motility and their Clinical Implications.* Pergamon Press, Stockholm, 1975.

81. HIGHSTEIN, S. M.: *Synaptic linkage of the vestibulo-ocular reflex pathways in the rabbit.* Mount Sinai J. Med. 41:144, 1974.

82. HIKOSAKA, D., AND MAEDA, M.: *Cervical effects on abducens motoneurons and their interaction with vestibulo-ocular reflex.* Exp. Brain Res. 18:512, 1973.

83. HIKOSAKA, O., AND KAWAKAMI, T.: *Inhibitory interneurons in the reticular formation and their relation to vestibular nystagmus.* Brain Res. 117:513, 1976.

84. HIXSON, W. C., AND NIVEN, J. I.: *Application of the system transfer function concept to a mathematical description of the labyrinth.* Bull. Med. Proj. MR005, 13-6001 Subtask 1, Reports No. 57 (1961) and 73 (1962), Naval School of Aviation Med., Pensacola, Florida.

85. HONRUBIA, V., ET AL.: *Experimental studies on optokinetic nystagmus. II. Normal humans.* Acta Otolaryngol. 65:441, 1968.

86. HONRUBIA, V., ET AL.: *The patterns of eye movements during physiologic vestibular nystagmus in man.* Trans. Am. Acad. Ophthalmol. Otolaryngol. 84:339, 1977.

87. HOOD, J. D., AND PFALTZ, C. R.: *Observations upon the effects of repeated stimulation upon rotational and caloric nystagmus.* J. Physiol. 124:130, 1954.

88. HOYT, W. F., AND DAROFF, R. B.: Supranuclear disorders of ocular control in man. In Bach-Y-Rita, P., Collins, C. C., and Hyde, J. E. (eds.): *The Control of Eye Movements.* Academic Press, New York, 1971.

89. HUIZINGA, E.: *On the tonic and the dynamic function of the cristae.* Acta Otolaryngol. 24:82, 1936.

90. HULK, J., AND JONGKEES, L. B. W.: *The normal cupulogram.* J. Laryngol. 62:70, 1948.

91. IGARASHI, M., ET AL.: *Nystagmus after experimental cervical lesions.* Laryngoscope 82:1609, 1972.

92. ITO, M.: The vestibulo-cerebellar relationships: vestibulo-ocular reflex arc and flocculus. In Naunton, R. F. (ed.): *The Vestibular System.* Academic Press, New York, 1975.

93. ITO, M., ET AL.: *Visual influence on rabbit horizontal vestibulo-ocular reflex presumably effected via the cerebellar flocculus.* Brain Res. 65:170, 1974.

94. JOHNSON, W. H., AND JONGKEES, L. B. W.: Motion sickness. In Kornhuber, H. H. (ed.): *Handbook of Sensory Physiology,* vol. VI, part 2. Springer-Verlag, New York, 1974.

95. DE JONG, P. T. V. M., ET AL.: *Ataxia and nystagmus induced by injection of local anesthetics in the neck.* Ann. Neurol. 1:240, 1977.

96. JONGKEES, L. B. W., AND GROEN, J. J.: *The nature of the vestibular stimulus.* J. Laryngol. 61:529, 1946.

97. JONGKEES, L. B. W.: *Which is the preferable method of performing the caloric test?* Arch. Otolaryngol. 49:594, 1949.

98. JONGKEES, L. B. W.: Pathology of vestibular sensation. In Kornhuber, H. H. (ed.): *Handbook of Sensory Physiology*, vol. VI, part 2. Springer-Verlag, New York, 1974.

99. JONGKEES, L. B. W.: Motion sickness. II. Some sensory aspects. In Kornhuber, H. H. (ed.): *Handbook of Sensory Physiology*, vol. VI, part 2. Springer-Verlag, New York, 1974.

100. KELLER, E. L.: *Participation of medial pontine reticular formation in eye movement generation in monkey.* J. Neurophysiol. 37:316, 1974.

101. KELLER, E. L., AND KAMATH, B. Y.: *Characteristics of head rotation and eye movement-related neurons in alert monkey vestibular nucleus.* Brain Res. 100:182, 1975.

102. DE KLEYN, A.: *Recherches quantitatives sur les positions compensatories l'oeil chez de lapin.* Arch. Neerl. Physiol. 7:138, 1922.

103. KONRAD, H. R., ET AL.: *The impulsive test in man.* Trans. Am. Acad. Ophthalmol. Otolaryngol. 82:ORL-232, 1976.

104. LACKNER, J. R.: *Visual rearrangement affects auditory localization.* Neuropsychology 11:29, 1973.

105. LACKNER, J. R.: *Induction of illusory self-rotation and nystagmus by a rotating sound-field.* Aviat. Space Environ. Med. 48:129, 1977.

106. LAU, C. G. Y., HONRUBIA, V., AND BALOH, R. W.: *The pattern of eye movement trajectories during physiological nystagmus.* Adv. Oto-Rhino-Laryngol. In Press.

107. LAU, C. G. Y., ET AL.: A linear model for visual and vestibular interaction. Aviat. Space Environ. Med. In Press.

108. LIDVALL, H. F.: *Mechanism of motion sickness as reflected in the vertigo and nystagmus responses to repeated caloric stimuli.* Acta Otolaryngol. 55:527, 1967.

109. LIEDGREN, S. R. C., ET AL.: *Representation of vestibular afferents in somatosensory thalamic nuclei of the squirrel monkey (Saimiri sciureus).* J. Neurophysiol. 39:601, 1976.

110. LIEDGREN, S. R. C., AND RUBIN, A. M.: *Vestibulo-thalamic projections studied with antidromic technique in the cat.* Acta Otolaryngol. 82:379, 1976.

111. LINDSLEY, D. B., SCHREINER, L. H., AND MAGOUN, H. W.: *An electromyographic study of spasticity.* J. Neurophysiol. 12:197, 1949.

112. LLINÁS, R., AND TERZUOLO, C. A.: *Mechanisms of supraspinal actions upon spinal cord activities. Reticular inhibitory mechanisms on alpha-extensor motoneurons.* J. Neurophysiol. 27:579, 1964.

113. LLINÁS, R., AND TERZUOLO, C. A.: *Mechanisms of supraspinal actions upon spinal cord activities. Recticular inhibitory mechanisms upon flexor motoneurons.* J. Neurophysiol. 28:413, 1965.

114. LORENTE DE NO, R.: *Ausgewahlte Kapitel aus der vergleichenden Physiologie des Labryrinthes. Die Augenmuskel-reflexe beim Kaninchen und ihre Grundlagen.* Ergebn. Physiol. 32:73, 1931.

115. LORENTE DE NÓ, R.: *Researches on labryinth reflexes.* Trans. Am. Otol. Soc. 22:287, 1932.

116. LORENTE DE NÓ, R.: *The regulation of eye positions and movements induced by the labyrinth.* Laryngoscope 42:233, 1932.

117. LORENTE DE NÓ, R.: *Anatomy of the eighth nerve. The central projection of the nerve endings of the internal ear.* Laryngoscope 43:1, 1933.

118. LORENTE DE NÓ, R.: *Vestibulo-ocular reflex arc.* Arch. Neurol. Psychiat. 30:245, 1933.

119. LORENTE DE NÓ, R., AND BERENS, C.: Nystagmus. In Piersol, G. M., and Bortz, E. L. (eds.): *Cyclopedia of Medicine, Surgery and Specialties,* vol. 9. F. A. Davis Co., Philadelphia, 1959.

120. LUND, S., AND POMPEIANO, O.: *Descending pathways with monosynaptic action on motoneurones.* Experientia 21:602, 1965.

121. MACH, E.: *Grundlinien der Lehre von den Bewegungsempfindungen.* Engelmann, Leipzig, 1875; Bonset, Amsterdam (translation), 1967.

122. MAEDA, M., SHIMAZU, H., AND SHINODA, Y.: *Nature of synaptic events in cat abducens motoneurons at slow and quick phase of vestibular nystagmus.* J. Neurophysiol. 35:279, 1972.

123. MAEKAWA, K., AND SIMPSON, J. I.: *Climbing fiber activation of Purkinje cells in the flocculus by impulses transferred through the visual pathway.* Brain Res. 39:245, 1972.

124. MAGNUS R.: *Körperstellung.* Springer-Verlag, Berlin, 1924.

125. MAGOUN, H. W., AND RHINES, R.: *An inhibitory mechanism in the bulbar reticular formation.* J. Neurophysiol. 9:165, 1946.

126. MARKHAM, C. H., AND CURTHOYS, I. S.: *Convergence of labyrinthine influences on units in the vestibular nuclei of the cat. II. Electrical stimulation.* Brain Res. 43:383, 1972.

127. McCABE, B. F.: *The quick component of nystagmus.* Laryngoscope 75:1619, 1965.

128. McCOUCH, G. P., DEERING, I. D., AND LING, T. H.: *Location of receptors for tonic neck reflexes.* J. Neurophysiol. 14:191, 1951.

129. MCNALLY, W. J., AND STUART, E. A.: *Physiology of the Labryinth. A manual prepared for graduates in medicine.* Am. Acad. Ophthalmol. Otolaryngol., McGill University and Royal Victoria Hospital, Montreal, 1967.

130. MEIRY, J. L.: *The vestibular system and human dynamic space orientation.* Sc.D. Thesis, M.I.T., June, 1965.

131. MEIRY, J. L.: Vestibular and proprioceptive stabilization of eye movements. In Bach-Y-Rita, P., Collins, C. C., and Hyde J. E. (eds.): *The Control of Eye Movements.* Academic Press, New York, 1971.

132. MELVILL-JONES, G.: *Predominance of anti-compensatory oculomotor responses during rapid head rotation.* Aerospace Med. 35:965, 1964.

133. MELVILL-JONES, G.: Organization of neural control in the vestibulo-ocular reflex arc. In Bach-Y-Rita, P., Collins, C. C., and Hyde, J. E. (eds.): *The Control of Eye Movements.* Academic Press, New York, 1971.

134. MELVILL-JONES, G., AND MILSUM, J. H.: *Characteristics of neural transmission from the semicircular canal to units in the vestibular nuclei of cats.* J. Physiol. 209:295, 1970.

135. MERTENS, R. A., AND COLLINS, W. E.: *Unilateral caloric habituation of nystagmus in the cat: Effects of rotation and bilateral caloric responses.* Acta Otolaryngol. 64:281, 1967.

136. MILES, F. A.: *Single unit firing patterns in the vestibular nuclei related to voluntary eye movements and passive body rotation in conscious monkeys.* Brain Res. 71:215 1974.

137. MILES, F. A., AND FULLER, J. H.: *Visual tracking and the primate flocculus.* Science 189:1000, 1975.

138. MILLER, E. F. 2ND: *Counterrolling of the human eye produced by head tilt with respect to gravity.* Acta Otolaryngol. 54:479, 1962.

139. MONEY, K. E.: *Motion sickness.* Physiol. Rev. 50:1, 1970.

140. MÜLLER, G. E.: *Über das Aubertsche Phändmen.* Z. Sinnesphysiol. 49:109, 1916.

141. NIVEN, J. I., CARROLL HIXSON, W., AND CORREIA, M. J.: An experimental approach to the dynamics of the vestibular mechanisms. In *Symposium on the Role of the Vestibular Organs in the Exploration of Space.* U.S. Government Printing Office, Washington, 1965.

142. NYBERG-HANSEN, R.: *Origin and termination of fibers from the vestibular nuclei descending in the medial longitudinal fasciculus. An experimental study with silver impregnation methods in the cat.* J. Comp. Neurol. 122:355, 1964.

143. NYBERG-HANSEN, R.: *Sites and mode of termination of fibers of the vestibulo-spinal tract in the cat. An experimental study with silver impregnation methods.* J. Comp. Neurol. 122:369, 1964.

144. NYBERG-HANSEN, R.: *Sites and mode of termination of reticulospinal fibers in the cat. An experimental study with silver impregnation methods.* J. Comp. Neurol. 124:71, 1965.

145. ORMSBY, C. C., AND YOUNG, L. R.: *Perception of static orientation in a constant gravitoinertial environment.* Aviat. Space Environ. Med. 47:159, 1976.

146. OSTERHAMMEL, P., TERKILDSEN, K., AND ZILSTORFF, K.: *Vestibular habituation in ballet dancers.* Acta Otolaryngol. 66:221, 1968.

147. PASIK, P., PASIK, T., AND BENDER, M. B.: *The pretectal syndrome in monkeys. II. Spontaneous and induced nystagmus in "lightening" eye movements.* Brain 92:871, 1969.

148. PENFIELD, W.: *Vestibular-sensation and the cerebral cortex.* Ann. Otol. 66:691, 1957.

149. PETERSON, B. W.: *Distribution of neural responses to tilting within vestibular nuclei of the cat.* J. Neurophysiol. 33:750, 1970.

150. POMPEIANO, O.: Cerebello-vestibular interrelations. In Kornhuber, H. H. (ed.): *Handbook of Sensory Physiology. The Vestibular System,* vol. VI, part 1. Springer-Verlag, New York, 1974.

151. POMPEIANO, O., AND BRODAL, A.: *Spino-vestibular fibers in the cat. An experimental study.* J. Comp. Neurol. 108:353, 1957.

152. PRECHT, W.: The physiology of the vestibular nuclei. In Kornhuber, H. H. (ed.): *Handbook of Sensory Physiology. The Vestibular System,* vol. VI, part 1. Springer-Verlag, New York, 1974.

153. PRECHT, W., AND SHIMAZU, H.: *Functional connections of tonic and kinetic vestibular neurons with primary vestibular afferents.* J. Neurophysiol. 28:1014, 1965.

154. PRECHT, W., SHIMAZU, H., AND MARKHAM, C. H.: *A mechanism of central compensation of vestibular function following hemilabyrinthectomy.* J. Neurophysiol. 29:996, 1966.

155. PROCTOR, L. R., AND FERNÁNDEZ, C.: *Studies on habituation of vestibular reflexes. IV. Effect of caloric stimulation in blindfolded cats.* Acta Otolaryngol. 56:500, 1963.

156. REINGOLD, D. B., HONRUBIA, V., AND WARD, P. H.: *Neurophysiologic correlates of nystagmus.* Trans. Am. Acad. Ophthalmol. Otolaryngol. 82:ORL-192, 1976.

157. ROBERTS, T. D. M.: *Neurophysiology of Postural Mechanisms.* Plenum Press, New York, 1967.

158. ROBINSON, D. A.: *The mechanics of human saccadic eye movement.* J. Physiol. 174:245, 1964.

159. ROBINSON, D. A.: *The oculomotor control system: A review.* Proc. IEEE 56:1032, 1968.

160. ROBINSON, D. A.: *Oculomotor unit behavior in the monkey.* J. Neurophysiol. 33:393, 1970.

161. ROBINSON, D. A.: Models of oculomotor neural organization. In Bach-Y-Rita, P., Collins, C. C., and Hyde, J. E. (eds.): *The Control of Eye Movements.* Academic Press, New York, 1971.

162. ROBINSON, D. A.: *The effect of cerebellectomy on the cat's vestibulo-ocular integrator.* Brain Res. 71:195, 1974.

163. ROBINSON, D. A.: Oculomotor control signals. In Lennerstrand, G., and Bach-Y-Rita, P. (eds.): *Mechanisms of Ocular Motility and Their Clinical Implications.* Pergamon Press, Oxford, 1975.

164. ROBINSON, D. A.: *Adaptive gain control of vestibuloocular reflex by the cerebellum.* J. Neurophysiol. 39:954, 1976.

165. RUBIN, A. M., ET AL.: *Vestibular-neck integration in the vestibular nuclei.* Brain Res. 96:99, 1975.

166. SADJADPOUR, K., AND BRODAL, A.: *The vestibular nuclei in man. A morphological study in the light of experimental findings in the cat.* J. Hirnforsch 10:299, 1968.

167. SCHMID, R., STEFANELLI, M., AND MIRA, E.: *Mathematical modeling. A contribution to clinical vestibular analysis.* Acta Otolaryngol. 72:292, 1971.

168. SCHUKNECHT, H. F.: *Pathology of the Ear.* Harvard University Press, Massachusetts, 1974.

169. SCHWINDT, P. C., RICHTER, A., AND PRECHT, W.: *Short latency utricular and canal input to ipsilateral abducens motoneurons.* Brain Res. 60:259, 1973.

170. SHERRINGTON, C. S.: *The Integrative Action of the Nervous System.* Yale University Press, New Haven, 1906.

171. SHIMAZU, H., AND PRECHT, W.: *Tonic and kinetic responses of cat's vestibular neurons to horizontal angular acceleration.* J. Neurophysiol. 28:991, 1965.

172. SHIMAZU, H., AND PRECHT, W.: *Inhibition of central vestibular neurons from the contralateral labyrinth and its mediating pathway.* J. Neurophysiol. 29:467, 1966.

173. SHIMAZU, H.: *Vestibulo-oculomotor relations: Dynamic responses.* Prog. Brain Res. 27:493, 1972.

174. SHINODA, Y., AND YOSHIDA, K.: *Dynamic characteristics of responses to horizontal head angular acceleration in vestibuloocular pathway in the cat.* J. Neurophysiol. 37:653, 1974.

175. SILLS, A. W., ET AL.: *A rapid optokinetic nystagmus test: Comparison with standard testing.* Trans. Am. Acad. Ophthalmol. Otolaryngol. 82:223, 1976.

176. SKAVENSKI, A. A., AND ROBINSON, D. A.: *Role of abducens neurons in vestibuloocular reflex.* J. Neurophysiol. 36:724, 1973.

177. SPARKS, D. L., AND TRAVIS, JR., R. P.: *Firing patterns of reticular formation neurons during horizontal eye movements.* Brain Res. 33:477, 1971.

178. SPIEGEL, E. A., AND PRICE, J. B.: *Origin of the quick component of labyrinthine nystagmus.* Arch. Otolaryngol. 20:576, 1939.

179. SPRAGUE, J. M., AND CHAMBERS, W. W.: *Regulation of posture in intact and decerebated cat. I. Cerebellum, reticular formation, vestibular nuclei.* J. Neurophysiol. 16:451, 1953.

180. STARK, L.: The control system for versional eye movements. In Bach-Y-Rita, P., Collins, C. C., and Hyde, J. E. (eds.): *The Control of Eye Movements.* Academic Press, New York, 1971.

181. SUGIE, N., AND MELVILL-JONES, G.: *Eye movement elicited by head rotation.* Bull. Electrotech. Lab. Japan 30:598, 1966.

182. SUZUKI, J.-I., COHEN, B., AND BENDER, M. B.: *Compensatory eye movements induced by vertical semicircular canal stimulation.* Exp. Neurol. 9:137, 1964.

183. SUZUKI, J.-I., TOKUMASU, K., AND GOTO, K.: *Eye movements from single utricular nerve stimulation in the cat.* Acta Otolaryngol. 68:350, 1969.

184. SUZUKI, J.-I., AND COHEN, B.: *Head, eye, body and limb movements from semicircular canal nerves.* Exp. Neurol. 10:393, 1964.

185. SZENTAGOTHAI, J.: *The elementary vestibulo-ocular reflex arc.* J. Neurophysiol. 13:395, 1950.

186. TAIT, J., AND MACNALY, W. J.: *Some features of the action of the utricular maculae (and of the associated action of the semicircular canals) of the frog.* Phil. Trans. B. 224:241, 1934.

187. TAKEMORI, S., AND SUZUKI, J.-I.: *Eye deviations from neck torsion in humans.* Ann. Otol. 80:439, 1971.

188. TAKEMORI, S., AND COHEN, B.: *Loss of visual suppression of vestibular nystagmus after flocculus lesions.* Brain Res. 72:213, 1974.

189. TARLOV, E.: Synopsis of current knowledge about ascending projections from the vestibular nuclei. In Naunton, R. (ed.): *The Vestibular System.* Academic Press, New York, 1975.

190. TERZUOLO, C. A., LLÍNAS, R., AND GREEN, K. T.: *Mechanisms of supraspinal sections upon spinal cord activities: distribution of reticular and segmental inputs in cat's alpha-motoneurons.* Arch. Ital. Biol. 103:635, 1965.

191. UEMURA, T., AND COHEN, B.: *Effects of vestibular nuclei lesions on vestibulo-ocular reflexes and posture in monkeys.* Acta Otolaryngol. Suppl. 315, 1973.

192. VAN EGMOND, A. A. J., GROEN, J. J., AND JONGKEES, L. B. W.: *The turning test with small regulable stimuli.* J. Laryngol. Otol. 62:63, 1948.

193. WAESPE, W., AND HENN, V.: *Neuronal activity in the vestibular nuclei of the alert monkey during vestibular and optokinetic stimulation.* Exp. Brain Res. 27:523, 1977.

194. WALSH, E. G.: *Role of the vestibular apparatus in the perception of motion on a parallel swing.* J. Physiol. 155:506, 1961.

195. WATZL, E., AND MOUNTCASTLE, V.: *Projection of vestibular nerve to cerebral cortex of the cat.* Am. J. Physiol. 159:594, 1949.

196. WARWICK, R.: Oculomotor organization. In Bender, M. B. (ed.): *The Oculomotor System.* John Wiley and Son, New York, 1964.

197. WESTHEIMER, G.: *Eye movement responses to a horizontally moving visual stimulus.* Arch. Ophthalmol. 52:932, 1954.

198. WESTHEIMER, G.: *Mechanism of saccadic eye movements.* Arch. Ophthalmol. 52:710, 1954.

199. WESTHEIMER, G., AND BLAIR, S. M.: *Functional organization of primate oculomotor system revealed by cerebellectomy.* Exp. Brain Res. 21:463, 1974.

200. WILSON, V. J., WYLIE, R. M., AND MARCO, L. A.: *Organization of the medial vestibular nucleus.* J. Neurophysiol. 31:166, 1968.

201. WILSON, V. J.: *Physiological pathways through the vestibular nuclei.* Int. Rev. Neurobiol. 15:27, 1972.

202. DE WIT, G.: *Seasickness.* Acta Otolaryngol. (Suppl. 108):1, 1953.

203. YOUNG, L. R.: *Developments in modeling visual-vestibular interactions.* Aerospace Med. Res. Lab., Wright-Patterson AFB, AMRL-TR-71-14, 1971.

204. YOUNG, L. R., AND SARK, L.: *Variable feedback experiments testing a sample data model for eye tracking movements.* IEEE Trans. Human Factors in Electronics HFE-4:28, 1963.

CHAPTER 4

Clinical Evaluation
of the Vestibular System

HISTORY

Dizziness is a nonspecific term that describes a sensation of altered orientation in space.[3, 17, 34, 72] Since visual, proprioceptive and vestibular signals provide the main source of information about the position of the head and body in space, damage to any of these systems can lead to a complaint of dizziness. The patient cannot distinguish the source of his dizziness, but certain features in the history help the examining physician determine if the vestibular system is involved (Table 2).

Table 2. Areas to be covered in the history of a patient complaining of dizziness

A. Character of dizziness	D. Associated symptoms
1. vertigo	1. nausea and vomiting
2. unsteadiness	2. blurred vision and oscillopsia
3. nonspecific lightheadedness, giddiness	3. auditory symptoms
	4. brain stem symptoms
B. Time course of dizziness	E. Predisposing factors
1. single bout lasting several days	1. infectious disease
2. recurrent bouts	2. trauma
3. continuous	3. surgery
	4. vascular disease
C. Precipitating factors	5. metabolic disease
1. head movements	6. developmental disorders
2. position change	7. drugs
3. coughing or sneezing	
4. loud noises	

Character of the Dizziness

The initial task is to obtain a description of what the patient means by dizziness. The patient should be encouraged to use other words (his own words) that describe the sensation and how this sensation interferes with his daily activities.

Dizziness Caused by Vestibular Lesions

By far the most common dizzy sensation associated with vestibular lesions is vertigo: an illusion of rotation. Damage to a semicircular canal or its afferent nerve decreases tonic activity from sensory cells all oriented in the same direction and produces a sensation similar to that experienced with physiologic stimulation, i.e. a sensation of angular rotation in the plane of the damaged canal. A lesion involving all the canals of one labyrinth produces a sensation of rotation in a plane determined by the balance of afferent signals from the contralateral canals (usually near the horizontal since the vertical canals partially cancel each other). An illusion of linear movement or tilting is rare probably because macular lesions decrease afferent activity from sensory cells oriented in multiple directions (see Fig. 20) producing a sensation unlike anything previously experienced by the patient.

The presence of vertigo indicates an imbalance in the vestibular system, but the absence of vertigo does not rule out a vestibular lesion. Other descriptions of the sensation associated with vestibular dysfunction include giddiness, swimming in the head, floating and drunkenness. The patient may describe dysequilibrium or loss of balance that occurs only when he is standing or walking and is unrelated to any abnormal head sensation.[2, 17] This suggests either symmetrical bilateral vestibular disease or involvement of proprioceptive and/or cerebellar pathways. Acute unilateral lesions in the deep paravertebral region of the neck may produce vertigo because of the resulting imbalance in the tonic neck proprioceptive signals arriving at the vestibular nuclei (see Neck-Vestibular Interaction, Chapter 3, and Cervical Vertigo, Chapter 7). Vertigo associated with cervical lesions is less severe than that associated with labyrinthine lesions, however, and it is compensated for more rapidly.[52]

Nonvestibular Dizziness

Many patients complain of dizziness when they first wear glasses, experiencing a vague feeling of disorientation often accompanied by headache.[1] Dizziness most frequently accompanies correction of astigmatism but also occurs after a change in magnification. A similar sensation is produced by imbalance in the extraocular muscles. After an acute ocular muscle paralysis, looking in the direction of the paralyzed muscles causes dizziness (in addition to diplopia), but within a short time the nervous system adapts to the altered spatial information. Dizziness associated with ocular defects is rarely severe and an illusion of movement does not occur.

Occasionally one can trace dizziness to disease involving multiple sensory systems, particularly in elderly patients or in patients with systemic disorders such as diabetes mellitus. A typical combination might include peripheral neuropathy resulting in diminished touch and proprioceptive input, decreased visual acuity (cataracts, glaucoma), and impaired hearing (as in presbycusis). In such patients an added vestibular impairment (from ototoxic drugs for example) can be devastating, making it impossible for them to walk without assistance. Patients with multisensory dizziness do poorly in the hospital—they are unable to adapt to the new surroundings because of their impaired sensory input. Not infrequently their complaint of dizziness will disappear when they return to familiar surroundings at home.

The nonspecific sensation of lightheadedness is most often associated with chronic anxiety and hyperventilation. The patient describes the feeling of an impending faint and often goes on to lose consciousness.[34, 70] Associated symptoms include: frequent sighing, air hunger, perioral numbness, paresthesias of the extremities, lump in the throat and tightness in the chest. Hyperventilation causes dizziness by lowering the carbon dioxide content of the blood producing constriction of the cerebral vasculature.[44] From a series of 125 patients presenting to a university neurological outpatient clinic with the complaint of dizziness, Drachman and Hart[34] found that, next to vestibular disorders, hyperventilation was the most common cause of dizziness (accounting for 23 percent of the patients).

Time Course of Dizziness

The time course of the dizziness is an important feature in distinguishing its cause. Dizziness associated with acute vestibular lesions is usually abrupt in onset, followed by decreasing intensity as compensation occurs. The rapidity of compensation depends on the patient's age, location of lesion and the functional status of the other body orienting systems. A young healthy patient suffering an acute peripheral vestibular insult is usually able to return to work in two to four weeks. With chronic vestibular disorders the dizziness may occur in brief paroxysms (seconds) related to sudden head movements or changes in head position, or in longer paroxysms (minutes to several hours) related to changes in fluid dynamics or blood circulation (see Chapter 7). Occasionally the patient experiences a mild background dizziness with superimposed episodic changes in intensity. Continuous dizziness without fluctuation for long periods of time is not typical of vestibular disorders.

Precipitating Factors

Events just prior to an episode of dizziness are important in determining the cause. Dizziness caused by vestibular lesions is usually worsened by rapid head movements since the new stimulus is sensed by the intact labyrinth and existing asymmetries are accentuated. Episodes may be precipitated by turning over in bed, sitting up from the lying position, extending the neck to look up, or bending over and straightening up. The types of positional dizziness are discussed in detail later, but in general the symptom suggests a vestibular disorder if postural changes in blood pressure and vertebral artery compression can be ruled out. Patients with a perilymph fistula have brief episodes of vertigo precipitated by changes in middle ear pressure (coughing, sneezing). Occasionally loud noises induce transient dizziness in patients with endolymphatic hydrops (Tulio phenomena).

Associated Symptoms

Autonomic symptoms such as nausea and vomiting commonly accompany dizziness caused by vestibular lesions while such symptoms are uncommon with other types of dizziness. Occasionally vegetative symptoms are the only manifestation of a vestibular lesion. Patients with symmetrical bilateral vestibular loss complain of blurred vision or oscillopsia when making rapid head movements or when walking because of impaired vestibulo-ocular reflexes.

Lesions of the vestibular end organ or vestibular nerve usually produce auditory symptoms while those of the vestibular nuclei and their connections result in symptoms related to brain stem dysfunction. Important auditory symptoms include hearing loss, tinnitus, a sensation of pressure or fullness in the ear, and pain in or about the ear. As with dizziness, the time course of the hearing loss is important. Fluctuating hearing loss and tinnitus are characteristic of Meniere's syndrome. Patients with this disease usually notice a buildup of pressure in the ear just prior to the onset of hearing loss, tinnitus and dizziness. Sudden, complete unilateral deafness and dizziness occurs with viral or bacterial labyrinthitis and vascular occlusion to the inner ear. A slow, progressive unilateral hearing loss strongly suggests the existence of a vestibular schwannoma or other cerebellopontine angle tumor. Brief episodes (minutes) of dizziness associated with transient brain stem and occipital lobe symptoms are characteristic of vertebrobasilar insufficiency. Such symptoms commonly include diplopia, hemianoptic field defects, drop attacks, dysarthia and ataxia. Dizziness in association with more prolonged (days) but reversible brain stem and optic nerve symptoms is typical of multiple sclerosis. Longstanding progressive brain stem symptoms are produced by an expanding mass lesion. Of note, hearing loss for pure tones is an unusual symptom of brain stem lesions even in the late stages.

Predisposing Factors

The patient's general state of health just prior to the onset of dizziness should be carefully investigated. Most severe systemic disorders are associated with a complaint of dizziness either due to partial involvement of all the body orienting systems or due to a decreased capacity of the CNS to deal with information from these systems (a type of multisensory dizziness). Some systemic disorders such as vasculitis, bacterial endocarditis and septicemia selectively affect the vestibular system by interfering with its blood supply. Such patients complain of severe vertigo, nausea and vomiting, typical of an acute peripheral vestibular loss. Patients with viral labyrinthitis and vestibular mononeuritis frequently report an upper respiratory tract illness either within two or three weeks before or at the time of onset of dizziness. Chronic middle ear infections may lead to bacterial labyrinthitis or serous labyrinthopathy and patients with bacterial meningitis can develop bacterial labyrinthitis through the direct CSF-perilymph connections.

Head injury commonly damages the delicate labyrinthine membranes with or without associated bone fracture. Labyrinthine trauma can result in a single prolonged episode of dizziness, or more commonly, recurrent episodes of positional dizziness. Surgery in or about the ear is a major cause of trauma to the labyrinthine membranes. Dizziness even follows surgery confined to the middle ear.

The medical history should focus on chronic medical illnesses that might predispose the patient to vestibular system damage, such as diabetes mellitus, atherosclerotic vascular disease, syphilis (congenital or acquired), and major allergies. Important disorders with a genetic predisposition include Meniere's syndrome, otosclerosis, neurofibromatosis and spinocerebellar degeneration. Congenital malformations of the inner ear are often associated with other congenital malformations.

Ototoxic drugs, such as the aminoglycosides and salicylates, occasionally cause vertigo, but more often produce imbalance from bilateral symmetrical vestibular end organ damage. Antihypertensive medications produce dizziness because of postural hypotension and associated transient cerebral ischemia. Anticoagulants can be associated with an acute inner ear hemorrhage, causing a dramatic onset of severe vertigo and nausea. Alcohol and phenytoin produce acute reversible dysequilibrium and chronic irreversible dysequilibrium from cerebellar degeneration. Numerous sedative drugs (barbiturates, antihistamines, diazepam) cause dizziness that is probably extravestibular in origin since it is not vertiginous or associated with impaired vestibular function.

EXAMINATION

The clinical evaluation of a patient suspected of having disease of the vestibular system should include a complete head, neck and neurologic examination. A few points deserve emphasis.

Ear

The neurotologist must be familiar with the normal anatomy of the external canal and tympanic membrane (see Chapter 2), must be capable of removing cerumen that interferes with visualization of the tympanic membrane and must be able to recognize certain disorders on inspection. Figure 49 illustrates the appearance of the tympanic membrane in a normal subject and in three common otologic disorders that may be associated with vestibular symptoms. The clinical features of each disorder are described in detail in Chapter 7.

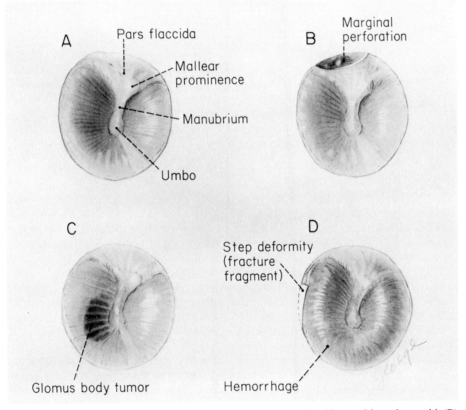

Figure 49. Appearance of the tympanic membrane in (A) a normal subject and in patients with (B) a superior marginal perforation and keratoma, (C) a tympanic glomus body tumor, and (D) a step deformity caused by a longitudinal temporal bone fracture.

While examining the ear, the pressure in the external canal is transiently increased and decreased using a pneumatic bulb attached to the otoscope. A positive fistula sign (severe vertigo and a transient burst of nystagmus) occurs in patients with a perforated tympanic membrane and erosion of the bony labyrinth (from chronic infection, surgery, trauma). The change in pressure is transmitted directly to the perilymph, compressing the membranous labyrinth and stimulating the semicircular canal cristae. The resulting nystagmus lasts from 10 to 20 seconds after the end of the stimulus. Lesser degrees of vertigo and nystagmus may occur in patients with an intact tympanic membrane and normal middle ear (Hennebert's sign). Hennebert first described this sign in patients with congenital syphilis[50] and subsequent investigators reported its occurrence in patients with Meniere's syndrome and other labyrinthine disorders.[61] Apparently fibrous adhesions between the medial surface of the stapedial footplate and the membranous labyrinth result in displacement of endolymph when the footplate moves. A similar mechanism could explain the production of dizziness by loud noises (Tulio phenomenon). Hennebert's sign is most often induced by negative pressure[61] presumably causing utriculofugal flow in the horizontal canal of the affected ear. The response is a slow ocular deviation (toward or away from the affected ear) followed by only 3 or 4 beats of nystagmus even with sustained pressure.

Posture and Equilibrium

As discussed in Chapter 3, the labyrinths influence spinal cord neurons through the lateral vestibulospinal tract, the reticulospinal tract and the descending medial longitudinal fascicles (MLF). Labyrinthine stimulation of the spinal cord increases extensor tonus and decreases flexor tonus, resulting in a facilitation of the antigravity muscles. Both otolith and semicircular canal signals influence spinal cord anterior horn cells, but the former are more important in maintenance of posture through counteraction of gravitational forces.

Past Pointing

Past pointing refers to a reactive deviation of the extremities caused by an imbalance in the vestibular system. One tests it by having the patient place his extended index finger on that of the examiner, close his eyes, raise the extended arm and index finger to a vertical position, and attempt to return his index finger to the examiner's. Consistent deviation to one side is past pointing.

Past pointing tests represent one of the earliest attempts to clinically assess vestibular function. In 1910 Bárány[12] published a review of pointing deviation produced by vestibular stimulation, and emphasized the importance of having the patient sit with eyes closed to avoid confusion with other orienting information. He attempted to improve the accuracy of the test by holding a disc in front of the subjects and having them repeatedly extend their index finger and touch the disc (producing a mark). With this technique, Bárány was able to demonstrate that caloric or rotatory stimulation consistently induced past pointing in the direction of the slow component of induced nystagmus. Cold caloric irrigation (inhibiting the horizontal ampullary nerve's spontaneous firing rate) resulted in past pointing toward the stimulated ear while warm caloric irrigation induced the opposite effect. As expected, patients with acute unilateral loss of labyrinthine function past pointed toward the damaged side. Bárány and numerous others emphasized that repeated testing shows a large variability, occasionally with the drift in the wrong direction. Subsequent investigators[64, 77] tried to improve test accuracy by eliminating tactile feedback and using small finger lamps that could be photographed, but the large variability among normal subjects and patients remained. Fukuda[39] introduced a vertical writing test to identify past pointing, but subsequent evaluation of his test suggested it was no more reliable than the more standard tests.[21]

It is apparent that results from a single pointing test can be misleading and should not be considered in isolation. Extralabyrinthine influences should be eliminated as much as possible by having the patient seated, with eyes covered and arms and index fingers extended throughout the test. The standard finger-to-nose test will not identify past pointing since joint and muscle proprioceptive signals permit accurate localization even when vestibular function is lost. Although patients with acute peripheral vestibular damage usually past point toward the side of loss, compensation rapidly corrects the past pointing and can even produce a drift to the other side. The cortical and subcortical neural pathways to the spinal anterior horn cells illustrated in Figure 45 apparently account for the compensation.

Postural Stability

Patients with damage to the vestibular system often suffer instability of the trunk and lower limbs, so that they sway back and forth or even fall to one side. In 1846 Romberg[68] noted that patients with proprioceptive loss from tabes dorsalis were unable to stand with feet together and eyes closed. Bárány[12] first emphasized the importance of vestibular influences in maintaining the Romberg position. As with past pointing he noted that patients with acute unilateral labyrinthine lesions swayed and fell toward the diseased side, that is, in the direction of the slow component of nystagmus. The Romberg test, like past pointing tests, however, was found to be rather insensitive for detecting chronic unilateral vestibular impairment and sometimes the patient would fall toward the intact ear. The so-called sharpened Romberg test is a more sensitive indicator of vestibular impairment.[37] For this test, the patient stands with feet aligned in the tandem heel-to-toe position with eyes closed and arms folded against the chest. Normal subjects can stand in this position for 30 seconds, while patients with unilateral or bilateral vestibular impairment rarely can sustain the position.

Although lower mammals consistently develop ipsilateral hypotonia of extensor muscles after labyrinthectomy, one rarely finds this in human patients. Occasionally, a slight asymmetry in posture is found with the ipsilateral upper extremity slightly flexed and abducted compared to the contralateral upper extremity. The clinically elicited deep tendon reflexes are also unaffected by vestibular lesions. Apparently other supraspinal influences on the anterior horn cells rapidly compensate for the loss of tonic vestibular signals.

The effect of vestibular lesions on postural righting reflexes has been studied extensively in the laboratory, but so far such testing has been of little clinical use. Righting reflexes can be induced by tipping or tilting a balance platform on which the subject is standing, sitting or kneeling.[57, 64] Patients with bilateral loss of vestibular function have marked difficulty maintaining the upright position, while patients with unilateral loss usually behave similarly to normal subjects.

Stepping Tests

Unterberger[80] was the first to systematically study the tendency of vestibular stimulation or unilateral vestibular lesions to induce blindfolded subjects to turn in the earth vertical axis when walking. The direction of turning coincided with the direction of past pointing and falling (in the direction of the slow component of nystagmus). Fukuda[38] obtained similar results by having subjects take 50 to 100 steps on the same spot and recording the angle of rotation as well as forward and backward movements. Both of these tests were performed with arms extended parallel and horizontal in front of the subject so that upper extremity deviation (past pointing) may have added to the tendency to rotate in a given direction Peitersen[66, 67] further modified the stepping test so that the blindfolded subject stepped with the arms folded and tried to stay in the center of two concentric circles drawn on the floor. The tests were performed in a quiet, darkened room to exclude orientation from auditory and visual clues. Despite these attempts to improve test precision, he found marked variability in the rotation angle from one subject to another and in the same subject on repeated testing.

Tandem gait tests are widely used as part of the routine neurologic examination and most clinicians readily recognize a normal and abnormal performance. When performed with eyes open, tandem walking is usually a test of cerebellar function since vision compensates for chronic vestibular and proprioceptive deficits. Acute vestibular lesions, however, may impair tandem walking even with eyes open. Tandem walking with eyes closed provides a good test of vestibular function, so long as cerebellar and proprioceptive function are intact. The blindfolded subject is asked to start with feet in the tandem position and arms folded against the chest and, at a comfortable speed, to make ten tandem steps beyond the first two starting steps. The number of steps without sidestepping is scored on three trials. Most normal subjects can take a minimum of 10 accurate tandem steps in three trials. Patients with acute or chronic vestibular system disease fail the test, but the direction of falling is not a reliable indicator of the side of the lesion.

Pathologic Nystagmus and Related Phenomena

Physiologic versus Pathologic Nystagmus

Nystagmus can be defined as a nonvoluntary, rhythmic oscillation of the eyes.[27] It usually has clearly defined fast and slow components alternating in opposite directions. By convention, the direction of the fast component defines the direction of nystagmus. Physiologic nystagmus refers to nystagmus that occurs in normal subjects while pathologic nystagmus implies an underlying abnormality. Table 3 lists the common varieties of physiologic and pathologic nystagmus. Spontaneous nystagmus refers to nystagmus that occurs with the patient seated, eyes in the primary position and without external stimulation such as movement of the head or surroundings. Nystagmus that is not present in the sitting position but present in some other head and body position is called positional nystagmus. This definition excludes nystagmus present in the sitting position that is modified by a change in position.

The term ocular nystagmus has been used to describe nystagmus that is nonvestibular in origin and is presumably caused by abnormalities in the visually controlled gaze mechanisms. Since the final expression of all nystagmus is ocular and since there are several types of nonvestibular nystagmus (see below), the term

Table 3. Common varieties of nystagmus

Physiologic	*Pathologic*
Rotatory induced	Spontaneous vestibular with fixation
Caloric induced	or Frenzel glasses
Optokinetic	Positional with fixation or Frenzel
End point	glasses
	Gaze paretic
	Rebound
	Fixation
	Congenital
	Dissociated

ocular nystagmus should be discarded. Similarly the terms central, neurologic and otologic nystagmus lack specificity and imply a separation that usually cannot be made.

Methods of Examination

The clinical examination for pathologic nystagmus should include a systematic study of 1) changes in eye position, 2) changes in fixation and 3) changes in head position. Omission of any of these three maneuvers may lead to overlooking the presence of nystagmus or misinterpreting its type.

To evaluate the effect of change in eye position, ask the patient to fixate with eyes in the midposition and 30 degrees to the right, left, up and down. Record the characteristic of nystagmus in each position. Since attempts to maintain horizontal eye deviation beyond 40 degrees may result in a low amplitude, high frequency nystagmus in the direction of gaze (so-called end point nystagmus) in normal subjects, extreme eye deviation should be avoided. Each eye position should be held for at least 20 seconds. First degree nystagmus refers to nystagmus that is

DIAGRAMS OF 3 COMMON VARIETIES OF NYSTAGMUS

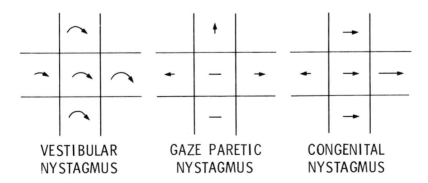

VESTIBULAR NYSTAGMUS   GAZE PARETIC NYSTAGMUS   CONGENITAL NYSTAGMUS

Figure 50. Method for describing the effect of eye position on nystagmus amplitude and direction. Arrows indicate direction of nystagmus (direction of fast component) in each eye position.

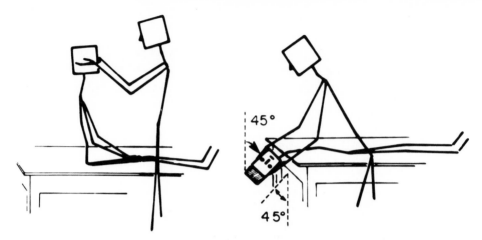

Figure 51. The positioning maneuver for inducing paroxysmal positional nystagmus. The patient is rapidly moved from the sitting to head-hanging position with the head 45 degrees below the horizontal and rotated 45 degrees to one side. (Reprinted from Neurology © 1972 by Harcourt Brace Jovanovich, Inc.)

present only on gaze in the direction of the fast component. Second degree nystagmus is present in the midposition and on gaze in the direction of the fast component and third degree nystagmus is present even on gaze away from the fast component. These terms are not applicable to all varieties of nystagmus and therefore can lead to confusion. A simple description can be rapidly summarized with a box diagram as illustrated in Figure 50. The size, shape and direction of the arrows provide information about the amplitude and direction of nystagmus in each ocular position.

Fixation affects different varieties of nystagmus in different ways. Vestibular nystagmus is inhibited by fixation, while gaze paretic, rebound and congenital nystagmus are all prominent with fixation. The effect of loss of fixation is easily studied with electronystagmography (ENG) and possibly represents the most important value of ENG testing (see Chapter 5). Frenzel glasses are useful for abolishing fixation in the office or at the bedside. They consist of +20 lenses mounted in a frame that contains a light source on the inside so that the patient's eyes are easily visualized. The light source can be powered by a battery, making the system completely portable.

Routinely, two types of positional testing are used: slow and rapid. With the first, one maneuvers the patient slowly into the supine, right lateral and left lateral positions. Positional nystagmus, induced by slow positioning, is persistent, low in frequency and often present only when fixation is inhibited. Paroxysmal positional nystagmus, on the other hand, is best induced by a rapid change from erect sitting to a supine head hanging left, center or right position (Figure 51). It is initially high in frequency (>5 beats/sec) and persists even when the patient is attempting to fixate. It depends on both the positioning maneuver and the final head hanging position.

Types of Pathologic Nystagmus

Table 4 summarizes the distinguishing characteristics, site of lesion and mechanism (where known) for the common varieties of pathologic nystagmus.

VESTIBULAR NYSTAGMUS.   A decrease in the spontaneous flow of action potentials from a single semicircular canal results in vestibular nystagmus in the plane of that canal with a slow conjugate deviation toward the damaged side interrupted by a quick corrective movement in the opposite direction. Since a selective loss of tonic afferent signals from one canal is unusual, vestibular nystagmus is usually rotatory because of the combined effects of altered vertical and horizontal canal input. The horizontal component is most prominent, however, because the components from the two vertical canals partially cancel each other. Gaze in the direction of the fast component increases the frequency and amplitude, while gaze in the opposite direction has the reverse effect (Alexander's law).

Although no completely reliable way exists of distinguishing vestibular nystagmus of peripheral origin (labyrinth and eighth nerve) from that of central nervous system origin, the latter is usually associated with other brain stem signs and is not effectively inhibited by fixation. The visual signals necessary to inhibit vestibular nystagmus are carried in the accessory optic tract to the inferior olives and midline cerebellum before arriving at the vestibular nuclei (see Visual-Vestibular Interaction, Chapter 3). If a CNS lesion involves any of these pathways, fixation will not suppress the vestibular nystagmus. The finding of an isolated vestibular nystagmus that fixation completely suppresses strongly suggests peripheral vestibular disease.

POSITIONAL NYSTAGMUS.   Since the time of Bárány, positional nystagmus has been attributed to lesions of the otoliths and their connections in the vestibular nuclei and cerebellum.[11,53,63] Recently, other mechanisms for the production of positional nystagmus have been proposed forcing a reexamination of traditional concepts. Theoretically, if one could alter a semicircular canal cupula so that its specific gravity no longer equaled that of the surrounding endolymph, the organ would become sensitive to changes in the direction of gravity and produce positional nystagmus. Several types of evidence suggest that both structural and metabolic factors can alter the specific gravity of the cupula and cause positional nystagmus (see Alcohol and Cupulolithiasis, Chapter 7).

Most investigators agree that two general categories of positional nystagmus can be identified on the basis of nystagmus regularity: paroxysmal and stationary positional nystagmus. Currently used classifications of positional nystagmus are confusing and difficult to apply in clinical practice, however. Some classifications are based on clinical observations obtained while the patient fixates while others are based on ENG recordings with eyes closed. Some investigators use slow positioning maneuvers while others employ only rapid positioning. These different methods make it difficult to compare classifications. Nylen[63] initially described three types of positional nystagmus based on visual inspection of nystagmus direction and regularity. Type 1, direction changing, and type 2, direction fixed, remained constant as long as the position was maintained. Type 3 was less clearly defined, comprising all paroxysmal varieties of positional nystagmus and some persistent varieties that did not fit into types 1 and 2. Numerous modifications of Nylen's classification have subsequently been proposed and the definition of each type has changed. In the most recent modification by Harrison and Ozsahinoglu,[48] type 1 comprises all varieties of persistent positional nystagmus, while types 2 and 3 are different varieties of paroxysmal positional nystagmus.

Paroxysmal Positional Nystagmus (PPN).   With this disorder the patient develops a burst of rotatory nystagmus after rapidly moving from the sitting to a head-hanging position (Fig. 51).[32] The response is not effectively inhibited by

111

Table 4. Types of pathologic nystagmus

Type	Characteristics	Location of Lesion	Mechanism
Spontaneous Vestibular			
Peripheral	Unidirectional, rotatory, inhibited with fixation except during acute stage of disease process	Labyrinth or eighth nerve	Imbalance in tonic labyrinthine signals
Central	Unidirectional, rotatory, decreased but not inhibited by fixation	Vestibular nuclei or their central connections	Imbalance of central vestibular signals
Paroxysmal Positional			
Peripheral	Unidirectional, high frequency, rotatory, 3 to 10 second latency, brief duration (<15 seconds), fatigues, prominent in only one head hanging position (with damaged ear down)	Labyrinth	Altered specific gravity of posterior semicircular canal cupula (see Cupulolithiasis, Chapter 7)
Central	Multidirectional, no latency, variable duration, does not fatigue, prominent in multiple positions	Brain stem or cerebellum	Unknown
Stationary Positional			
Peripheral	Direction fixed or changing, inhibited with fixation except during acute stage	Labyrinth or eighth nerve	Imbalance in tonic labyrinthine signals
Central	Direction fixed or changing, not inhibited with fixation	Brain stem or cerebellum	Imbalance of central vestibular signals
Gaze Paretic	High frequency, small amplitude, always in direction of gaze, loss of fixation decreases frequency and increases amplitude	Symmetric—nonspecific nervous system dysfunction, asymmetric—brain stem and/or cerebellum usually on side of larger amplitude	Impaired ocular position maintenance

	Description	Anatomic Location	Mechanism
Rebound	Like gaze paretic except slowly disappears as eccentric position is maintained and then may reverse direction	Cerebellum	Unknown
Fixation	Present in midposition, most prominent with fixation, may change direction with change in gaze position	Vertical—caudal brain stem and midline cerebellum, horizontal—lateral brain stem and cerebellum	Asymmetry in tonic pursuit signals
Congenital	High frequency, variable waveform, never purely vertical, decreased with convergence, most prominent with fixation, longstanding	Unknown	Unknown
Periodic Alternating	Spontaneous periodic changes in direction, can have features of fixation or congenital nystagmus	Caudal brain stem when acquired	Unknown
Dissociated MLF	Larger amplitude in abducting eye, rounded waveform in adducting eye	MLF	Unknown
Monocular	Uniocular oscillations	Brain stem or long-standing uniocular visual loss	Unknown
See-Saw	One eye rises and intorts; other falls and extorts	Tegmentum	Unknown

fixation, and can be elicited during the routine physical examination. The most common variety of PPN (called benign paroxysmal positional nystagmus by Dix and Hallpike)[32] usually has a 3 to 10 second latency before onset and rarely lasts longer than 15 seconds. The nystagmus is prominent in only one head hanging position and a burst of nystagmus in the reverse direction usually occurs when the patient moves back to the sitting position. Another key feature is that the patient experiences severe vertigo with the initial positioning, but with repeated positioning the vertigo and nystagmus rapidly disappear.

In most cases, PPN with the features just described is caused by vestibular end organ disease.[32, 48] It can be the only finding in an otherwise healthy individual, or it may be associated with other signs of peripheral vestibular damage, such as vestibular nystagmus and unilateral caloric hypoexcitability. In those instances that an abnormality is identified on caloric testing, PPN will invariably occur when the patient is positioned with the damaged ear down. PPN is a common sequella of head injury, viral labyrinthitis and occlusion of the vasculature to the inner ear. In the majority of cases, however, it occurs as an isolated symptom of unknown cause.

Rapid positional testing can induce a burst of nystagmus in normal subjects from stimulation of the semicircular canals in the plane of movement. Depending on the speed of movement and excitability of the subject's semicircular canals, variable magnitudes of nystagmus are produced. This positioning nystagmus can be differentiated from PPN, however, since it reaches peak magnitude during or immediately after the positioning maneuver, whereas PPN reaches its peak 5 to 15 seconds after the final position is reached.

Another variety of PPN has been associated with brain stem and cerebellar lesions.[22, 46, 48] This type does not decrease in amplitude or duration with repeated positioning, does not have a clear latency and usually lasts longer than 30 seconds. The direction is unpredictable and may be different in each position. The presence or absence of associated vertigo is not a reliable diagnostic feature.

Stationary Positional Nystagmus (SPN). Unlike PPN, SPN is seldom seen without the aid of ENG or Frenzel glasses to inhibit fixation, and is dependent on the final head position rather than the positioning maneuver. SPN remains as long as the position is maintained, although it may fluctuate in frequency and amplitude. Vertigo is usually not associated with the nystagmus. SPN may be unidirectional in all positions or direction changing in different positions. Not infrequently, patients with PPN have SPN of opposite direction after the PPN disappears, or if the position is reached very slowly. Despite earlier reports to the contrary,[63] it is now generally accepted that direction changing and direction fixed SPN are most common with peripheral vestibular disorders,[13, 23, 48] although both occur with central lesions. Their presence only indicates a dysfunction in the vestibular system without localizing value, thus they have the same significance as vestibular nystagmus. As with vestibular nystagmus, however, lack of suppression with fixation and signs of associated brain stem dysfunction suggest a central lesion.

GAZE PARETIC NYSTAGMUS. Patients with gaze paretic nystagmus are unable to maintain conjugate eye deviation away from the midposition. The drift back to the center (slow component) is regularly interrupted by a quick corrective movement toward the periphery (fast component). Gaze paretic nystagmus is always in the direction of gaze. As the gaze angle increases, the amplitude of nystagmus increases. Gaze nystagmus is readily visible on inspection, even though it may be less than half a degree in amplitude. In contrast to vestibular nystagmus, the frequency and slow component velocity of gaze paretic nystagmus decrease with loss of fixation, although the amplitude usually increases.

The site of abnormality in gaze paretic nystagmus can be at the neuromuscular level or in the multiple brain centers controlling conjugate gaze (frontal and occipital lobes, brain stem and cerebellum). Symmetrical gaze paretic nystagmus (equal amplitude to left and right) is commonly produced by ingestion of drugs such as phenobarbital, phenytoin, alcohol and diazepam. With these agents high frequency, small amplitude nystagmus (< 2 degrees) is found in all directions of gaze except down gaze. For unknown reasons, downbeat gaze paretic nystagmus is uncommon. A rough correlation exists between nystagmus amplitude and blood drug level.[40, 58] The nystagmus initially appears at extreme horizontal gaze positions (for example 40 degrees deviation). In addition to its association with drug ingestion, gaze paretic nystagmus is commonly found in patients with myasthenia gravis, multiple sclerosis and cerebellar atrophy.[10, 27]

Asymmetric horizontal gaze paretic nystagmus always indicates a structural brain lesion. When it is caused by a focal lesion of the brain stem or cerebellum, the larger amplitude nystagmus is usually directed toward the side of the lesion.[7, 59] Large cerebellopontine angle tumors commonly produce asymmetric gaze paretic nystagmus from compression of the brain stem and cerebellum (Bruns' nystagmus). Some patients with large vestibular schwannomas develop a combination of asymmetric gaze paretic nystagmus from brain stem compression and vestibular nystagmus from eighth nerve compression.[7] The larger amplitude gaze paretic nystagmus is directed toward the lesion and the vestibular nystagmus occurs only when fixation is inhibited. Asymmetric gaze paretic nystagmus may be present during the recovery from gaze paralysis (either cortical or subcortical in origin) in which case it is large in amplitude and low in frequency and present in only one direction of gaze (the direction of the previous gaze paralysis).

REBOUND NYSTAGMUS. Rebound nystagmus is a type of gaze paretic nystagmus that either disappears or reverses direction as the gaze position is held.[51] With gaze to the right or left, a high frequency nystagmus develops in the direction of gaze and then slowly disappears. After a brief latent period the nystagmus may reverse directions with the second phase being of lower frequency but lasting longer than the primary phase. This nystagmus reversal occurs in approximately one third of the cases. In most cases, the nystagmus decays, but does not reverse direction. When the eyes are returned to the midposition, another burst of nystagmus is initiated in the direction of the return saccade.

Rebound nystagmus has been reported to occur in patients with cerebellar atrophy and focal structural lesions of the cerebellum.[10, 51] It is the only variety of nystagmus considered specific for cerebellar involvement.

FIXATION NYSTAGMUS. Fixation nystagmus is defined as midposition nystagmus that is most prominent with fixation. The fact that it does not increase in magnitude when fixation is inhibited clearly differentiates it from the more common midposition vestibular nystagmus. Gaze in the direction of the fast component usually increases nystagmus frequency and amplitude, although the reverse has been observed.[25, 84] When gaze is directed approximately 15 to 30 degrees off-center in the direction opposite to that of the fast component, a null region is reached and the nystagmus is minimal or absent. Gaze beyond this null region may

115

result in a reversal of the nystagmus direction. Vertical and horizontal fixation nystagmus have similar features.[42] In some cases the nystagmus waveform is pendular in the midposition and converts to a jerk type on lateral or vertical gaze.

Since fixation nystagmus is associated with impaired smooth tracking in the direction of the fast component Zee and coworkers[84] proposed that damage to the normally balanced smooth pursuit system results in a slow drift of the eyes from the midposition (slow component) interrupted by corrective saccades to permit refixation (fast component). Although many areas of the brain are involved in the production of smooth pursuit eye movements, fixation nystagmus is found only with structural lesions of the brain stem and cerebellum. Smooth pursuit signals are carried to the vestibular nuclei via the inferior olives and midline cerebellum (see Visual-Vestibular Interaction, Chapter 3) and interruption of these signals might produce fixation nystagmus in a manner analogous to the way that interruption of labyrinthine signals to the vestibular nuclei produces vestibular nystagmus.[42]

Vertical (upbeat and downbeat) fixation nystagmus has been reported in patients with multiple sclerosis, brain stem and cerebellar infarction, infiltrating tumors of the brain stem and cerebellum, familial cerebellar degeneration, pontine myelinolysis, and alcohol nutritional cerebellar degeneration. [16, 25, 29, 42, 49, 69, 81] Downbeat fixation nystagmus is particularly common with Arnold-Chiari congenital malformation. Of 27 cases of primary position downbeat nystagmus reported by Cogan, 8 had the Arnold-Chiari malformation.[25] The reason for this association of Arnold-Chiari malformation with the downbeat variety of fixation nystagmus is unknown. Although it has been suggested on clinical grounds that primary position upbeat nystagmus is specific for anterior vermian involvement,[29] 2 patients studied at necropsy had lesions involving the inferior olives in the caudal brain stem.[42, 69] Horizontal fixation nystagmus occurs in patients with multiple sclerosis, familial cerebellar degeneration, brain stem infarction (lateral medullary plate syndrome), and cerebellar pontine angle tumors (unpublished observation). Aschoff and coworkers[5] found pendular horizontal fixation nystagmus in 4 percent of their patients with multiple sclerosis.

CONGENITAL NYSTAGMUS. Congenital nystagmus resembles acquired fixation nystagmus in several ways. It is usually present with the eyes open in midposition and a null region exists to the right or left of the center, where the nystagmus is minimal or absent. Occasionally, the null region is near the midposition so that nystagmus occurs only on gaze deviation. Congenital nystagmus is almost always highly dependent on fixation, disappearing or decreasing with loss of fixation. In some instances a slow nystagmus in the reverse direction is recorded with the eyes closed. One common variety, called latent congenital nystagmus, occurs only when either eye is covered, permitting monocular fixation. The resulting nystagmus beats toward the fixating eye. Latent congenital nystagmus is commonly associated with other congenital ocular defects, such as a comitant squint and alternating hyperphoria.

Several characteristic clinical features help distinguish congenital nystagmus from acquired nystagmus.[27] It is usually horizontal, occasionally rotatory, but never purely vertical, and convergence may diminish or eliminate the nystagmus. It is often associated with an inversion of the optokinetic response. Different waveforms characterize congenital nystagmus, varying from a pendular to sawtooth pattern with many variations in between. Different waveforms occur in the same patient as eye position is varied. Gaze in the direction of the fast component converts a pendular nystagmus to a sawtoothed (jerk) nystagmus. Many different waveforms may be seen in members of the same family with congenital nystagmus.[83] The frequency of congenital nystagmus is usually greater than 2 beats per second, and at times reaches 5 to 6 beats per second.[83] Nystagmus of this high frequency is unusual other than on a congenital basis.

The pathophysiologic mechanism of congenital nystagmus is poorly understood. Convincing evidence exists that the slow component causes the target to slip from the fovea and that the fast component brings the target back to the fovea.[31, 83] The slow component is not the result of, but the cause of, decreased vision. Maneuvers designed to decrease the target slippage (fitting glasses with prisms and extraocular muscle surgery) improve visual acuity.[31, 65] Patients with congenital nystagmus can make normal velocity saccades, suggesting that the extraocular muscles and orbital mechanics are normal.[83]

PERIODIC ALTERNATING NYSTAGMUS (PAN). PAN is nystagmus that periodically changes direction without a change in eye or head position.[9] Cycle length varies between 1 and 6 minutes with null periods between each half cycle varying from 2 to 20 seconds. The nystagmus slowly builds in intensity, reaching a peak slow component velocity near the center of each half cycle before slowly decreasing. PAN has been reported in association with such varied conditions as encephalitis, brain stem ischemia, demyelinating disease, syringobulbia, syphilis, trauma and as a congenital condition.[9, 30] The waveform seen with acquired PAN is the usual sawtoothed pattern, while that associated with the congenital variety frequently is pendular. Unlike patients with other forms of congenital nystagmus, patients with congenital PAN frequently complain of oscillopsia since they are unable to adapt to the constantly changing direction of nystagmus. PAN is usually present with fixation, although cases have been reported in which PAN occurs only with loss of fixation.[79]

Necropsy studies of three patients with acquired PAN revealed diffuse brain stem involvement with a predilection for the caudal brain stem.[54] Three reported cases have been associated with downbeat nystagmus, further suggesting a caudal brain stem dysfunction.[54] The pathophysiologic mechanism for production of PAN is unknown. PAN cycles can be altered in both phase and magnitude by a vestibular stimulus (rotatory or caloric), suggesting that the PAN rhythm is not the result of an independent CNS pacemaker, but rather a response pattern of the central vestibulo-oculomotor reflex arc.[9]

DISSOCIATED NYSTAGMUS (DISCONJUGATE NYSTAGMUS). The most common variety of dissociated nystagmus, *MLF nystagmus,* is produced by a lesion of the medial longitudinal fascicle (MLF), and is also called internuclear ophthalmoplegia. With early MLF lesions, the eyes appear to move conjugately, but the abducting eye on the side opposite the MLF lesion develops a regular small-amplitude high-frequency nystagmus in the direction of gaze. With more extensive MLF lesions, the adducting eye lags behind and develops a low amplitude nystagmus while the abducting eye overshoots the target and develops large amplitude nystagmus that has a characteristic "peaked" waveform.[8] MLF nystagmus can be bilateral or unilateral, depending on the extent of MLF involvement. Bilateral MLF nystagmus is most commonly seen with demyelinating disease, while unilateral MLF nystagmus most often accompanies vascular disease of the brain stem.[28, 47] Cogan and Wray reported on several children in the first decade of life in whom MLF nystagmus was a prominent early sign of brain stem tumors.[26] Patients with myasthenia gravis develop dissociated nystagmus similar to MLF nystagmus (*pseudo MLF nystagmus*), because of unequal impairment of neuromuscular transmission in adducting and abducting muscles.[43, 74] Unlike MLF nystagmus, the dissociated nystagmus with myasthenia progressively increases in amplitude as the gaze position is maintained.[74] An edrophonium chloride test should be administered to patients with isolated MLF nystagmus to exclude myasthenia gravis.

Several different lesions of the posterior fossa lead to dissociated rotatory nystagmus with horizontal and vertical components varying in each eye. The nystagmus is synchronized, however, in that the fast component occurs at exactly the same time in both eyes. Tumors, vascular disease and demyelinating disease of the brain stem produce this form of dissociated nystagmus.[24] Frequently the eye on the side of the lesion shows the largest amplitude oscillation. *Monocular nystagmus* results from similar posterior fossa lesions; this unusual form of dissociated nystagmus also has been reported with such varied entities as congenital syphilis, meningitis, optic nerve glioma, cerebral trauma, unilateral amblyopia and high refractive error.[33, 62] As might be expected, patients with these forms of nystagmus frequently complain of oscillopsia.

See-saw nystagmus is an unusual type of dissociated nystagmus in which one eye rhythmically rises and intorts while the other eye falls and extorts. It may be congenital, but most often is produced by acquired lesions near the optic chiasm, particularly those producing a bitemporal field defect and decreased central visual acuity.[4] Lesions reported in association with see-saw nystagmus include craniopharyngiomas, syringobulbia, brain stem infarction and diffuse choroiditis.[36, 56] Westheimer and Blair[82] produced an ocular movement pattern similar to see-saw nystagmus by stimulating the brain stem tegmentum in alert monkeys. Since all the sellar and parasellar tumors reported with see-saw nystagmus have been large enough to compress the upper brain stem, the tegmentum could have been involved.

Summary of Pathologic Nystagmus Classification

The flow chart in Figure 52 summarizes the classification of pathologic nystagmus. Different varieties are identified by a systematic study of the effect of loss of fixation, gaze deviation and change in head position. If nystagmus is present while the patient is seated and fixating on a target in the midposition, it is either vestibular, fixation or congenital nystagmus. Fixation is then inhibited with Frenzel glasses in order to differentiate these three varieties. Vestibular nystagmus increases in amplitude and frequency whereas fixation and congenital nystagmus either remain unchanged or decrease in frequency and amplitude. Congenital nystagmus is distinguished from acquired fixation nystagmus on the basis of its presence since infancy, high frequency and variable waveform.

If nystagmus is not present in the midposition either with or without fixation, maintained gaze deviation may reveal gaze paretic, rebound, dissociated or congenital nystagmus. Gaze paretic nystagmus is conjugate and persists as long as the gaze position is held, and the fast component is always in the direction of gaze. Rebound nystagmus decays as the gaze deviation is held and recurs transiently when the eyes return to the midposition. Dissociated nystagmus is nonconjugate, while congenital nystagmus is longstanding and high in frequency.

A change to the supine, lateral or head hanging position induces positional nystagmus. Paroxysmal positional nystagmus occurs after a rapid position change, while stationary positional nystagmus depends only on the final position.

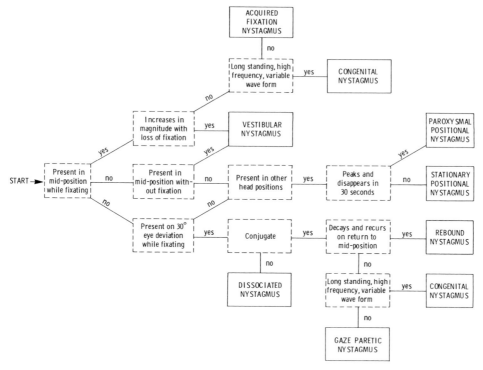

Figure 52. Flow chart summarizing pathologic nystagmus identification. (From Baloh, R. W.: *Pathologic nystagmus: A classification based on electro-oculographic recordings.* Bull. L. A. Neurol. Soc. 41:120, 1976, with permission.)

Related Phenomena

AMBLYOPIC NYSTAGMUS. Although patients with severely impaired vision can have many different types of spontaneous eye movement, a clear etiologic connection between loss of visual acuity and nystagmus is lacking. Blind patients frequently have wandering eye movements that are irregular in frequency and amplitude and occur in every possible direction. The associated ocular defects frequently present in patients with congenital nystagmus are not the cause of the nystagmus.[83] Of historical interest, coal miners who worked in dark mines for many years developed nystagmus (miner's nystagmus) that was dependent on the degree of illumination; it was most prominent in darkness and decreased or disappeared in strong light (the opposite of congenital nystagmus).[73] Some miners developed oscillopsia and vertigo with the nystagmus, suggesting the possibility of vestibular system involvement. Methane poisoning and/or poor nutrition may have caused the vestibular system damage. Since this phenomenon has apparently disappeared with improved mining conditions, the pathogenic mechanism may never be known.

VOLUNTARY NYSTAGMUS. Some normal subjects are able to produce rapid oscillations of the eyes at will, apparently because of an unusual ability to manipulate the convergence system. The main significance of these ocular gymnastics is that they may be mistaken for pathologic nystagmus. High in frequency (90 to 1,380 cycles per minute), low in amplitude (2 to 5 degrees), these horizontal pendular movements cannot be maintained for more than 20 to 30 seconds because of fatigue.[18, 19] Several siblings in the same family often produce voluntary nystagmus, and Keyes reported voluntary nystagmus in two generations of the same family, suggesting a dominant mode of inheritance.[55] Keyes proposed that the term "voluntary nystagmus" be replaced by "voluntary ocular oscillations" since nystagmus by definition is nonvoluntary.

CONVERGENCE RETRACTION NYSTAGMUS.   This dramatic oculomotor disorder results from lesions involving the tectal and pretectal region of the midbrain. When the patient attempts to make a voluntary saccade upward, he develops co-contraction of all extraocular muscles and the eyes rhythmically retract and converge (apparently because of the superior power of the medial recti).[41] Similar phenomena can be produced when the fast phase (involuntary saccade) of optokinetic or vestibular nystagmus is directed upward.[71] Convergence retraction nystagmus is usually associated with other signs of midbrain dysfunction (impaired upward gaze, pupillary abnormalities, accommodative spasm, retraction of the lids, vertical diplopia and skew deviation) constituting Parinaud's syndrome. This syndrome is most frequently produced by pinealomas, but is also associated with other tumors and vascular lesions involving the tectal or pretectal area.

OCULAR DYSMETRIA, SQUARE WAVE JERKS AND OCULAR FLUTTER.   These phenomena are found in patients with cerebellar lesions, all three frequently coexisting in the same patient. Ocular dysmetria refers to conjugate overshooting and undershooting of the target with voluntary saccades. This is analogous to the limb dysmetria frequently seen in the finger-to-nose test in patients with cerebellar lesions. Square wave jerks are a type of fixation instability with frequent saccadic eye movements away from the target followed after a characteristic delay time of approximately 200 msec by saccades returning to the target. These involuntary saccades are nonrhythmic and of varying amplitude. Finally, ocular flutter represents a burst of to-and-fro saccades occurring either spontaneously or after a saccade overshoots the target. This burst of saccades frequently lacks the characteristic delay normally present between serial saccades. Each of these phenomena probably represents a release of the brain stem saccade generating system from the normal cerebellar controlling influence.[10, 35]

OPSOCLONUS.   Opsoclonus is a rare eye movement disorder in which the eyes are constantly making random conjugate saccades of unequal amplitude in all directions. The phenomenon occurs with several different types of CNS disease and probably represents a mixed group of eye movement disorders.[14] The abnormal eye movements are most prominent immediately before or after a refixation, and are only slightly affected by inhibition of fixation. One variety of opsoclonus probably represents a continuum with square wave jerks and ocular flutter.[35] Other more dramatic varieties of opsoclonus have been reported in patients with brain stem encephalitis and as a remote effect of systemic carcinoma.[14] Necropsy examination in some of these cases revealed no involvement of the cerebellum. Recently, opsoclonus was found in several workers exposed to the pesticide, Kepone.[78] Cerebellar signs were variable, but all workers demonstrated a tremor of the extremities typical of essential tremor.

OCULAR BOBBING.   Ocular bobbing consists of abrupt, nonrhythmic, conjugate, downward jerks of the eyes, followed by a slow return to midposition. Typical cases are associated with a complete paralysis of spontaneous and reflex horizontal eye movements. Ocular bobbing usually represents an ominous prognostic sign since it results from massive pontine damage, either intrinsic (hemorrhage, infarction, tumor) or from extrinsic compression (cerebellar hemorrhage, uncal herniation), very often culminating in death.[20, 75]

OCULAR MYOCLONUS. This is a rhythmic oscillation of the eyes associated with synchronous oscillation of the palate. An associated rhythmic oscillation of the pharynx, larynx, mouth, tongue, diaphragm, extremities and intercostal muscles may also occur.[45, 60] The eye movements are frequently disconjugate, with the amplitude of excursion varying with eye position (usually greatest on extreme lateral gaze). The oscillations occur in any direction and are usually pendular or rotatory. The frequency varies from 1 to 3 per second, and the eye movements continue with loss of fixation. Ocular myoclonus disappears with sleep, but reappears during REM sleep.[76] Ocular and palatal myoclonus is seen in association with lesions disrupting the connections between the cerebellar dentate nucleus, the red nucleus, and the inferior olivary nucleus (Guillain-Mollaret triangle). It most commonly accompanies vascular lesions, but also occurs with tumors and degenerative disease.

REFERENCES

1. ADLER, R. H.: *Ocular vertigo*. Trans. Am. Acad. Ophthalmol. Otolaryngol. 46:271, 1941.

2. ALPERS, B. J.: *Vertigo: Its neurological features*. Trans. Am. Acad. Ophthalmol. Otolaryngol. 46:38, 1941.

3. ALPERS, B. J.: *Vertigo and Dizziness*. Grune and Stratton, Inc., New York, 1958.

4. ARNOTT, F. J., AND MILLER, S. J. H.: *See-saw nystagmus*. Trans. Ophthalmol. Soc. U. K. 90:483, 1970.

5. ASCHOFF, J. C., CONRAD, B., AND KORNHUBER, H. H.: *Acquired pendular nystagmus with oscillopsia in multiple sclerosis: A sign of cerebellar nuclei disease*. J. Neurol. Neurosurg. Psychiat. 37:570, 1974.

6. BALOH, R. W.: *Pathologic nystagmus: A classification based on electro-oculographic recordings*. Bull. L. A. Neurol. Soc. 41:120, 1976.

7. BALOH, R. W., ET AL.: *Cerebellar-pontine angle tumors. Results of quantitative vestibulo-ocular testing*. Arch. Neurol. 33:507, 1976.

8. BALOH, R. W., YEE, R. D., AND HONRUBIA, V.: *Internuclear ophthalmoplegia. I. Saccades and dissociated nystagmus*. Arch. Neurol. In press.

9. BALOH, R. W., HONRUBIA, V., AND KONRAD, H. R.: *Periodic alternating nystagmus*. Brain 99:11, 1976.

10. BALOH, R. W., KONRAD, H. R., AND HONRUBIA, V.: *Vestibulo-ocular function in patients with cerebellar atrophy*. Neurology 25:160, 1975.

11. BÁRÁNY, R.: *Diagnose von krankheitserscheinungen im Bereiche des Otolithen-apparates*. Acta Otolaryngol. 2:434, 1921.

12. BÁRÁNY, R.: *Neue Untersuchungsmethoden, die Beziehungen zwischen Vestibular-apparat, Kleinhirn, Grosshirn and Rückenmark betreffend*. Wien. med. Wschr. 60:2033, 1910.

13. BARBER, H. O.: *Positional nystagmus: testing and interpretation*. Ann. Otol. Rhinol. Laryngol. 73:838, 1964.

14. BELLUS, S. N.: *Opsoclonus: Its clinical value*. Neurology 25:502, 1975.

15. BENDER, M. B., FELDMAN, M., AND ATKIN, A.: Optic illusions in lesions of the vestibular system. In: *Proceedings of the International Symposium on Vestibular and Oculomotor Problems*. Nippon Hoechst., Tokyo, 1965.

16. BENDER, M. B., AND GORMEN, W. F.: *Vertical nystagmus on direct forward gaze with vertical oscillopsia*. Ann. J. Ophthalmol. 32:967, 1949.

17. BLACK, O.: *Vestibular causes of vertigo.* Geriatrics 30:123, 1975.
18. BLAIR, C. J., GOLDBERG, M. F., AND VON NORDEN, G. K.: *Voluntary nystagmus.* Arch. Ophthalmol. 77:349, 1976.
19. BLUMENTHAL, H.: *Voluntary nystagmus.* Neurology 23:223, 1973.
20. BOSCH, E. P., KENNEDY, S. S., AND ASCHENBRENER, C. A.: *Ocular bobbing: The myth of its localizing value.* Neurology 25:949, 1975.
21. BRUNIA, C. H. M., AND HOPPENBROUWERS, T.: *In search of tonic cervical reflexes. An evaluation of Fukuda's vertical writing test.* Acta Otolaryngol. 61:547, 1966.
22. CAWTHORN, T., AND HINCHCLIFFE, R.: *Positional nystagmus of the central type as evidence of subtentorial metastases.* Brain 84:415, 1961.
23. COATS, A. C.: Electronystagmography. In Bradford, L. (ed.): *Physiological Measures of the Audio-Vestibular System.* Academic Press, New York, 1975.
24. COGAN, D. G.: *Dissociated nystagmus with lesions in the posterior fossa.* Arch. Ophthalmol. 70:121, 1963.
25. COGAN, D. G.: *Downbeat nystagmus.* Arch Ophthalmol. 80:757, 1968.
26. COGAN, D. G., AND WRAY, S. H.: *Internuclear ophthalmoplegia: An early sign of brain stem tumors.* Neurology 20:629, 1970.
27. COGAN, D. G.: *Neurology of the Ocular Muscles.* Charles C Thomas, Springfield, Illinois, 1956.
28. COGAN, D. G., KUBIK, S. C., AND SMITH, W. L.: *Unilateral internuclear ophthalmoplegia: Report of eight clinical cases and one post-mortem study.* Arch. Ophthalmol. 44:783, 1950.
29. DAROFF, R. B., AND TROOST, T.: *Upbeat nystagmus.* JAMA 225:312, 1973.
30. DAVIS, D. G., AND SMITH, J. L.: *Periodic alternating nystagmus.* Am. J. Ophthalmol. 72:757, 1971.
31. DELL'OSSO, L. F., FLYNN, J. T., AND DAROFF, R. B.: *Hereditary congenital nystagmus. An intrafamilial study.* Arch. Ophthalmol. 92:366, 1974.
32. DIX, M. R., AND HALLPIKE, C. S.: *The pathology, symptomatology, and diagnosis of certain disorders of the vestibular system.* Ann. Otol. Rhinol. Laryngol. 61:987, 1951.
33. DONIN, J. F.: *Acquired monocular nystagmus in children.* Can. J. Ophthalmol. 2:212, 1967.
34. DRACHMAN, D. A., AND HART, C. W.: *An approach to the dizzy patient.* Neurology 22:323, 1972.
35. ELLENBERGER, C., KELTNER, J. L., AND STROUD, M. B.: *Ocular dyskinesia in cerebellar disease: evidence for the similarity of opsoclonus, ocular dysmetria and flutter-like oscillations.* Brain 95:685, 1972.
36. FEIN, J. M., AND WILLIAMS, R. D. B.: *See-saw nystagmus.* J. Neurol. Neurosurg. Psychiat. 32:265, 1969.
37. FREGLY, A. R.: Vestibular ataxia and its measurement in man. In Kornhuber , H. H. (ed.): *Handbook of Sensory Physiology,* vol. VI, part 2. Springer-Verlag, New York, 1974.
38. FUKUDA, T.: *The stepping test: Two phases of the labyrinthine reflex.* Acta Otolaryngol. 50:95, 1959.
39. FUKUDA, T.: *Vertical writing with eyes covered: A new test of vestibulospinal reaction.* Acta Otolaryngol. 50:26, 1959.
40. GALLAGHER, B. B., ET AL.: *Primidone, dipenylhydantoin and phenobarbital. Aspects of acute and chronic toxicity.* Neurology 23:145, 1973.
41. GAY, A. J., BRODKEY, J., AND MILLER, J. E.: *Convergence retraction nystagmus: an electromyographic study.* Arch. Ophthalmol. 70:456, 1963.
42. GILMAN, N., BALOH, R. W., AND TOMIYASU, U.: *Primary position upbeat nystagmus. A clinical pathological study.* Neurology 27:294, 1977.
43. GLASER, J. S.: *Myasthenic pseudo-internuclear ophthalmoplegia.* Arch. Ophthalmol. 75:365, 1966.
44. GOTCH, F., MEYER, J. S., AND YASUYUKI, T.: *Cerebral effects of hyperventilation in man.* Arch. Neurol. 12:410, 1965.
45. GUILLAIN, G.: *The syndrome of synchronous and rhythmic palato-pharyngo-laryngo-oculo-diaphragmatic myoclonus.* Proc. Roy. Soc. Med. 31:1031, 1938.
46. HALLPIKE, C. S.: *Vertigo of central origin.* Proc. Roy. Soc. Med. 55:364, 1962.

47. HARRIS, W.: *Ataxic nystagmus: A pathognomonic sign in disseminated sclerosis.* Brit. J. Ophthalmol. 28:40, 1944.

48. HARRISON, M. S., AND OZSAHINOGLU, C.: *Positional vertigo.* Arch. Otolaryngol. 101:675, 1975.

49. HART, D. J. C., AND SANDERS, M. D.: *Downbeat nystagmus.* Trans. Ophthalmol. Soc. U.K. 90:483, 1970.

50. HENNEBERT, C.: *A new syndrome in hereditary syphilis of the labyrinth.* Presse Med. Belg. Brux 63:467, 1911.

51. HOOD, J. D., KAYAN, A., AND LEECH, J.: *Rebound nystagmus.* Brain 96:507, 1973.

52. DEJONG, P. T. V. M., ET AL.: *Ataxia and nystagmus induced by injection of local anesthetics in the neck.* Ann. Neurol. 1:240, 1977.

53. JONGKEES, L. B. W.: *On positional nystagmus.* Acta Otolaryngol. (Suppl. 159):78, 1961.

54. KEANE, J. R.: *Periodic alternating nystagmus with downward beating nystagmus. A clinico-anatomical case study of multiple sclerosis.* Arch. Neurol. 30:399, 1974.

55. KEYES, M. J.: *Voluntary nystagmus in two generations.* Arch. Neurol. 29:63, 1973.

56. KINDER, R. S. L., AND HOWARD, G. M.: *See-saw nystagmus.* Am. J. Dis. Child. 106:331, 1963.

57. KITAHARA, M.: *Acceleration registrography. A method of examinations concerned with the labyrinthine righting reflex.* Ann. Otol. 74:203, 1965.

58. KUTT, H., ET AL.: *Diphenylhydantoin metabolism, blood levels and toxicity.* Arch. Neurol. 11:642, 1964.

59. LUNDBORG, T.: *Diagnostic problems concerning acoustic tumors.* Acta Otolaryngol. (Suppl. 99):1, 1952.

60. MCCARTHY, W.: *Ocular and palatal myoclonus.* Arch. Ophthalmol. 55:580, 1956.

61. NADOL, J. B.: *Positive Hennebert's sign in Meniere's disease.* Arch. Otolaryngol. 103:524, 1977.

62. NATHANSON, M., BERGMAN, P. S., AND BERKER, M. B.: *Monocular nystagmus.* Am. J. Ophthalmol. 40:685, 1955.

63. NYLEN, C. O.: *Positional nystagmus. A review and future prospects.* J. Laryngol. Otol. 64:295, 1950.

64. NYMAN, H.: *A graphic registration of tipping and pointing reaction.* Acta Otolaryngol. (Suppl. 60):1, 1945.

65. PARKS, M. M.: *Congenital nystagmus surgery: Symposium on nystagmus.* Ann. Orthopt. J. 23:35, 1973.

66. PEITERSEN, E.: Measurement of vestibulo-spinal responses in man. In Kornhuber, H. H. (ed.): *Handbook of Sensory Physiology,* vol. VI, part 2. Springer-Verlag, New York, 1974.

67. PEITERSEN, E.: *Vestibulospinal reflexes. X. Theoretical and clinical aspects of the stepping test.* Arch. Otolaryngol. 85:192, 1967.

68. ROMBERG, M. H.: *Lehrbuch der Nervenkrankheiten des Menschen.* A. Dunker, Berlin, 1946.

69. SCHATZ, N., SCHLEZINGER, N., AND BERRY, R.: *Vertical upbeat nystagmus on downward gaze: A clinical pathological correlation (Abstract).* Neurology 25:380, 1975.

70. SINGER, E. P.: *The hyperventilation syndrome in clinical medicine.* New York J. Med. 58:1494, 1958.

71. SMITH, J. L., ET AL.: *Nystagmus retractorius.* Arch. Ophthalmol. 62:864, 1959.

72. SPECTOR, M.: Incidence of various types of dizziness. In Spector, M. (ed.): *Dizziness and Vertigo.* Grune and Stratton, New York, 1967.

73. SPIEGEL, E. A., AND SOMMER, I.: *Neurology of the Eye, Ear, Nose and Throat.* Grune and Stratton, New York, 1944.

74. SPOONER, J. W., AND BALOH, R. W.: *Eye movement fatique in myasthenia gravis. (Abstract).* Neurology 27:345, 1977.

75. SUSAC, J. O., ET AL.: *Clinical spectrum of ocular bobbing.* J. Neurol. Neurosurg. Psychiat. 33:771, 1970.

76. TAHMOUSH, A. J., BROOKS, J. E., AND KELTNER, J. L.: *Palatal myoclonus associated with abnormal ocular and extremity movements.* Arch. Neurol. 27:431, 1972.

77. TALPIS, L.: *Zur Methode der grafischen Registrierung des Zerge-und Einstellungsversuches, der Armtonus und Abweichreaktion.* Arch. Ohr.-Nas.-u. Kehlk.-Heilk. 116:255, 1927.

78. TAYLOR, J. R., ET AL.: *Neurologic disorder induced by Kepone: Preliminary report (Abstract).* Neurology 26:538, 1976.
80. UNTERBERGER, S.: *Neue objectiv registrierbare Vestibularis—Körperdrehreaktion, erhalten durch Treten auf der Stelle: Der "Tretversuch."* Arch. Ohr.-Nas.-u. Kehlk.-Heilk. 145:478, 1938.
81. VICTOR, M., ADAMS, R. D., AND MANCALL, E. L.: *A restricted form of cerebellar cortical degeneration occurring in alcoholic patients.* Arch. Neurol. 1:678, 1959.
82. WESTHEIMER, G., AND BLAIR, M.: *The ocular tilt reaction—a brain stem oculomotor routine.* Invest. Ophthalmol. 14:833, 1975.
83. YEE, R. D., ET AL.: *A study of congenital nystagmus: Waveforms.* Neurology 26:326, 1976.
84. ZEE, D., FRIENDLICH, A., AND ROBINSON, D.: *The mechanism of downbeat nystagmus.* Arch. Neurol. 30:227, 1974.

CHAPTER 5

Electronystagmography

METHOD OF RECORDING EYE MOVEMENTS

Electro-oculography (EOG) is the simplest and most readily available system for recording eye movements.[23, 28, 46, 48] With this technique, a voltage surrounding the orbit is measured whose magnitude is proportional to the amplitude of the eye movement. When used for evaluating vestibular function the technique has been termed electronystagmography (ENG) and often the terms EOG and ENG are used interchangeably. ENG provides a permanent record for comparison with nystagmus recorded in other patients. Because of the transient nature of many types of nystagmus, a permanent record is invaluable. By comparing clinical observation with paper recordings, both students and experienced clinicians become more efficient in recognizing different varieties of nystagmus. With ENG, one can quantify the slow component velocity, frequency and amplitude of spontaneous or induced nystagmus and the changes in these measurements brought about by loss of fixation (either with eyes closed, or eyes open in darkness). Of equal importance, voluntary saccadic and pursuit eye movements can be accurately measured.

Principle of ENG

The principle of ENG is illustrated in Figure 53.[28] The pigmented layer of the retina maintains a negative potential with regard to the surrounding tissue by means of active ion transport. Because of the sclera's insulating properties the cornea becomes positive in relation to the retina (analogous to a capacitor). The potential difference between the cornea and retina, known as the corneoretinal potential, acts as an electric dipole, oriented in the direction of the long axis of the eye. In relation to a remote location, an electrode placed in the vicinity of the eye becomes more positive when the eye rotates towards it and less positive when it rotates in the opposite direction. The maximum sensitivity is obtained when the eye movement is in the plane of a line joining the center of the pupil with the center of the electrode. In this case, the measured voltage is proportional to the sine of the angle of motion.[36]

Recordings are usually made with a three electrode system using differential amplifiers. Two of the (active) electrodes are placed on each side of the eye and

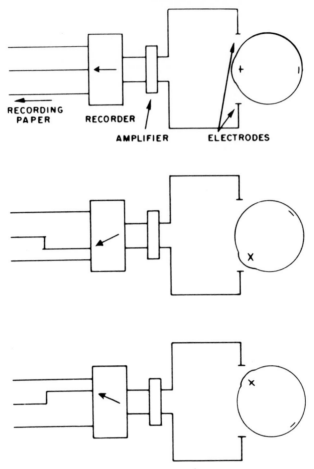

Figure 53. Principle of electronystagmography (ENG). (From Coats, A. C.: Electronystagmography. In Bradford, L. (ed.): *Physiological Measures of the Audio-Vestibular System*. Academic Press, New York, 1975, with permission.)

the reference (ground) electrode somewhere remote from the eyes. The two active electrodes measure a potential change of equal amplitude but opposite direction. The difference in potential between these electrodes is amplified and used to control the displacement of a pen-writing recorder or similar device to produce a permanent record. Since the differential amplifiers monitor the difference in voltage between the two active electrodes, remote electric signals (electrocardiographic or electroencephalographic for example) arrive at the electrodes with approximately equal amplitude and phase and cancel out.

The corneoretinal potential on which the ENG is based varies with the amount of light striking the retina, with the maximum light-adapted potential being approximately twice that of the dark-adapted potential. Therefore, the ENG signal must be calibrated frequently and major shifts in room lighting should be avoided.

The sensitivity and frequency response of the ENG equipment varies from one laboratory to another.[28, 49] Many commercially available recorders have sensitivities of between 2 and 5 degrees of eye rotation with an upper frequency cutoff

126

of 15 Hz. With properly designed amplification, ENG can consistently record eye rotation of 0.5 degree, although one occasionally encounters a patient with a high noise-to-signal ratio (particularly elderly patients), limiting the sensitivity to 1 to 2 degrees. Even at its best, the sensitivity of ENG is less than that of direct visual inspection (approximately 0.1 degree) and therefore visual inspection for small amplitude eye movements remains an important part of the examination. With all electronic equipment one must tailor the frequency response so that interfering signals (for example 60 cycle hum and muscle potentials) are removed with the least possible interference with the desired event. In order to accurately reproduce the high frequency transients of eye movement recordings (nystagmus fast components and saccades), we have found that the upper frequency cutoff must be at least 25 Hz and preferably 35 Hz.

Electrode Placement

The plane of the recording electrodes defines the plane of recorded eye movements. Electrodes attached medial and lateral to the eye will record the horizontal components of eye movement; those above and below the eye, the vertical components. A ground electrode is placed on the center of the forehead or on the auricle. Frequently the horizontal component of both eyes is summed by placing an electrode lateral to each eye (bitemporal recording). This has the advantage of increasing the signal-to-noise ratio but it has the disadvantage of camouflaging disconjugate eye movements. The vertically aligned electrodes sense the voltage associated with both vertical eye and lid movement so that the recording represents a summation of these two movements.[24] For this reason, ENG cannot be used for detailed study of the waveform of vertical eye movements. In most instances, however, it is adequate for clinical assessment of vertical eye movement disorders.

Interpreting the Recording

By convention, for horizontal recordings, eye movements to the right are displayed so that they produce upward pen deflection and those to the left produce downward deflection. For vertical recordings upward and downward eye movements produce upward and downward deflections, respectively. In order to interpret ENG recordings, calibration must be performed so that a standard angle of eye deviation is represented by a known amplitude of pen deflection. Calibration is performed by having the patient maintain his gaze on a series of dots or lights 10 to 20 degrees on each side of and above and below the central fixation point. Once this relationship is established the amplitude, duration, and velocity of recorded eye movements can be easily calculated. Figure 54 illustrates the relationship between components of a typical beat of nystagmus as recorded with ENG. Values chosen for each component are those commonly seen with vestibular nystagmus recorded in the dark. The fast component moves to the left, so by convention the nystagmus is to the left. A 10 degree fast component would have an average velocity (a/fd) of approximately 100 deg/sec. The slow component velocity (a/sd) is usually much slower (in this case 10 deg/sec). It is approximately the product of amplitude times frequency as long as the fast duration is small compared to the slow duration.

Although the magnitude of each nystagmus measurement shown in Figure 54 can be calculated directly from the polygraph recording, such a procedure is

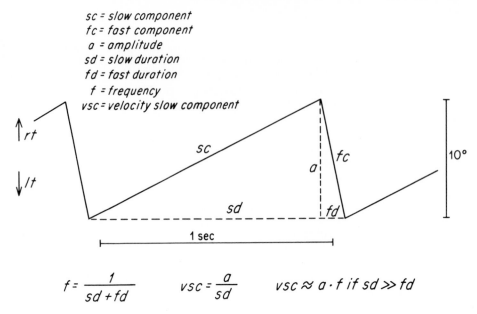

$$f = \frac{1}{sd + fd} \qquad vsc = \frac{a}{sd} \qquad vsc \approx a \cdot f \; if \; sd \gg fd$$

Figure 54. A single beat of vestibular nystagmus recorded with ENG.

tedious and therefore subject to error. Digital computers are ideally suited for making such measurements. After analogue to digital conversion of the data, a digital computer, using a programmed algorithm, calculates the amplitude, duration and velocity of each of the slow and fast components.[62] In our laboratory, the nystagmus algorithm identifies the minimum and maximum voltages of each nystagmus beat and computation of the nystagmus parameter values is made under the assumption that the nystagmus waveform is accurately represented by straight lines connecting the minumum and maximum points. Plots of nystagmus slow component velocity against time are particularly useful for quantifying the magnitude of induced nystagmus (see Figs. 60 and 61).

Recommended Test Battery

ENG can be used to evaluate any type of eye movement disorder, and the testing procedure should be flexible enough to deal with any such abnormality encountered. It is useful, however, to have a standard test battery that will at least screen all areas of potential abnormality (Table 5). The test battery should include: 1) recording for pathologic nystagmus, 2) tests of vestibulo-ocular reflex function and 3) tests of visual ocular control.

RECORDING PATHOLOGIC NYSTAGMUS

The same systematic search for pathologic nystagmus outlined in the previous chapter should be conducted during the ENG examination. Recording with eyes closed or with eyes opened in darkness is more effective than Frenzel glasses for identifying vestibular and positional nystagmus. Approximately 20 percent of normal subjects have spontaneous nystagmus[47,53,74] and as many as 75 percent

Table 5. Recommended ENG test battery

A. Recording for pathologic nystagmus
   1. Fixation at midposition
   2. Fixation inhibited with eyes closed or eyes open in darkness (mental arithmetic to maintain alertness)
   3. Gaze held 30 degrees right, left, up and down for 1 minute in each position
   4. Rapid and slow positional changes

B. Vestibulo-ocular reflex function
   1. Bithermal caloric stimulation—30 and 44 degrees C water infused into each ear for 40 seconds, eyes open behind Frenzel glasses or in darkness, continuous mental arithmetic to maintain alertness, minimum of 5 minutes between each stimulus.
   2. Sinusoidal rotation (0.05 Hz, 30-120 deg/sec)
      a. in darkness with eyes open
      b. lights on stationary background and
      c. lights on and fixation point moving with rotatory chair. Continuous mental arithmetic to maintain alertness

C. Visual-ocular control
   1. Saccades: 5 to 40 degree saccades induced in each direction, target can be either a series of dots or lights.
   2. Smooth pursuit: target moves sinusoidally with maximum velocity approximately 30 deg/sec
   3. Optokinetic nystagmus: stripes move clockwise and counterclockwise at constant velocity (20 to 40 deg/sec).

have positional nystagmus[22] when tested with eyes closed. Apparently the vestibular system is unable to completely stabilize the position of the eyes when visual signals are removed. If the average slow component velocity of spontaneous vestibular or positional nystagmus exceeds 3 deg/sec, however, it is a sign of vestibular impairment (p <0.05).[63]

The effect of change in ocular position and fixation on vestibular nystagmus is illustrated with the ENG recordings in Figure 55.[6] The patient was tested three days after and again two weeks after a left labyrinthectomy. On the initial recording, nystagmus is present with fixation although it is much more prominent without fixation. On the subsequent recording, nystagmus only occurs when eye closure removes fixation. This pattern is typical of an acute peripheral vestibulopathy of any cause. As a general rule, nystagmus with fixation (nystagmus seen on routine neurologic examination) disappears within one to two weeks after the occurrence of an acute peripheral vestibular lesion. By contrast, vestibular nystagmus can be recorded with eyes closed for as long as 5 to 10 years after an acute peripheral vestibular lesion.[65] In some patients vestibular nystagmus emerges only when they are mentally alerted (for example when performing serial 7 subtractions from 100).

Changes in head position with respect to gravity generally alter the direction and magnitude of vestibular nystagmus. A patient tested four weeks after the onset of an acute left sided labyrinthitis did not have nystagmus with eyes open, but with eyes closed he developed a right beating vestibular nystagmus in the sitting position (Fig. 56).[6] In the supine position, the nystagmus increased in frequency and amplitude, beating down and to the right. The right lateral position (affected ear up) accentuated the vertical component, while the left lateral position (affected ear down) increased the horizontal component. The head-hanging

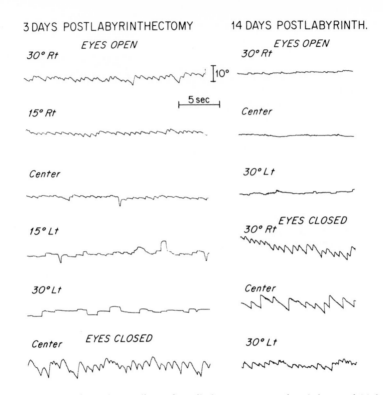

Figure 55. Bitemporal horizontal recordings of vestibular nystagmus taken 3 days and 14 days after the patient underwent a left labyrinthectomy. Nystagmus with eyes open disappears by 14 days but nystagmus with eyes closed remains prominent. (From Baloh, R. W.: *Pathologic nystagmus: A classification based on electro-oculographic recordings.* Bull. L.A. Neurol. Soc. 41:120, 1976, with permission.)

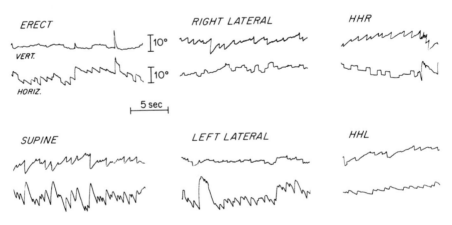

Figure 56. Effect of change in position on vestibular nystagmus. Vertical component is accentuated in the right lateral position (affected ear up) and horizontal component is accentuated in the left lateral position (affected ear down). All recordings (bitemporal horizontal and monocular vertical) are with eyes closed. (From Baloh, R. W.: *Pathologic nystagmus: A classification based on electro-oculographic recordings.* Bull. L.A. Neurol. Soc. 41:120, 1976, with permission.)

130

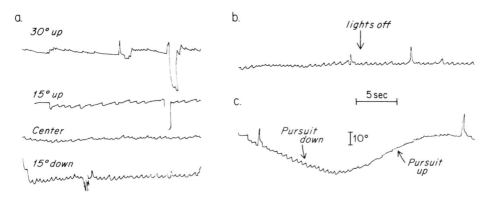

Figure 57. Monocular vertical recordings of downbeat fixation nystagmus. (a) The midposition nystagmus increases on downward gaze and decreases on upward gaze. Gaze 30° up changes nystagmus direction. (b) Loss of fixation has little effect on the nystagmus. (c) Downward smooth pursuit is impaired. (From Baloh, R. W.: *Pathologic nystagmus: A classification based on electro-oculographic recordings.* Bull. L.A. Neurol. Soc. 41:120, 1976, with permission.)

positions accentuated the vertical components. This pattern of positional change with vestibular nystagmus frequently occurs after an acute unilateral vestibulopathy and can be explained on the basis of utriculocupular interaction on the remaining intact side[39] (see Interaction of Semicircular Canal and Otolith Induced Eye Movements, Chapter 3). The effects of positional change on longstanding vestibular nystagmus of peripheral and central origin is less predictable, however, and one cannot consistently identify the abnormal side on the basis of positional information alone.

Figures 57 and 58 illustrate how ENG can help differentiate congenital and fixation nystagmus from vestibular nystagmus.[6] The downbeat fixation nystagmus (Fig. 57) increases in frequency and amplitude with downward gaze but reverses

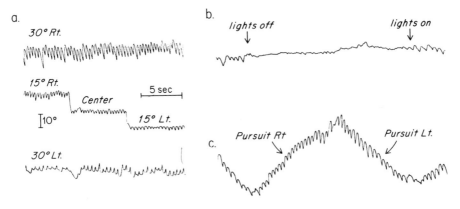

Figure 58. Bitemporal horizontal recordings of congenital nystagmus. (a) Pendular nystagmus in the midposition becomes a right beating jerk nystagmus on gaze to the right. A null region is between 15° and 30° to the left. (b) Loss of fixation inhibits the nystagmus. (c) The congenital nystagmus is superimposed on attempted smooth pursuit. (From Baloh, R. W.: *Pathologic nystagmus: A classification based on electro-oculographic recordings.* Bull. L.A. Neurol. Soc. 41:120, 1976, with permission.)

direction on 30 degrees upward gaze. Loss of fixation does not change nystagmus frequency or amplitude. Downward smooth pursuit is impaired while upward pursuit is relatively maintained. The waveform of the congenital nystagmus (Fig. 58) is rounded in the midposition without a clear slow and fast component, but with 30 degrees gaze to the right a saw-toothed waveform develops with the fast component to the right. When fixation is inhibited by darkness, the congenital nystagmus almost disappears. The markedly impaired horizontal smooth pursuit in both directions is typical of congenital nystagmus. By comparison, vestibular nystagmus does not change direction with change in gaze position, increases with loss of fixation and usually does not impair smooth pursuit.

TESTS OF VESTIBULO-OCULAR REFLEX FUNCTION

The ultimate goal of vestibulo-ocular reflex testing is to determine if the labyrinthine end organs and the nervous system pathways are functioning normally. A normal response is obtained only when all components of the reflex arc are intact (see Nystagmus, Effect of Experimental Lesions, Chapter 3).

Caloric Testing

Mechanism of Stimulation

The caloric test uses a nonphysiologic stimulus (water or air) to induce endolymphatic flow in the semicircular canals by creating a temperature gradient from one side of the canal to the other[61] (Fig. 59). Irrigation of the external auditory canal with water or air that is below or above body temperature transfers a temperature gradient from the external auditory canal to the internal ear by conduction. The horizontal semicircular canal develops the largest temperature gradient because it lies closest to the source of temperature change. Since the other two canals are relatively remote from the external canal, caloric stimulation of the vertical canals is unreliable. The endolymph circulates because of the difference in its specific gravity on the two sides of the canal if the semicircular canal being investigated is either in or near the vertical plane. Caloric testing of horizontal semicircular canal function is usually performed with the patient in the supine position, head tilted 30 degrees up (placing the horizontal canals in the vertical plane—see Fig. 19). With the warm caloric stimulus illustrated in Figure 59, the column of endolymph nearest the middle ear rises because of its decreased density. This causes the cupula to deviate toward the utricle (ampullopetal flow) and produces horizontal nystagmus with the fast component directed toward the stimulated ear. A cold stimulus produces the opposite effect on the endolymph column causing ampullofugal endolymph flow and nystagmus directed away from the stimulated ear (COWS—cold opposite, warm same). If the same test is repeated with the patient lying on his abdomen so that the horizontal canal is reversed in the vertical plane (so that the direction of the gravity vector with relation to the head is reversed) the direction of nystagmus induced by warm and cold stimulation will be reversed.

The caloric test is the most widely used clinical test of vestibulo-ocular reflex function. The two main reasons for its clinical usefulness are: 1) each labyrinth can be stimulated individually, and 2) the stimulus is easy to apply without requiring complex equipment. Several limitations of the test must be appreciated if one

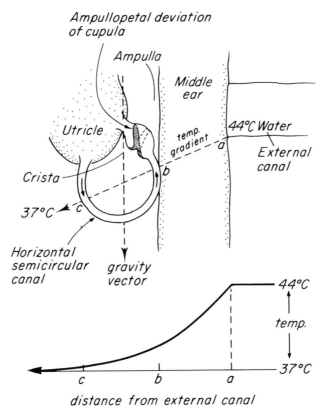

Figure 59. Mechanism of caloric stimulation of the horizontal semicircular canal. (See text for details).

is to properly assess the results. The slow component velocity and duration of caloric induced nystagmus are dependent not only on the relationship between the temperature gradient vector and gravity vector, but also on the blood flow to the skin, length of transmission pathway from the tympanic membrane to the horizontal canal, and heat conductivity of the temporal bone.[2] If local blood flow to the skin is decreased (from vasoconstriction due to pain or anxiety), the maximum slow component velocity of the response decreases (from decreased heat conductivity through skin), but its duration is prolonged (from delayed heat transfer). Patients with infection or fluid in the middle ear and mastoid air cells may have an increased caloric response (increased maximum slow component velocity) because of the increased heat conductivity from the external to inner ear. A thickened temporal bone on the other hand, would produce the opposite effect because of decreased bone heat conductivity. Some of these factors no doubt underlie the large variability of caloric responses measured in normal subjects and explain the occasional unexpected increase or decrease in caloric response found in patients with temporal bone disease.

Test Methodology

Since the time when Bárány introduced irrigation of the external auditory canal with a large volume of cold water as a method of evaluating the function of each

133

labyrinth separately, numerous modifications of the caloric test have been proposed.

ICE WATER TESTS. Because of its availability, ice water (approximately 0°C) has been used to obtain a rapid assessment of vestibular function in the office setting.[35] The volume of ice water used varies from 50 cc to less than 1 cc. When small volumes (5 cc or less) are used, the stimulus may not reach the eardrum (injection into the canal wall or cerumen) and a false impression of vestibulo-ocular reflex malfunction is obtained. To avoid the problems of inadequate stimulation, at least 10 cc of ice water should be used. Ice water calorization lacks sensitivity since patients with normal response to ice water caloric testing frequently demonstrate asymmetry in response to the bithermal test (described below). As a general rule, ice water testing can provide only gross information about the symmetry of vestibular function.[35] Ice water testing should not be used as a preliminary step to bithermal testing since it frequently produces prominent subjective symptoms making the patient less willing to cooperate with the more precise testing. When bithermal testing does not produce a response, ice water can then be used as a massive stimulus to determine if any function remains.

BITHERMAL TESTS. Bithermal caloric stimulation, introduced by Fitzgerald and Hallpike,[38] has received the widest acceptance and represents a significant step in the development of reliable clinical caloric testing. Each ear is irrigated for a fixed duration (40 seconds) at a constant flow rate of water that is 7 degrees below body temperature (30°C) and 7 degrees above body temperature (44°C). A five minute rest period is given between each stimulus to avoid additive effects. The major advantages of this type of testing are: 1) both ampullopetal and ampullofugal endolymph flow are serially induced in each horizontal semicircular canal; 2) the caloric stimulus is highly reproducible from patient to patient; and 3) the test is tolerated by most patients. The major limitation is the need for constant temperature baths and plumbing to maintain continuous circulation of the water through the infusion hose.

INHIBITION OF FIXATION. The magnitude of caloric induced nystagmus is highly dependent on the degree of fixation permitted during the test procedure. Four different fixation conditions have been used for caloric testing: 1) eyes open and fixating; 2) eyes open, Frenzel glasses; 3) eyes open, total darkness; and 4) eyes closed. Without eye movement recording devices, obviously only the first two conditions can be used. Comparison of these four conditions in normal subjects reveals a consistently lower coefficient of variation (standard deviation/mean) for response measurements when the test is performed with eyes open either behind Frenzel glasses or in total darkness.[13]

When caloric testing is performed with fixation (as initially described by Fitzgerald and Hallpike),[38] two separate systems are being evaluated: 1) the vestibulo-ocular reflex, and 2) the smooth pursuit system (see Visual-Vestibular Interaction, Chapter 3). Some normal subjects completely suppress caloric induced nystagmus with fixation,[13] whereas patients with impaired smooth pursuit (such as patients with cerebellar atrophy) may show no difference in caloric-induced nystagmus with or without fixation.[68] This finding is predicted by the visual-vestibular interaction model shown in Figure 41. Eye closure and the associated upward deviation of the eyes causes periodic suppression of induced nystagmus and rounding of the saw-toothed pattern, making it more difficult to quantify with ENG.[13] In addition, patients with CNS lesions frequently have horizontal deviation of the eyes on closure changing the induced nystagmus according to Alexander's law.[29] To avoid these uncontrollable variables, caloric testing should be performed with eyes open, but fixation must be inhibited (Frenzel glasses or darkness). For a brief period during the test, fixation is permitted to evaluate the functional status of the smooth pursuit system.

Results of Bithermal Caloric Testing in Normal Subjects

The response to caloric stimulation is assessed in several ways. The simplest method is to measure the duration of nystagmus after each infusion, using a stopwatch. Prior to the development of ENG, this was the only practical way to quantify caloric test results. Now, however, it is possible to accurately record multiple response measurements. Figure 60 illustrates an ENG recording of a normal caloric response. The subject was supine, head elevated 30 degrees, and eyes open behind Frenzel glasses in a semidarkened room. Two hundred fifty cc of 44°C water were infused into the left ear during the 40 seconds marked on the figure resulting in ampullopetal endolymph flow in the left horizontal semicircular canal and left-beating horizontal nystagmus. The nystagmus began just before the end of stimulation, reached a peak approximately 40 seconds post stimulus, and then slowly decayed over the next 2 to 3 minutes. Below the ENG tracing, nystagmus slow component velocity, slow component amplitude and frequency are plotted versus time. Each measurement demonstrates beat-to-beat variability but as is typically the case, the velocity of the slow components shows the least variability.

The peak value of slow component velocity, slow component amplitude and frequency along with the duration of response are the measurements most commonly used for quantifying the caloric response. Table 6 lists the normal range for each of these measurements after the four stimuli in a standard bithermal test. The large variability in each response measurement is apparent, with the standard deviation varying from approximately 25 percent of the mean value of nystagmus duration to 50 percent of that of maximum slow component velocity. The scatter of each response measurement was tested for normality and only nystagmus duration was found to follow a normal distribution. Therefore, the normal range (mean

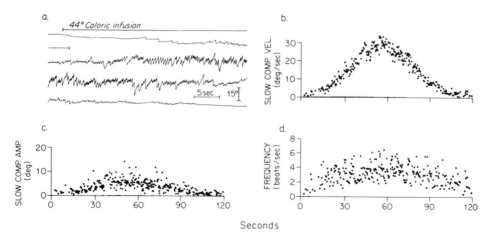

Seconds

Figure 60. Caloric response produced by infusion of 250 cc of 44°C water into the left ear of a normal subject (bitemporal ENG recording). The frequency (a), slow component velocity (b) and amplitude (c) were computed for each nystagmus beat by a digital computer algorithm.

Table 6. Caloric responses in normal subjects (N = 44)

		Duration (sec)	Max slow component velocity (deg/sec)	Max slow component amplitude (deg)	Max frequency (beats/sec)
		Absolute Value Measurements			
L 30°C	*(U)	130 ± 30	15.3 ± 7.7	5.9 ± 2.4	2.9 ± 0.6
	**(L)	—	1.2 ± .21	.81 ± .19	.46 ± .10
	***NR	70 – 190	5.5 – 38	3.1 – 9.7	0.3 – 5.5
R 30°C	(U)	136 ± 34	14.5 ± 6.7	5.3 ± 2.0	3.0 ± .58
	(L)	—	1.2 ± .23	.71 ± .17	.48 ± .09
	NR	68 – 204	5.0 – 43	2.1 – 8.1	0.6 – 5.4
L 44°C	(U)	121 ± 30	21.3 ± 11.7	6.4 ± 2.8	3.5 ± .73
	(L)	—	1.3 ± .25	.80 ± .18	.55 ± .08
	NR	61 – 181	6.2 – 62	3.3 – 9.3	1.2 – 6.0
R 44°C	(U)	123 ± 26	21.0 ± 12.0	6.5 ± 3.0	3.9 ± .72
	(L)	—	1.3 ± .28	.78 ± .21	.58 ± .08
	NR	71 – 175	5.6 – 74	2.8 – 9.2	1.4 – 6.2
		Difference Measurements (%)			
Vestibular	(U)	3.8 ± 7	1.7 ± 11	−4.1 ± 10	3.4 ± 6
Paresis	(NR)	−14 – +14	−22 – +22	−20 – +20	−12 – +12
Directional	(U)	−1.3 ± 6	2.7 ± 14	5.3 ± 12	0.2 ± 7
Preponderance	NR	−12 – +12	−28 – +28	−24 – +24	−14 – +14

*(U) = untransformed data **(L) = $\log_{10}$ transformed data ***(NR) = Normal range (mean ± 2 S.D.), transformed data used when necessary to produce normal distribution. For vestibular paresis and directional preponderance the mean difference was assumed to be zero.

± 2 standard deviations) for the other measurements was calculated after log transformation of the data (after producing a normal distribution for each measurement).

Because of the large intersubject variability in caloric responses, intrasubject measurements have been found to be more useful clinically. The *vestibular paresis* formula $\dfrac{(R30° + R44°) - (L30° + L44°)}{R30° + R44° + L30° + L44°} \times 100$ compares the right-sided responses with the left-sided responses and the *directional preponderance* formula $\dfrac{(R30° + L44°) - (R44° + L30°)}{R30° + L44° + R44° + L30°} \times 100$ compares nystagmus to the right with nystagmus to the left in the same subject. In both of these formulas the difference in response is reported as a percentage of the total response. As suggested earlier, the absolute magnitude of caloric response depends on several physical factors unique to each subject that are unrelated to actual semicircular canal function. Dividing by the total response normalizes the measurements to remove the large variability in absolute magnitude of normal caloric responses.

Table 6 (lower half) lists the normal range for the difference formulas calculated with each of the four common response measurements.[63] The mean value is not significantly different from zero in each case, indicating that caloric responses are symmetrical with regard to side and nystagmus direction in normal subjects. The difference measurements were normally distributed and therefore the normal range could be determined without requiring transformation. Using maximum slow component velocity as an example, a vestibular paresis is defined as greater than 22 percent asymmetry between left and right-sided response and a directional preponderance as greater than 28 percent asymmetry between left and right beating nystagmus. It is apparent that the standard deviations of these intrasubject measurements are lower than those of the intersubject measurements. The normal range values given in Table 6 are comparable to those reported by other investigators (see Table 5 in reference 63) but it must be emphasized that each laboratory should establish its own normal range because of the many methodologic variables discussed earlier.

Results of Bithermal Caloric Testing in Patients

Table 7 summarizes the abnormalities found on caloric testing, their meaning in terms of location of lesion, and the mechanism by which each abnormality is produced.

UNILATERAL PERIPHERAL LESIONS. Of the four caloric response measurements listed in Table 6, maximum slow component velocity is most useful for identifying unilateral peripheral vestibular lesions. Figure 61 summarizes the velocity profile after each stimulus of a bithermal caloric test in a patient with a right viral labyrinthitis. The maximum slow component velocity and nystagmus duration values for each response are easily determined from these plots. None of these values falls below the normal range given in Table 6, although there is an obvious asymmetry in response on the two sides. When the vestibular paresis formula is calculated using nystagmus duration $\dfrac{(115 + 90) - (135 + 110)}{450} \times 100$

$= -9\%$, it is not outside the normal range. On the other hand, when it is calculated

using maximum slow component velocity $\dfrac{(30 + 40) - (15 + 15)}{100} \times 100 = -40\%$,

a highly significant ($p < 0.01$) asymmetry is documented. Therefore, despite the fact that the normal range is narrower for nystagmus duration, maximum slow component velocity is more sensitive in identifying a vestibular paresis. Similar testing in 35 patients clinically suspected of having unilateral peripheral vestibular lesions (end organ or eighth nerve) revealed that the maximum slow component velocity of induced nystagmus identified approximately three times as many abnormalities as the duration of response.[14] The difference formulas consistently identified more abnormalities than absolute magnitude values and a vestibular paresis occurred four times as frequently as a directional preponderance.[14]

The finding of a vestibular paresis with any of the response measurements suggests impairment of the unilateral vestibular system that can be located anywhere from the end organ to the vestibular nerve root entry zone in the brain stem. It is almost certainly a sign of unilateral peripheral vestibular disease if there are no associated brain stem signs. Animal studies support this clinical impression. Uemura and Cohen[71] studied caloric responses after various focal lesions in and around the vestibular nuclear complex in monkeys and found that a vestibular paresis occurred only with lesions involving the eighth nerve root entry zone. Focal lesions in different vestibular nuclei did not produce a vestibular paresis.

A directional preponderance on caloric testing occurs with peripheral end organ and eighth nerve lesions and with central vestibular lesions (from brain stem to

Table 7. Interpreting the results of bithermal caloric testing

Caloric Abnormality	Definition	Location of Lesion	Mechanism
Vestibular paresis	>22% asymmetry between right and left sided maximum slow component velocity	Unilateral labyrinth, eighth nerve including root entry zone	Unilateral decrease in afferent signals to the vestibular nuclei.
Directional preponderance	>28% asymmetry between left beating and right beating maximum slow component velocity	Peripheral or central vestibular system	Interaction of spontaneous nystagmus with caloric induced nystagmus
Bilateral decreased responses	Maximum slow component velocity below normal range	Bilateral labyrinth, eighth nerve including root entry zones	Bilateral decrease in afferent signals to the vestibular nuclei
Hyperactive responses	Maximum slow component velocity above normal range	Cerebellum	Loss of normal inhibitory influence of cerebellum on the vestibular nucleus
Dysrhythmia	Marked variability in nystagmus amplitude without change in slow component velocity profile	Cerebellum	Loss of cerebellar control on pontine saccade center
Impaired fixation suppression	Fixation does not produce at least 50% decrease in maximum slow component velocity	Inferior olives, midline cerebellum	Interruption of visual signals carried to the vestibular nuclei via the midline cerebellum
Perverted nystagmus	Vertical or oblique nystagmus resulting from horizontal canal stimulation	Pontomedullary region	Disturbance of commissural fibers between the vestibular nuclei
Disconjugate nystagmus	Different amplitude and waveform of nystagmus in each eye	Intrinsic brain stem, usually MLF	Interruption of pathways connecting sixth and third nuclei

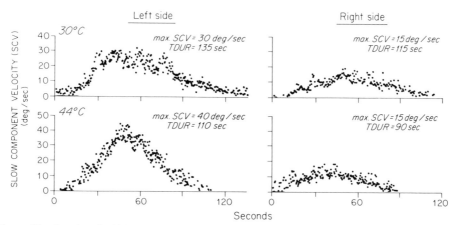

Figure 61. Results of a bithermal caloric test in a patient with a right viral labyrinthitis. SCV, slow component velocity, TDUR, duration of response.

cortex).[14] It indicates an imbalance in the vestibular system and is usually associated with spontaneous vestibular nystagmus; the velocity of the slow components of the spontaneous nystagmus adds to that of caloric induced nystagmus in the same direction and subtracts from that of caloric induced nystagmus in the opposite direction. The average slow component velocity of pathologic vestibular nystagmus correlates ($p < 0.01$) with the directional preponderance percentage in patients with vestibular lesions.[26, 63] Occasional exceptions occur, however, where the spontaneous nystagmus moves in the direction opposite to that of the directional preponderance, or when a directional preponderance is not associated with spontaneous nystagmus.

The need to distinguish between end organ and eighth nerve lesions is a common clinical problem. Partial lesions of the eighth nerve should not, in theory, affect the duration of induced nystagmus since it is related to the time course of cupular deflection and not to the ability of the nerve fibers to transmit action potentials. On the other hand, end organ lesions involving the cupula and hair cells should affect all responses (including duration). Unfortunately, this turns out not to be a reliable way of differentiating end organ from eighth nerve lesions. Lesions involving the eighth nerve can reduce the duration of nystagmus, while end organ lesions (particularly in the early stages) frequently result only in decreased maximum slow component velocity (see Fig. 61). The magnitude of the caloric asymmetry is of some help in differentiating nerve from end organ lesions. A complete or nearly complete unilateral paralysis is more commonly associated with nerve lesions than with labyrinthine lesions.

BILATERAL PERIPHERAL LESIONS. The vestibular paresis and directional preponderance formulas are often of no use in evaluating patients with bilateral vestibular lesions since caloric responses may be symmetrically depressed. As with unilateral vestibular lesions, maximum slow component velocity is the most sensitive measure of bilateral decreased vestibular function.[14] This is not surprising since in normal subjects the maximum velocity of the slow components of induced nystagmus changes with slight changes in the temperature of the caloric stimulus while the duration of response remains relatively fixed for changes in water temperature within a range of $\pm 10°C$ from body temperature.[42] Because of the wide range of normal values for maximum slow component velocity, the

139

patient's value may decrease several fold before falling below the normal range. For this reason serial measurements in the same patient are needed if one hopes to identify early bilateral vestibular impairment (such as from the ototoxic effects of drugs).

CENTRAL VESTIBULAR LESIONS. *Changes in Magnitude of Response.* As suggested earlier, patients with central nervous system lesions may exhibit a vestibular paresis on caloric testing if the lesion involves the root entry zone of the vestibular nerve. The most common central causes of a vestibular paresis are multiple sclerosis, lateral brain stem infarction and infiltrating gliomas (see Chapter 7). Each disease produces other brain stem signs so that the finding of a vestibular paresis is not likely to be misinterpreted as a sign of peripheral vestibular dysfunction. In rare cases, a massive brain stem infarction or diffusely infiltrating glioma leads to bilaterally decreased caloric responses.

Lesions of the cerebellum can lead to increased caloric responses, possibly because of loss of the normal inhibitory influence of the cerebellum on the vestibular nuclei.[5] Because of the wide range of normal caloric responses, however, it is unusual for any of the responses to exceed the normal upper range. Patients with cerebellar atrophy demonstrate a wide range of caloric responses.[5] Those with Friedreich's ataxia often have bilaterally decreased caloric responses because of involvement of the vestibular nerve and ganglia, while those with olivopontocerebellar degeneration have decreased, normal or even increased responses, depending on which areas of the medulla and pons are involved. Increased caloric responses, when they do occur, are usually found in patients with "clinically pure" cerebellar atrophy.

Abnormalities in the Pattern of Response. Patients with cerebellar lesions also develop dysrhythmic caloric responses.[59] Dysrhythmia refers to a marked beat-to-beat variability in nystagmus amplitude without any change in the slow component velocity profile. The cerebellum is important for controlling the amplitude of nystagmus fast components, and loss of this control with cerebellar lesions may lead to a disorganized nystagmus pattern. Unfortunately, from a diagnostic point of view, caloric dysrhythmia also occurs in normal subjects when they are tired and inattentive. As will be shown in the next section, rotatory stimuli are better suited than caloric stimuli for examining the pattern of induced nystagmus.

Visual-Vestibular Interaction. As suggested earlier, the degree of nystagmus suppression resulting from fixation during caloric testing is used to evaluate the integrity of the smooth pursuit system. Although the anatomic pathways for visual-vestibular interaction (Fig. 40) have been elucidated only recently, the clinical observation that central nervous system lesions alter fixation suppression of caloric induced nystagmus was made years ago. Demanez[34] proposed an ocular fixation index defined as $\dfrac{\text{amplitude} \times \text{frequency (eyes open)}}{\text{amplitude} \times \text{frequency (eyes closed)}} \times 100$ to quantify fixation suppression of caloric induced nystagmus. The ocular fixation index is measured after the lights are turned on during the middle of the caloric response and the patient is asked to fixate on a dot on the ceiling. Since the amplitude and frequency of the caloric induced nystagmus is constantly changing it is important that the fixation period occur near the time of maximum response to obtain the best estimate of fixation suppression.

Ledoux and Demanez[50] rarely found an ocular fixation index greater than 50 percent in normal subjects and patients with peripheral vestibular lesions, whereas 82 percent of a series of patients with CNS lesions had an ocular fixation index greater than 50 percent. The CNS diseases included such varied entities as epilepsy, supratentorial tumors and polioencephalitis. Takemori[68] found that the ratio of maximum slow component velocity of caloric induced nystagmus in light and darkness provided a more sensitive index of visual suppression than nystagmus frequency multiplied by amplitude. The average visual suppression level in normal human subjects and rhesus monkeys was approximtely 50 percent, that is, the maximum slow component velocity in light with fixation was one-half that in darkness. The mean visual suppression in 22 normal adults was 48 ± 10 percent. Monkeys with midline cerebellar lesions and a small series of patients with different varieties of disease affecting the cerebellum demonstrated decreased visual suppression of caloric responses.[67, 68]

Perverted Nystagmus. Vertical or oblique nystagmus produced by caloric stimulation of the horizontal semicircular canals is called perverted nystagmus. Uemura and Cohen[71] found perverted caloric nystagmus in rhesus monkeys after producing unilateral focal lesions in the rostral medial vestibular nucleus. Warm caloric stimulation on the intact side produced downward nystagmus and cold stimulation produced upward diagonal nystagmus. The investigators atttributed their findings to a disturbance of the commissural fibers between the vestibular nuclei. Perverted nystagmus with caloric stimulation has been reported with many different lesions of the posterior fossa usually in the region of the floor of the fourth ventricle (near the vestibular nuclei).[40]

Rotatory Testing

With rotatory testing, the patient is seated in a chair that rotates about its vertical axis. His head is fixed so that the angular rotation occurs in the plane of one of the semicircular canal pairs (usually with the head tilted 30 degrees forward in the plane of the horizontal canals). Rotatory tests of the canal ocular reflexes have not been widely accepted as part of the routine vestibular examination[1] for two reasons: 1) rotatory stimuli affect both labyrinths simultaneously compared to the selective stimulation of one labyrinth possible with caloric tests; and 2) expensive bulky equipment is required in order to generate precise rotatory stimuli. Rotatory tests do have several advantages, however. Multiple, graded stimuli can be applied in a relatively short period of time, and rotatory testing is usually less bothersome to patients than caloric testing. Unlike caloric testing, a rotatory stimulus to the semicircular canals is unrelated to physical features of the external ear or temporal bone so that a more exact relationship between stimulus and response is possible. According to the pendulum model introduced in Chapter 2, the slow component velocity of induced nystagmus should be proportional to the deviation of the cupula which in turn is proportional to the intensity of stimulation. As will be demonstrated in the following sections, this model's applicability to different forms of stimulation is remarkably consistent and provides a rational approach to the evaluation of clinical rotatory testing.

Background

Three types of angular acceleration have been used to clinically evaluate the vestibulo-ocular reflex: 1) impulsive, 2) constant and 3) sinusoidal. Historically, each type of stimulation has been popular at different times for different reasons. Bárány in 1907[21] introduced an impulsive rotatory test in which the chair on which the patient was seated was manually rotated 10 times in 20 seconds and then suddenly stopped with the patient facing the observer. The function of the semicircular canals in the plane of rotation was assessed by measuring the duration of visually monitored nystagmus after clockwise (CW) and counterclockwise (CCW) rotation. In normal subjects an average of 22 seconds was required for cessation of the postrotatory nystagmus, but intersubject variability was large. With this method the magnitude of stimulus was uncertain because of the difficulty in manually maintaining a constant velocity and producing the same impulse of deceleration in every test. In addition, the response to the initial acceleration was often not completed before the deceleration began, resulting in an interaction between the acceleration and deceleration responses.

Van Egmond, Groen and Jongkees[73] attempted to improve the reliability of the impulsive test by slowly bringing the patient to different constant velocities with subliminal acceleration. They introduced the term *cupulogram* for the plot of postrotatory sensation and nystagmus duration versus the magnitude of the sudden change in velocity and called the test sequence cupulometria (see Fig. 48). For the range of impulses used (≤60 deg/sec) the duration of postrotatory nystagmus was proportional to the log of the impulse intensity.[45]

As ENG techniques became available for recording nystagmus during rotation (per rotatory nystagmus), rotatory tests using constant and sinusoidal acceleration became popular in several clinical laboratories. Montadon[54, 55] introduced a constant acceleration test in which the patient was slowly brought to a constant angular velocity (90 deg/sec) and then after a period at constant speed (3 minutes), slowly decelerated to zero velocity. The *nystagmus threshold* was determined (the rate of acceleration and deceleration at which the nystagmus was first observed) by administering a series of different constant accelerations (0.5 to 9 deg/sec^2). In normal subjects this value was approximately 1 deg/sec^2 while in patients with vestibular disease values of 6 or 7 deg/sec^2 or more were obtained. Subsequent investigation suggested that the difference in nystagmus threshold between acceleration and deceleration could be more accurately determined by presenting a constant acceleration stimulus just above threshold (2 deg/sec^2) and measuring the delay before the onset of nystagmus in each direction.[57] This type of test permitted a rapid assessment of the symmetry in nystagmus threshold between CW and CCW stimulation.

Nystagmus threshold measurements rely on the identification of the first beat of nystagmus (first fast component) after the beginning of a constant acceleration stimulus. As discussed in Chapter 3, several factors determine the threshold of fast components. Particularly important is the eye position in the orbit when the slow movement of the vestibulo-ocular reflex begins. Threshold measurements therefore are not simply an assessment of the reflex threshold but rather an assessment of the interaction of the vestibular signal with the fast component generating centers in the pontine reticular formation.

Several investigators have suggested that a sinusoidal rotatory stimulus is a more efficient and quantitative stimulus than impulsive or constant acceleration.[31, 51, 56] A sinusoidal stimulus is defined by two simple variables: 1) the period of oscillation and 2) the amplitude of oscillation, both of which can be controlled with relatively simple mechanical devices. The *torsion swing test* was popularized in France as a simple reproducible method of generating sinusoidal acceleration in the clinic setting. With this test the patient is seated in a chair whose rotation is mechanically controlled by the action of a calibrated spring.[72] When the chair is deviated from its equilibrium position, it returns to that position with a damped sinusoidal oscillation. This stimulus alternately deviates the cupula in ampullopetal and ampullofugal directions, producing nystagmus that alternates direction with each half cycle of rotation. Most commonly maximum or average slow component velocity and maximum frequency are used to quantify the response during each half cycle. The torsion swing provides a reproducible stimulus in that responses to CW and CCW rotation can be compared in a given subject; the stimulus intensity, however, is dependent on the weight and distribution of mass in the chair and so varies from subject to subject.

Relationship Between Stimulus and Response

Over the past few decades motorized rotatory chairs have been designed to produce angular acceleration that can be precisely controlled; techniques have improved so that multiple response measurements can be accurately monitored. Figure 62 illustrates the nystagmus response of a normal subject to the three basic types of angular acceleration. The subject was rotated in the plane of the horizontal semicircular canals with eyes opened in complete darkness while he performed continuous mental arithmetic to maintain alertness.[20] Each stimulus produced a peak angular velocity of 120 deg/sec.

The slow component velocity profile for each stimulus can be predicted by the pendulum model for cupular deviation discussed in Chapter 2. Note the similarity between these profiles and the time course of cupular deviation illustrated in Figure 23. The difference in the predicted and recorded responses is largely due to the peripheral adaptation phenomenon (see Characteristics of Primary Afferent Responses, Chapter 3). The impulsive response best illustrates the effect of adaptation on the induced nystagmus. Instead of slowly returning to the baseline as would be predicted by the pendulum model, the velocity of the slow components reverses direction and then slowly returns to the baseline. Reversals of this type

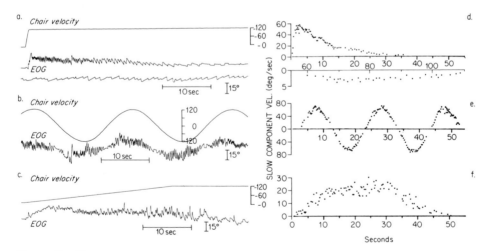

Figure 62. Nystagmus recording (left side) and slow component velocity profile (right side) after three types of angular acceleration each resulting in a maximum angular velocity of 120 deg/sec. With the impulsive stimulus (a) the change in velocity occurs in less than 1 second with an acceleration of approximately 140 deg/sec². The sinusoidal stimulus (b) has a frequency of 0.05 Hz (20 sec/cycle) and a maximum acceleration of 38 deg/sec². The constant acceleration stimulus (c) is 4 deg/sec² for 30 seconds.

consistently occur in normal subjects when the impulse change in angular velocity is greater than 120 deg/sec.

Results in Normal Subjects

Although several features of the nystagmus induced by each type of stimulus could be used as a measure of response, as in the case of caloric testing, maximum slow component velocity is most useful for distinguishing normal from abnormal reactions.[20] Figure 63 illustrates normative data for a series of impulsive and sinusoidal changes in angular velocity. The test conditions are identical to those described for Figure 62 except a series of stimuli of different intensity in the CW and CCW directions are administered. For both types of rotatory stimulus the log of maximum slow component velocity increases linearly with the log of stimulus intensity (as predicted by the pendulum model). The coefficient of variation (standard deviation/mean) for maximum slow component velocity after the rotatory stimuli in normal subjects is approximately one-half the coefficient of variation after caloric stimuli (see Table 6) suggesting that caloric stimuli are less precise than rotatory stimuli. Even with precisely controlled rotatory stimuli, however, there is still large variation in the vestibulo-ocular reflex function measured in normal subjects.[20] The variability in response is not related to the type of rotatory stimulus since it is almost identical for the impulsive and sinusoidal rotatory stimuli. Factors such as stress, fatigue, level of mental alertness, and habituation all contribute to the variability (see Nystagmus Habituation, Chapter 3).

The variance associated with difference measurements comparing CW and CCW responses in the same subject is much less than the variance in response between subjects. This is illustrated in Figure 64 where the normalized difference between CW and CCW maximum slow component velocity for the 44 normal subjects is plotted against stimulus intensity for the impulsive and sinusoidal tests.

The normalized difference formula $\left(\dfrac{CW - CCW}{CW + CCW} \times 100 \right)$ is analogous to the

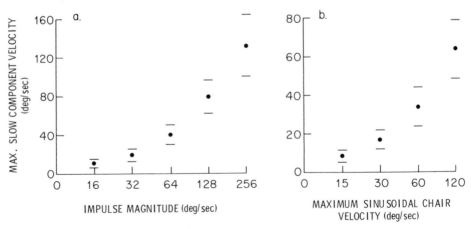

Figure 63. Average maximum slow component velocity (± 1 standard deviation) produced by a series of (a) impulsive and (b) sinusoidal rotatory stimuli in 44 normal subjects. (See text for details).

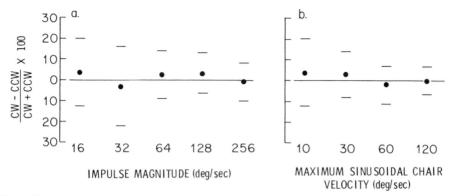

Figure 64. Average normalized difference (± 1 standard deviation) between clockwise and counterclockwise maximum slow component velocity plotted against stimulus intensity for the impulsive (a) and sinusoidal (b) rotatory test (same subjects as in Fig. 69).

directional preponderance formula used with caloric testing. The mean value for the normalized difference between CW and CCW responses is approximately zero at each stimulus intensity demonstrating that CW and CCW responses are symmetrical in normal subjects.

Results in Patients

UNILATERAL PERIPHERAL LESIONS. Patients with unilateral loss of vestibular function have asymmetric responses to rotatory stimuli because of the difference in excitation and inhibition with ampullopetal and ampullofugal stimulation of the intact labyrinth (see Ewald's second law, Chapter 2). The asymmetry is most pronounced after high intensity stimuli. Figure 65 illustrates the results of impulsive rotatory testing in a typical patient with only one functioning labyrinth (left acoustic neuroma).[8] The induced nystagmus is symmetrical after low intensity stimuli but is significantly (p <0.01) asymmetric after high intensity stimuli. The 256 deg/sec CCW impulse produced ampullofugal endolymph flow in the intact right labyrinth and as expected the induced nystagmus had a decreased maximum slow component velocity compared to the induced nystagmus after 256 deg/sec CW impulse.

Figure 66 summarizes the results of similar testing in 11 patients with only one functioning labyrinth.[15] All had complete loss of caloric response on the damaged side (including after stimulation with ice water). In 6 patients the vestibular nerve was sectioned at the time of surgery and 5 were clinically diagnosed as having peripheral labyrinthine disease (3 labyrinthitis, 1 vascular occlusion and 1 vestibulopathy of unknown cause). The maximum slow component velocity of the nystagmus induced by ampullopetal and ampullofugal endolymph flow in the intact labyrinth (Fig. 66a) and the normalized difference between responses to ampullopetal and ampullofugal endolymph flow (Fig. 66b) are plotted against the intensity of impulse. It is apparent that as the intensity of impulsive stimulus increased the amount of asymmetry in response increased. The maximum slow component velocity of the nystagmus induced by ampullofugal flow was not abnormal in every case because of the large normal range. The normalized difference measurements for the 256 deg/sec impulses were significantly (p <0.05) abnormal in every patient, however. Results were indistinguishable in patients with eighth

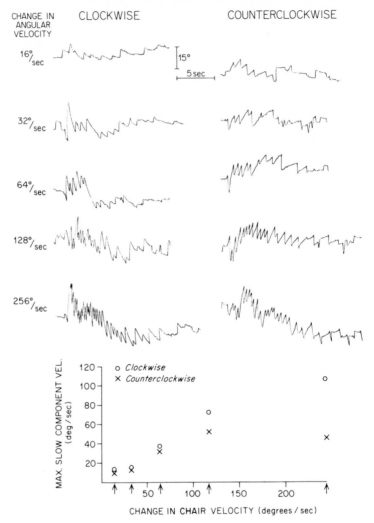

Figure 65. Responses to a series of impulse changes in angular velocity in a patient with a left cerebellopontine angle tumor. Graph represents maximum slow component velocity for each response. (From Baloh, R. W., et al.: *Cerebellar-pontine angle tumors. Results of quantitative vestibulo-ocular testing.* Arch. Neurol. 33:507, 1976, with permission.)

nerve and labyrinthine lesions and in those with and without spontaneous vestibular nystagmus. Sinusoidal rotatory testing in the same patients gave identical results.

Although rotatory testing consistently identifies complete unilateral peripheral vestibular paralysis it infrequently identifies partial peripheral vestibular lesions. Of 25 patients with peripheral vestibular disease who manifested significant (p <0.05) but less than complete unilateral paralysis on bithermal caloric testing only 10 had significantly asymmetric responses on impulsive rotatory testing.[20] Again, the higher intensity stimuli identified more abnormalities than the low intensity stimuli.

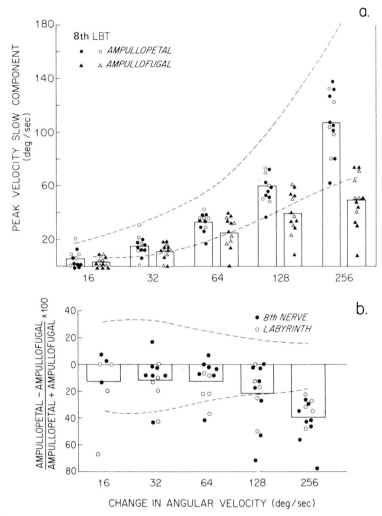

Figure 66. (a) Peak slow component velocity of nystagmus induced by impulses of acceleration resulting in ampullopetal and ampullofugal endolymph flow in the horizontal semicircular canal of the intact labyrinth in 6 patients with unilateral eighth nerve section (8th) and 5 patients with unilateral labyrinthine (LBT) disease (2 of the eighth nerve patients were tested before and after surgery and both results are included). Vertical range bars represent the mean patient response for each stimulus. (b) Percentage difference in peak slow component velocity between ampullopetal and ampullofugal endolymph flow in same patients shown in (a). Vertical range bars represent the mean difference in patient responses. At the lower magnitude of stimulation several patients did not produce measurable nystagmus accounting for the decreased number of data points. The normal range is given by the dashed lines. (From Baloh, R. W., Honrubia, V., and Konrad, H. R.: *Ewald's second law reevaluated.* Acta Otolaryngol. 83:475, 1977, with permission.)

BILATERAL PERIPHERAL LESIONS. Rotatory stimuli are ideally suited for testing patients with bilateral peripheral vestibular lesions since both labyrinths are stimulated simultaneously and the degree of remaining function is accurately quantified. Because the variance associated with normal rotatory responses is less than that associated with caloric responses, diminished function is identified earlier. Artificially decreased caloric responses on both sides occasionally occur in patients with angular, narrow external canals or with thickened temporal bones. Since the intensity of rotatory stimuli is unrelated to these physical features, rotatory induced nystagmus is normal in such patients.[20] Frequently, patients with absent response to bithermal caloric stimulation have decreased but recordable rotatory induced nystagmus, particularly at higher stimulus intensities. The ability to identify remaining vestibular function even if minimal is an important advantage of rotatory testing, particularly when the physician is contemplating ablative surgery or monitoring the effects of ototoxic drugs. By using precisely graded rotatory stimuli on a serial basis he can recognize ototoxic effects earlier than by using the less precise caloric stimulus.

CENTRAL VESTIBULAR LESIONS. As with lesions of the peripheral vestibular structures, lesions of the central vestibulo-ocular reflex pathway can lead to a decrease or asymmetry in the velocity of the slow components of nystagmus induced by rotatory stimuli. Lesions involving the nerve root entry zones and vestibular nuclei may be indistinguishable from peripheral vestibular lesions. The spectrum of abnormality associated with central lesions, however, is more diverse than a simple decrease in the slow component velocity of induced nystagmus. The highly organized pattern of nystagmus usually produced by rotatory stimuli in normal subjects may be disorganized so that an abnormal relationship exists between the onset of slow and fast components. Although the vestibulo-ocular reflex pathways are intact, because of impaired fast components the waveform of induced nystagmus is distorted. Since the nervous system modifies the nystagmus response with relation to visual and proprioceptive signals, central lesions may impair the interaction of these different sensory signals.

Changes in Nystagmus Pattern. Sinusoidal stimuli are ideally suited for studying the pattern of induced nystagmus. Figure 67 illustrates the responses to sinusoidal rotation (eyes open in darkness) in (a) a normal subject, (b) a patient with cerebellar atrophy, (c) a patient with a left pontine lesion (glioma), and (d) a patient with a bilateral lesion of the medial longitudinal fascicle (MLF). In the normal subject the eyes alternately deviate in the direction of the fast component for each half cycle of induced nystagmus. As discussed in Chapter 3, the eye position in the orbit for initiation of fast components is near the midline. Fast components (saccades) are generated in the parapontine reticular formation, and the cerebellum controls the amplitude of both voluntary and involuntary saccades. In the patient with cerebellar atrophy the nystagmus pattern is disorganized with fast components occurring in random fashion causing marked beat-to-beat variability in amplitude. This type of abnormality has been termed *nystagmus dysrhythmia* and is commonly found in patients with all varieties of cerebellar lesions. Patients with dysrhythmic vestibular nystagmus also demonstrate dysmetria of voluntary saccades, as will be discussed in the next section.

The patient with a left pontine lesion (Fig. 67c) could not produce voluntary or involuntary saccades (fast components) to the left so that during the half cycle which normally produces left beating nystagmus the eyes tonically deviated to the right. In patients with bilateral pontine lesions the eyes tonically deviate to the right and left with each half cycle of rotation because of the complete absence of fast components.

The patient with a bilateral MLF lesion (Fig. 67d) demonstrates a dissociation in fast components between the two eyes. When either "paretic" adducting eye is required to make a fast component the nystagmus beats are rounded because of a

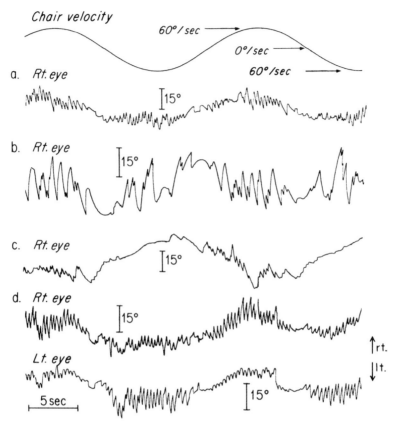

Figure 67. Nystagmus response to sinusoidal rotation of 0.05 Hz, with a maximal velocity of 60 deg/sec in (a) normal subject, and in patients with (b) cerebellar atrophy, (c) left pontine glioma and (d) bilateral MLF lesion caused by multiple sclerosis.

decrease in the frequency of action potentials arriving at the medial rectus neurons via the damaged MLF. Abducting fast components, however, are normal, because the abducting muscles (abducens nuclei) receive their innervation for fast components directly from the parapontine region with no involvement of the MLF. Frequently the abducting fast components are actually too large. The oculomotor control centers attempt to overcome the block at the MLF by increasing the innervation sent from the parapontine centers to the oculomotor neurons.[19] Since, according to Herring's law, this increased innervation is sent equally to both medial and lateral rectus oculomotor neurons, the difference in amplitude between adducting and abducting fast components is further magnified.

Visual-Vestibular Interaction. Experimental studies in animals suggest that loss of the normal cerebellar inhibiting influence on the vestibular nuclei may result in the production of hyperactive vestibulo-ocular reflex responses.[37] Figure 68a summarizes the results of sinusoidal rotatory testing (eyes open in darkness) in a series of patients with different varieties of cerebellar atrophy. A wide spectrum of response was obtained but the majority of values were within normal limits. The responses of the 3 patients with Friedreich's ataxia were near or below the lower normal range probably on the basis of associated vestibular nerve

149

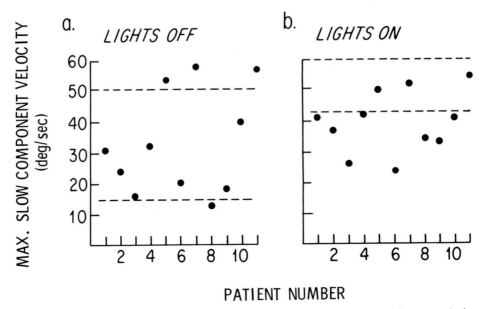

PATIENT NUMBER

Figure 68. Maximum slow component velocity induced by sinusoidal rotation (0.05 Hz, max velocity 60 deg/sec) in darkness (a) and in the light (b) in 11 patients with cerebellar atrophy. The clinical diagnoses were: olivopontocerebellar degeneration (1,2,6), Friedreich's ataxia (3,8,9), ataxia-telangiectasia (7), alcohol cerebellar degeneration (10) and cerebellar degeneration of unknown cause (4,5,11).

atrophy. The 3 patients with significantly increased responses all had "clinically pure" cerebellar syndromes without signs of associated brain stem and/or peripheral nerve involvement.

In contrast to the results of rotatory testing in darkness, patients with cerebellar atrophy usually have impaired rotatory induced nystagmus when they are tested in the light and can fixate on a surrounding stationary optokinetic drum (Fig. 68b). Because of the synergistic effect of the visual and vestibular stimuli, normal subjects more than double the magnitude of induced nystagmus when tested in light compared to darkness. Visual-vestibular interaction is impaired in patients with cerebellar lesions and therefore they cannot properly use visual signals to increase their vestibulo-ocular reflex response (see Visual-Vestibular Interaction, Chapter 3).

Visual-vestibular interaction can also be tested by rotating the patient in the dark and then in the light with a fixation point moving with the rotatory chair (for example, the extended thumb). The ratio $\dfrac{\text{maximum slow component velocity in light}}{\text{maximum slow component velocity in dark}}$ × 100 is a rotatory ocular fixation index analogous to the caloric ocular fixation index introduced in the previous section. Patients with cerebellar lesions are unable to inhibit vestibular signals with visual fixation and therefore have an increased index (usually greater than 0.5). The rotatory index overcomes several of the difficulties associated with the caloric index since the slow component velocity of induced nystagmus with and without fixation can be measured at exactly the same point in the response cycle and several cycles can be averaged, increasing the reliability of the measurement.

150

Table 8. Summary of visual ocular control abnormalities produced by focal neurologic lesions

Location of Lesion	Saccades	Smooth Pursuit	Optokinetic Nystagmus
Unilateral peripheral vestibular	Normal	Transient contralateral impairment	Transient contralateral decreased SCV*
Cerebello-pontine angle	Ipsilateral dysmetria	Progressive ipsilateral or bilateral impairment	Progressive ipsilateral or bilateral decreased SCV
Diffuse cerebellar	Bilateral dysmetria	Bilateral impairment	Bilateral decreased SCV
Intrinsic brain stem	Decreased maximum velocity, increased delay time	Ipsilateral or bilateral impairment	Ipsilateral or bilateral decreased SCV, disconjugate
Basal ganglia	Hypometria,, increased delay time (bilateral)	Bilateral impairment	Bilateral decreased SCV
Frontoparietal cortex	Contralateral hypometria	Normal	Normal
Parieto-occipital cortex	Normal	Ipsilateral impairment	Ipsilateral decreased SCV

* slow component velocity

TESTS OF VISUAL OCULAR CONTROL

The central vestibulo-ocular connections are highly integrated with the visual ocular stabilizing pathways, and both systems share the final common pathway of the oculomotor neurons (see Organization of Visual-Ocular Control, Chapter 3). If the efferent limb of the vestibulo-ocular reflex arc is damaged, visually controlled eye movements are also abnormal, whereas if the afferent limb of the reflex is damaged, visually controlled eye movements are usually normal. Because ENG techniques used for quantifying the vestibulo-ocular reflex can be used for quantification of visually controlled eye movements, an important "bonus" of information is obtained with little increased effort. Table 8 summarizes the types of saccade, smooth pursuit and optokinetic abnormalities commonly associated with focal lesions of the nervous system.

Saccadic Eye Movements

Methods of Testing and Results in Normal Subjects

One induces voluntary saccades by asking the patient to look back and forth between two targets held directly in front of him (which can be the examiner's index fingers). The examiner, with practice, can visually appreciate gross slowing or overshooting and undershooting of the induced saccades. He can obtain a more accurate assessment of saccades, however, by using precise targets and recording

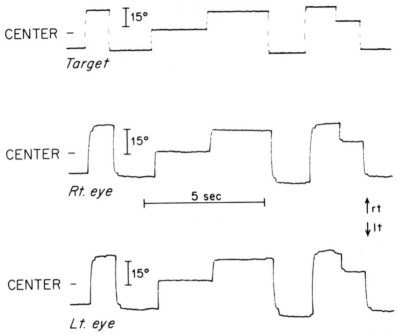

Figure 69. Saccadic eye movements induced in a normal subject by a target moving in steps of random amplitude (3 to 36 degrees) and changing intervals between jumps (0.5 to 2.5 seconds).

induced saccades with either ENG or other eye movement recording systems.[3, 4, 7] The targets can be a series of dots or lights separated by known angular degrees or a dot of light generated on a screen and moved through a series of stepwise jumps of different amplitude. The ENG recording in Figure 69 illustrates the high speed and accuracy of saccadic eye movements induced in a normal subject by a target moving in steps of random amplitude. Normal subjects consistently undershoot the target for jumps larger than 20 degrees, requiring a second small corrective saccade to achieve the final position.[11] Overshoots of the target are rare. A characteristic delay time of approximately 200 msec occurs between each target jump and induced saccade.

Results in Patients

Slowing of saccadic eye movements results from lesions anywhere from the pretectal and parapontine saccade-pulse-generating centers to the extra ocular muscles.[16] Lesions involving these pathways slow both voluntary and involuntary saccades. Damage to the oculomotor neurons, oculomotor nerves and extraocular muscles causes slowing of saccades when the paretic muscle is the agonist required to generate the sudden increase in force necessary to rapidly move the globe. Saccade slowing is often seen before clinical examination reveals the presence of strabismus.[52, 64] Saccade slowing produced by myasthenia gravis (impaired transmission at the myoneural junction) increases with fatigue (repetitive saccades) and is reversed when the patient is given intravenous edrophonium.[12] Lesions of the MLF result in slowing of adducting saccades made by the medial rectus on the side of the lesion (Fig. 70).[18]

152

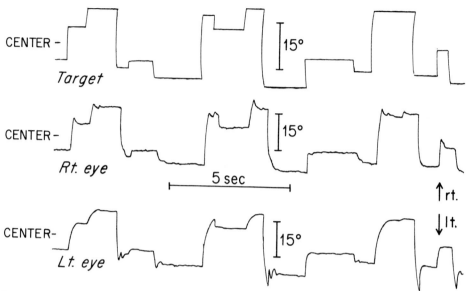

Figure 70. Saccadic eye movements in a patient with a bilateral MLF lesion caused by multiple sclerosis. Bilateral slowing of adducting saccades is visually apparent. Abducting saccades overshot the target because the oculomotor control centers attempted to overcome the MLF block by increasing the innervation to the agonist medial and lateral rectus motoneurons. (From Baloh, R. W., Yee, R. D., and Honrubia, V.: *Internuclear ophthalmoplegia. I. Saccades and dissociated nystagmus.* Arch. Neurol. In press, with permission.)

The brain stem pulse-generating centers are affected by focal disease or by a nonspecific, diffuse neuronal dysfunction. Reversible saccade slowing is produced by fatigue and by ingestion of alcohol or tranquilizers.[41, 48, 76] This apparently results from impaired transsynaptic conduction in the neuronal networks needed to generate the pulse increase in firing for horizontal and vertical saccades. Patients with Huntington's chorea and progressive supranuclear palsy develop permanent slowing of saccades due to degeneration of the same neuronal networks.[66, 70] Focal disease of the pretectal or parapontine region produces selective slowing of vertical and horizontal saccades, respectively. Focal lesions of one parapontine center produce ipsilateral saccade slowing. The pretectal regions for upward and downward saccades are probably separate (downward saccade center rostral to the upward center) but are so close that lesions usually involve both. Complete destruction of the saccade-pulse-generating centers results in complete absence of saccadic eye movements (voluntary and involuntary).[44] Patients with such a dysfunction produce only a slow tonic deviation of the eyes with vestibular or optokinetic stimuli because of the absence of fast components (see Fig. 67c).

Damage to the supranuclear control of the bran stem saccade-generating centers is not associated with saccade slowing but rather with an alteration in the accuracy or initiation (reaction time) of saccades.[16] Patients with Parkinson's disease exhibit delayed saccade reaction time and hypometria of voluntary saccades.[16, 32] Impaired saccade accuracy is most prominent with cerebellar disorders.[5, 78] Both overshooting and undershooting of the target occur, requiring several corrective saccades to attain the target position (saccade dysmetria). The velocity of these saccades is normal unless the brain stem is also involved. Disorders of the cortical saccade control centers also affect the accuracy of saccades.

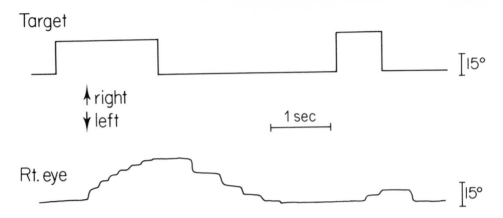

Figure 71. Hypometric saccades in a patient with ataxia-telangiectasia. Note the prolonged delay time (approximately 500 msec) for initiation of the first saccade after target jump. (From Baloh, R. W., Yee, R. D., and Boder, E.: *Ataxia-telangiectasia. Quantitative analysis of eye movements in six cases.* Neurology. In press, with permission.)

Complete removal of one hemisphere or presence of a large frontoparietal lesion results in hypometria of horizontal saccades made in the contralateral direction.[16, 69] Vertical saccades are unaffected.

Patients with congenital oculomotor apraxia[77] and ataxia-telangiectasia[17] exhibit prolonged reaction time for the initiation of voluntary saccades and use a series of hypometric saccades to produce refixations (Fig. 71). Nystagmus fast components (involuntary saccades) are normal in amplitude but the eyes deviate in the direction of the slow component rather than in the direction of the fast component. To compensate for the impaired voluntary saccades these patients often use head thrusts to perform refixations. Since their vestibulo-ocular reflex is intact the head thrusts produce contraversive deviation of the eyes necessitating an overshoot of the head thrust in order to obtain fixation. Fixation is then maintained as the head is slowly returned on line with the target. The site of the anatomic defect that produces these abnormalities in voluntary saccades is unknown.

Smooth Pursuit

Methods of Testing and Results in Normal Subjects

The examining physician can test smooth pursuit eye movements by slowly moving his finger or pencil back and forth and asking the patient to follow it as well as possible. The target should be moved as smoothly as possible and the movement should not be too fast (about one-half cycle per second is an ideal rate). A more exact relationship between velocities of target and eye is determined by using more precise targets and ENG.[10] A pendulum hanging from the ceiling or a metronome provides an inexpensive, reproducible sinusoidally moving target. Projection of a moving dot on a screen offers more precise control of the target over a series of velocities. Figure 72b illustrates a polygraph recording of smooth pursuit in a normal subject as he follows a sinusoidally moving dot on a modified television set (0.3 Hz, maximum excursion 36 degrees). The accuracy of smooth

154

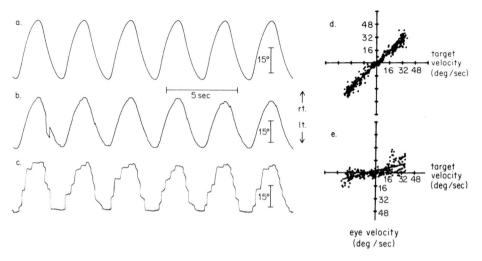

Figure 72. Smooth pursuit of a target moving with a sinusoidal waveform (a) in a normal subject (b) and a patient with cerebellar atrophy (c). In (d) and (e) eye velocity is plotted against target velocity (both sampled 10 times per second) after saccades have been removed for the normal subject and the patient respectively.

pursuit is quantified by repeatedly sampling eye and target velocity and plotting the two velocities against each other (Fig. 72d). A computer algorithm makes the comparison between eye and target velocity after saccade waveforms have been removed. The slope of this eye-target velocity relationship (in this case 0.95) represents the gain of the smooth pursuit system. The mean gain determined from similar plots in 25 normal subjects was 0.95 ± 0.07.

Results in Patients

Patients with impaired smooth pursuit require frequent corrective saccades to keep up with the target and produce so-called cogwheel or saccadic pursuit (Fig. 72c). As expected, the gain of the smooth pursuit system (Fig. 72e) is markedly decreased in such patients. It must be emphasized that normal subjects may intermix saccades with smooth pursuit movements particularly if they are inattentive or fatigued or if the target velocity exceeds the limit of the smooth pursuit system. Therefore, quantitative analysis of intersaccade eye velocity is a more reliable way for assessing the accuracy of smooth pursuit than observing the frequency of superimposed saccades.

Impaired smooth pursuit is of limited localizing value since it occurs with disorders throughout the CNS. Acute lesions of the peripheral labyrinth transiently impair smooth pursuit contralateral to the lesion when the eyes are moving against the tonic vestibular imbalance.[16] This asymmetry in smooth pursuit disappears in a few weeks despite the persistence of vestibular nystagmus in darkness. Just as they affect saccadic eye movements, tranquilizing drugs, alcohol and fatigue also impair smooth pursuit eye movements.[43, 58] Rashbass[58] found that barbiturates impair smooth pursuit before affecting saccadic eye movements, suggesting an increased sensitivity of the smooth pursuit system. Patients with diffuse cortical disease[60] (degenerative or vascular), basal ganglia disease[16, 32] (Parkinson's disease and Huntington's chorea) and diffuse cerebellar disease[5] consistently have bilaterally impaired smooth pursuit movements. Focal disease of one cerebellar hemisphere or one side of the brain stem usually produces ipsilateral impairment of smooth pursuit[8, 25, 30, 75] although large cerebellopontine angle tumors are frequently associated with bilaterally impaired smooth pursuit.[8] Focal cortical lesions in the parieto-occipital region impair ipsilateral smooth pursuit.[16]

Optokinetic Nystagmus

Methods of Testing and Results in Normal Subjects

The simplest optokinetic stimulus is a striped cloth that can be moved across the patient's visual field in each direction. While the patient stares at the cloth the amplitude of induced nystagmus in each direction is compared. This type of test permits identification of absent or markedly asymmetric optokinetic nystagmus.

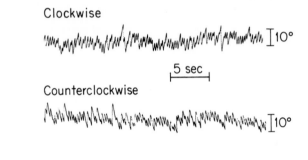

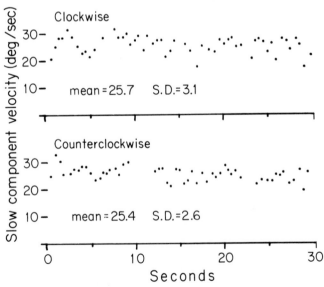

Figure 73. Bitemporal ENG recordings of optokinetic nystagmus in a normal subject. Drum speed 30 deg/sec.

156

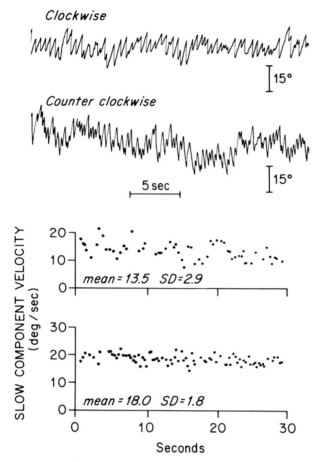

Figure 74. Abnormal optokinetic nystagmus in a patient with a right cerebellopontine angle tumor (drum speed 30 deg/sec). When the drum moved clockwise (toward the tumor) the average slow component velocity is more than 3 standard deviations below the normal mean. The response to counterclockwise drum movement is 2 standard deviations below the normal mean (borderline abnormal).

The test sensitivity is improved by using an optokinetic stimulus of known velocity and a method for recording the induced nystagmus. Figure 73 shows an ENG recording of nystagmus induced by a striped optokinetic drum completely surrounding the subject and moving at an angular velocity of 30 deg/sec. A plot of slow component velocity for each nystagmus beat is beneath the tracings. The mean slow component velocity was 25.7 and 25.4 for clockwise and counterclockwise stimuli, respectively. The average values ± 1 standard deviation obtained from similar testing in 30 normal subjects were 24.2 ± 2.7 and 24.5 ± 2.9, respectively. As in the case of rotatory testing the symmetry between clockwise and counterclockwise responses in any single subject shows less variability than that seen between subjects (mean difference $\dfrac{CW - CCW}{CW + CCW}$ in the 30 normal subjects was 0.01 ± 0.08).

157

Results in Patients

Abnormalities of optokinetic nystagmus result from lesions affecting either or both the smooth pursuit and saccade system. Alterations in the slow component are most commonly seen. Symmetrically decreased slow component velocity is produced by diffuse disease of the cortex, diencephalon, brain stem and cerebellum.[16] As with smooth pursuit, transient unilaterally decreased slow component velocity occurs when the optokinetic stimulus moves contralateral to an acute labyrinthine lesion (in the direction of associated pathologic vestibular nystagmus).[16] Optokinetic nystagmus is usually normal in patients with chronic labyrinthine disease (even in those patients with prominent pathologic vestibular nystagmus in darkness).[27] Focal lateralized disease of the brain stem and cerebellum results in impaired optokinetic nystagmus when the stimulus moves toward the damaged side (Fig. 74). When a cerebellopontine angle tumor impairs optokinetic nystagmus the tumor is compressing the brain stem and/or cerebellum.[8,25] Subcortical parieto-occipital lesions impair optokinetic nystagmus when the stimulus moves toward the damaged hemisphere.[16,44] Lesions of the occipital lobe, even though associated with a hemianoptic field defect, often are not associated with grossly impaired optokinetic nystagmus[44] possibly because pursuit pathways that generate the nystagmus slow components leave the optic tract to enter the brain stem prior to reaching the occipital lobes. Further studies are needed in such patients, using precise stimuli and quantification of responses, to confirm this clinical impression.

Patients who are unable to produce saccadic eye movements because of brain stem lesions involving the saccade-pulse-generating centers only produce a slow tonic deviation of the eyes in the direction of the optokinetic stimulus. Although patients with saccade-slowing produce optokinetic nystagmus, the waveform is rounded and the amplitude and slow component velocity are decreased[19] similar to the vestibular nystagmus illustrated in Figure 67d. The delayed ending of the slow corrective fast component subtracts from the initial part of the slow component in the opposite direction.[33] The many causes of saccade slowing were outlined in detail in the previous section.

REFERENCES

1. Aschan, G.: *Clinical vestibular examinations and their results.* Acta Otolaryngol. (Suppl. 224):56, 1967.
2. Baertschi, A. J., Johnson, R. N., and Hanna, G. R.: *A theoretical and experimental determination of vestibular dynamics in caloric stimulation.* Biol. Cybern. 20:175, 1975.
3. Baloh, R. W., et al.: *Quantitative measurement of saccade amplitude, duration, and velocity.* Neurology 25:1065, 1975.
4. Baloh, R. W., et al.: *The saccade velocity test.* Neurology 25:1071, 1975.
5. Baloh, R. W., Konrad, H. R., and Honrubia, V.: *Vestibulo-ocular function in patients with cerebellar atrophy.* Neurology 25:160, 1975.
6. Baloh, R. W.: *Pathologic nystagmus: A classification based on electro-oculographic recordings.* Bull. L.A. Neurol. Soc. 41:120, 1976.
7. Baloh, R. W., Kumley, W. E., and Honrubia, V.: *Algorithm for analyses of saccadic eye movements using a digital computer.* Aviat. Space Environ. Med. 47:523, 1976.
8. Baloh, R. W., et al.: *Cerebellar-pontine angle tumors. Results of quantitative vestibulo-ocular testing.* Arch. Neurol. 33:507, 1976.
9. Baloh, R. W., Honrubia, V., and Konrad, H. R.: *Periodic alternating nystagmus.* Brain 99:11, 1976.
10. Baloh, R. W., et al.: *Quantitative measurement of smooth pursuit eye movements.* Ann. Otol. Rhinol. Laryngol. 85:111, 1976.

11. BALOH, R. W., AND HONRUBIA, V.: *Reaction time and accuracy of the saccadic eye movements of normal subjects in a moving-target task.* Aviat. Space Environ. Med. 47:1165, 1976.
12. BALOH, R. W., AND KEESEY, J. C.: *Saccade fatigue and response to edrophonium for the diagnosis of myasthenia gravis.* Ann. N.Y. Acad. Sci. 274:631, 1976.
13. BALOH, R. W., ET AL.: *Caloric testing. I. Effect of different conditions of ocular fixation.* Ann. Otol. Rhinol. Laryngol. 86(Suppl. 43):1, 1977.
14. BALOH, R. W., SILLS, A. W., AND HONRUBIA, V.: *Caloric testing. III. Patients with peripheral and central vestibular lesions.* Ann. Otol. Rhinol. Laryngol. 86(Suppl. 43):24, 1977.
15. BALOH, R. W., HONRUBIA, V., AND KONRAD, H. R.: *Ewald's second law reevaluated.* Acta Otolaryngol. 83:475, 1977.
16. BALOH, R. W., HONRUBIA, V., and SILLS, A.: *Eye-tracking and optokinetic nystagmus. Results of quantitative testing in patients with well-defined nervous system lesions.* Ann. Otol. Rhinol. Laryngol. 86:108, 1977.
17. BALOH, R. W., YEE, R. D., AND BODER, E.: *Ataxia-telangiectasia. Quantitative analysis of eye movements in six cases.* Neurology. In press.
18. BALOH, R. W., YEE, R. D., AND HONRUBIA, V.: *Internuclear ophthalmoplegia. I. Saccades and dissociated nystagmus.* Arch. Neurol. In press.
19. BALOH, R. W., YEE, R. D., AND HONRUBIA, V.: *Internuclear ophthalmoplegia. II. Smooth pursuit, optokinetic nystagmus and the vestibulo-ocular reflex.* Arch. Neurol. In press.
20. BALOH, R. W., SILLS, A. W., AND HONRUBIA, V.: *Impulsive and sinusoidal rotatory testing. A comparison with results of caloric testing.* Laryngoscope. In press.
21. BÁRÁNY, R.: *Physiologie and Pathologie des Bogengangsapparates beim Menschen.* Deuticke, Vienna, 1907.
22. BARBER, H. O., AND WRIGHT, G.: Positional nystagmus in normals. Adv. Otol. Rhinol. Laryngol. 19:276, 1973.
23. BARBER, H. O., STOCKWELL, C. W.: *Manual of electronystagmography.* The C. V. Mosby Co., St. Louis, 1976.
24. BARRY, W., AND MELVILL-JONES, G.: *Influence of eye lid movement upon electro-oculographic recording of vertical eye movements.* Aerospace Med. 36:855, 1965.
25. BENITEZ, J. T.: *Eye tracking and optokinetic tests: Diagnostic significance in peripheral and central vestibular disorders.* Laryngoscope 80:834, 1970.
26. COATS, A. C.: *Directional preponderance and spontaneous nystagmus.* Ann. Otol. Rhinol. Laryngol. 75:1135, 1966.
27. COATS, A. C.: *Central and peripheral optokinetic asymmetry.* Ann. Otol. Rhinol. Laryngol. 77:938, 1968.
28. COATS, A. C.: Electronystagmography. In Bradford, L. (ed.): *Physiological Measures of the Audio-Vestibular System.* Academic Press, New York, 1975.
29. COGAN, D. G.: *Neurologic significance of lateral conjugate deviation of the eyes on forced closure of the lids.* Arch. Ophthalmol. 39:37, 1948.
30. COVERA, J., TORRES-COURTNEY, G., and LOPES-RIOS, G.: *The neurological significance of alterations of pursuit eye movements and the pendular eye tracking test.* Ann. Otol. 82:855, 1973.
31. CRAMER, R. L., DOWD, P. J., and HELMS, D. B.: *Vestibular responses to oscillations about the yaw axis.* Aerospace Med. 34:1031, 1963.
32. DEJONG, J. D., and MELVILL-JONES, G.: *Akinesia, hypokinesia and bradykinesia in the oculomotor system of patients with Parkinson's disease.* Exp. Neurol. 32:58, 1971.
33. DELL'OSSO, L. F., ROBINSON, D. A., AND DAROFF, R. B.: Optokinetic asymmetry in internuclear ophthalmoplegia. Arch. Neurol. 31:138, 1974.
34. DEMANEZ, J. P.: *L'influence de la fixation oculaire sur le nystagmus postcalorique.* Acta Oto-Rhino-Laryngol. Belgica 22:7, 1968.
35. EVIATAR, A., AND EVIATAR, L.: *A critical look at the "cold calorics."* Arch. Otolaryngol. 99:361, 1974.
36. FENN, W. O., AND HURSH, J. B.: *Movements of the eyes when the lids are closed.* Amer. J. Physiol. 118:8, 1937.
37. FERNÁNDEZ, C. AND FREDRICKSON, J. M.: *Experimental cerebellar lesions and their effect on vestibular function.* Acta Otolaryngol. (Supp. 192):52, 1964.
38. FITZGERALD, G., AND HALLPIKE, C. S.: *Studies in human vestibular function: I. Observations of the directional preponderance of caloric nystagmus resulting from cerebral lesions.* Brain 65:115, 1942.
39. FLUUR, E.: *Interaction between the utricles and the horizontal semicircular canals. IV. Tilting of human patients with acute unilateral vestibular neuritis.* Acta Otolaryngol. 76:349, 1973.

40. FREDRICKSON, J. M., AND FERNÁNDEZ, C.: *Vestibular disorders in fourth ventricle lesions*. Arch. Otolaryngol. 80:521, 1964.
41. GENTLES, W., AND LLEWELLYN-THOMAS, E.: *Effect of benzodiazepines upon saccadic eye movements in man*. Clin. Pharmacol. Ther. 12:563, 1971.
42. HENRIKSSON, N. G.: *Speed of the slow component and duration in caloric nystagmus*. Acta. Otolaryngol. (Suppl. 125):14, 1955.
43. HOLZMAN, P. S., ET AL.: *Smooth-pursuit eye movements, and diazepam, CPZ, and secobarbital*. Psychopharmacologia 44:111, 1975.
44. HOYT, W. F., AND DAROFF, R. B.: Supranuclear disorders of ocular control in man. In Bach-Y-Rita, P., Collins, C. C., and Hyde, J. E. (eds.): *The Control of Eye Movements*. Academic Press, New York, 1971.
45. HULK, J., AND JONGKEES, L. B. W.: *The turning test with small regulable stimuli. II. The normal cupulogram*. J. Laryngol. Otol. 62:70, 1948.
46. JONGKEES, L. B. W., AND PHILIPZOON, A. J.: *Electronystagmography*. Acta Otolaryngol. (Suppl. 189):55, 1964.
47. KAMEI, T., AND KORNHUBER, H. H.: *Spontaneous and head shaking nystagmus in normals and in patients with central lesions*. Can. J. Otolaryngol. 3:372, 1974.
48. KRIS, C.: Electro-oculography. In Glasser, O. (ed.): *Medical Physiology*, vol. 3. Year Book Medical Publishers, Inc., Chicago, 1960.
49. KTONAS, P. Y., BLACK, F. O., SMITH, J. R.: *Effect of electronic filters on electronystagmographic recordings*. Arch. Otolaryngol. 101:413, 1975.
50. LEDOUX, A., AND DEMANEZ, J. P.: "Ocular fixation index" in the caloric test. Contribution of the nystagmographic diagnosis of central diseases. In Stahle, J. (ed.): *Vestibular Function on Earth and in Space*. Pergamon Press, New York, 1970.
51. MATHOG, R. H.: *Testing of the vestibular system by sinusoidal angular acceleration*. Acta Otolaryngol. 74:96, 1972.
52. METZ, H. S., ET AL.: *Ocular saccades in lateral rectus palsy*. Arch. Ophthalmol. 84:453, 1970.
53. MILOJEVIC, B.: *Electronystagmographical study of vertigo*. Pract. Oto-Rhino-Larnygol. 29:85, 1967.
54. MONTANDON, A.: *A new technique for vestibular investigation*. Acta Otolaryngol. 39:594, 1954.
55. MONTANDON, A., AND RUSSBACH, A.: *L'epreune giratoire liminaire*. Pract. Oto-Rhino-Laryngol. 17:224, 1955.
56. NIVEN, J. J., HINSON, C., AND CORREIA, M. J.: An experimental approach to the dynamics of the vestibular mechanisms. In: *Symposium on the Role of the Vestibular Organs in the Exploration of Space*. Pensacola, Florida. NASA SP-77:43, 1965.
57. OOSTERVELD, W. J.: The threshold value for stimulation of the horizontal semicircular canals. In Busby, D. W. (ed.): *Recent Advances in Aerospace Medicine*. D. Reidel Publishing Co., Dordrecht-Holland, 1970.
58. RASHBASS, C.: *The relationship between saccadic and smooth tracking eye movements*. J. Physiol. 159:326, 1961.
59. RIESCO-MCCLURE, J., AND STROUD, M.: *Dysrhythmia in the post-caloric nystagmus. Its clinical significance*. Laryngoscope 70:697, 1960.
60. RODIN, E. A.: *Impaired ocular pursuit movements*. Arch. Neurol. 10:327, 1964.
61. SCHMALTZ, G.: The physical phenomena occurring in the semicircular canals during rotatory and thermic stimulation. Proc. Roy. Soc. Med. 25:359, 1932.
62. SILLS, A. W., HONRUBIA, V., AND KUMLEY, W. E.: *Algorithm for the multi-parameter analysis of nystagmus using a digital computer*. Aviat. Space Environ. Med. 46:934, 1975.
63. SILLS, A. W., BALOH, R. W., AND HONRUBIA, V.: *Caloric testing. II. Results in normal subjects*. Ann. Otol. Rhinol. Laryngol. 86(Suppl. 43):7, 1977.
64. SOLINGEN, L. D., ET AL.: *Subclinical eye movement disorders in patients with multiple sclerosis*. Neurology 27:614, 1977.
65. STAHLE, J.: Electronystagmography—its value as a diagnostic tool. In Wolfson, R. J. (ed.): *The Vestibular System and Its Diseases*. University of Pennsylvania Press, Philadelphia, 1968.
66. STARR, A.: *A disorder of rapid eye movements in Huntington's chorea*. Brain 90:545, 1967.
67. TAKEMORI, S., AND COHEN, B.: *Loss of visual suppression of vestibular nystagmus after flocculus lesions*. Brain Res. 72:213, 1974.
68. TAKEMORI, S.: *Visual suppression test*. Ann. Otol. Rhinol. Laryngol. 86:80, 1977.
69. TROOST, B. T., WEBER, R. B., AND DAROFF, R. B.: *Hemispheric control of eye movements. II. Quantitative analysis of smooth pursuit in a hemispherectomy patient*. Arch. Neurol. 27:449, 1972.

160

70. TROOST, B. T., AND DAROFF, R. B.: *The ocular motor defects in progressive supranuclear palsy.* Ann. Neurol. 2:397, 1977.
71. UEMURA, T., AND COHEN, B.: *Effects of vestibular nuclei lesions on vestibulo-ocular reflexes and posture in monkeys.* Acta Otolaryngol. (Suppl. 315):1, 1973.
72. VAN DE CALSEYDE, P., AMPE, W., AND DEPONDT, M.: *The damped torsion swing test. Quantitative and qualitative aspects of the ENG pattern in normal subjects.* Arch. Otolaryngol. 100:449, 1974.
73. VAN EGMOND, A. A. J., GROEN, J. J., AND JONGKEES, L. B. W.: *The turning test with small regulable stimuli. I. Method of examination: cupulometria.* J. Laryngol. Otol. 2:63, 1948.
74. VISSER, S. L.: *Some aspects of evaluating electronystagmographic examination in clinical neurology.* Psychiat. Neurol. Neurochir. 66:24, 1963.
75. VON NOORDEN, G. K., AND PREZIOSI, T. J.: *Eye movement recordings in neurological disorders.* Arch. Ophthalmol. 76:162, 1966.
76. WILKINSON, I. M. S., KIME, R., AND PURNELL, M.: *Alcohol and human eye movement.* Brain 97:785, 1974.
77. ZEE, D. S., YEE, R. D., AND SINGER, H. S.: *Congenital ocular motor apraxia.* Brain 100:581, 1977.
78. ZEE, D. S., ET AL.: *Ocular motor abnormalities in hereditary cerebellar ataxia.* Brain 99:207, 1976.

CHAPTER 6

Clinical Evaluation of Hearing

TYPES OF HEARING LOSS

Hearing disorders can be classified as conductive, sensorineural and central based on the anatomic site of lesion.[3, 8] *Conductive hearing loss* is caused by lesions involving the external or middle ear. The tympanic membrane and ossicles act as a transformer, amplifying airborne sound and efficiently transferring it to the inner ear fluid (see Middle Ear, Chapter 2). If this normal pathway is obstructed, transmission may occur across the skin and through the bones of the skull (bone conduction) but at the cost of considerable energy loss. Patients with conductive hearing loss can hear loud speech in a noisy background better than soft speech in a quiet background since their deficit is impaired amplification, not discrimination.

Sensorineural hearing loss results from lesions of the cochlea and/or the auditory division of the eighth cranial nerve. As suggested in Chapter 1, the sensory cells of the cochlea are force transducers converting sound energy in the inner ear fluid to action potentials in the auditory nerve. Since different frequency tones stimulate sensory cells at different positions along the spiral basilar membrane the cochlea mechanically analyzes the frequency content of sound. Patients with lesions of the cochlea and its afferent nerve cannot understand loud speech mixed with background noise and may be annoyed by loud speech.

Central hearing disorders are caused by lesions of the central auditory pathways: the cochlear and dorsal olivary nuclear complexes, inferior colliculi, medial geniculate bodies, auditory cortex in the temporal lobes and their interconnecting afferent and efferent fiber tracts.[4] As a rule, patients with central lesions do not develop impaired hearing levels for pure tones and can understand speech as long as it is clearly spoken in a quiet environment. If the patient's task is made more difficult with the introduction of background noise or competing messages his performance may deteriorate markedly.

EXAMINATION OF HEARING

Rapid Qualitative Tests

A quick test for hearing loss in the speech range is to observe the response to spoken commands at different intensities (whispering, talking, shouting). The examiner must be careful to prevent the patient from reading his lip movement. Tuning fork tests permit a rough assessment of the hearing level for pure tones of known frequency. The clinician can use his own hearing level as a reference standa d. The *Rinne test* compares the patient's hearing by air conduction with that by bone conduction. The fork (preferably 512 cps) is first held against the mastoid process until the sound fades, then is placed one inch from the ear. Normal subjects can hear the fork about twice as long by air as by bone conduction. In patients with conductive hearing loss bone conduction is greater than air conduction. The *Weber test* compares the patient's hearing by bone conduction in the two ears. The fork is placed at the center of the forehead or on a central incisor and the patient is asked where he hears the tone. A normal subject hears the tone equally in both ears and localizes the sound to the center of his head. Bone conduction is equal in both ears in a patient with a unilateral conductive loss but since competing airborne noise is blocked by the conductive defect he hears the tone louder in the abnormal ear. Patients with unilateral sensorineural hearing loss lateralize the tone to the normal ear because bone conduction is impaired in the damaged ear.

Audiometry

Table 9 summarizes the results of audiometric testing in patients with conductive, sensorineural and central hearing loss.

Tests Requiring Subjective Responses

Pure tone testing is the nucleus of most auditory examinations.[3, 8] Pure tones at selected frequencies are presented by means of either earphones (air conduction) or a vibrator pressed against the mastoid portion of the temporal bone (bone conduction). The minimal level that the subject can hear is determined for each frequency. In order for the audiologist to quantify the magnitude of hearing loss, normal hearing levels are defined by an international standard. These levels approximate the intensity of the faintest sound that can be heard by normal ears. A patient's hearing level is the difference in decibels (db) between the faintest pure tone that he can hear and the normal reference level given by the standard. Two speech tests are routinely used. The speech reception threshold is the intensity at which the patient can correctly repeat 50 percent of the words presented and therefore is a test of hearing sensitivity reflecting the hearing level for pure tones in the speech range. The speech discrimination test is a measure of the patient's ability to understand speech when it is presented at a level that is easily heard by normal subjects. In patients with eighth nerve lesions speech discrimination may be severely reduced even when pure tone thresholds are normal or near normal, whereas in patients with cochlear lesions discrimination tends to be proportional to the magnitude of hearing loss.[7]

Important manifestations of sensorineural lesions are diplacusis and recruitment which commonly occur with cochlear lesions, and tone decay which usually occurs with eighth nerve involvement. With diplacusis the tonal quality of a pure tone is distorted so that it may sound like a complex mixture of tones. Binaural diplacusis occurs when the two ears are affected unequally so that the same frequency has a different pitch in each ear, and the patient hears double. Monaural diplacusis refers to the unusual situation where two tones or a tone and a noise are heard simultaneously in one ear. With recruitment the sensation of loudness

Table 9. Results of audiometric testing with different types of hearing loss

Type of Hearing Loss	Pure Tone	Speech Discrimination	Drum Mobility (tympanometry)	Stapedius Reflex	Special Tests
Conductive	Air–abnormal Bone–normal	Normal	Decreased	Normal except with ossicular chain fixation	—
Sensorineural					
Labyrinth	Air and bone abnormal	Relatively preserved	Normal	Normal except with profound loss	Recruitment Diplacusis Tone decay
Eighth nerve	Air and bone abnormal	Impaired early	Normal	Abnormal	
Central	Air and bone normal	Normal	Normal	May be abnormal with brain stem lesions	Unable to understand distorted speech and competing messages

grows at an abnormally rapid rate as the intensity of a sound is increased so that faint or moderate sounds cannot be heard while the loudness of loud sounds changes relatively little. The inability to maintain perception of a continuous tone presented above auditory threshold is called tone decay. Patients with conductive or cochlear lesions are usually able to hear a continuous tone for at least 60 seconds while the tone rapidly decays for patients with eighth nerve lesions.

Recruitment is usually measured by the alternate binaural loudness balance test (if the hearing loss is unilateral).[8, 11] This test compares the loudness for tones of varying intensity as perceived by the diseased ear and the normal ear. Recruitment is present if smaller increases in stimulus intensity are required in the poorer ear than in the better ear to maintain equal loudness. Tone decay is tested by presenting a tone at a prescribed suprathreshold level and asking the patient to respond as long as he hears the tone.[2, 5, 13] Special tests for central auditory lesions assess the patient's ability to understand distorted speech or speech that is presented to one ear with a competing message in the other ear.[6, 10]

Tests Using Objective Measurements

By inserting probes in the external canal that present a tone and then measuring the sound pressure level, the audiologist can assess the acoustic impedance of the middle ear.[9] Two types of impedance measurement are routinely used: tympanometry and stapedius reflex measurement. Tympanometry, the measurement of impedance as a function of ear canal air pressure, is primarily useful for detection of middle ear disorders, stapedius reflex measurements for identifying lesions of the eighth nerve and/or brain stem.[12, 16] The stapedius muscle contracts and tightens the ossicular chain to protect the inner ear from excessively loud noises. The magnitude of the acoustic impedance change is an indirect measure of the strength of contraction of the stapedius muscle. The reflex arc consists of the 1) auditory nerve, 2) brain stem interneurons and 3) facial nerve.[1] If the middle ear structures are intact, loss of the stapedius reflex suggests a lesion in this reflex arc.

Measurement of auditory evoked responses is a promising new functional test of the peripheral and central auditory pathways.[14, 15] In the initial 10 msec following a click signal, a sequence of low amplitude (nanovolt) potentials can be recorded from scalp electrodes. By using a series of clicks and computer averaging techniques 7 reproduceable potentials have been identified. These "far field" potentials reflect the electric events generated in the auditory nerve, brain stem nuclei and interconnecting tracts. Lesions of these pathways alter the amplitude and/or latency of the evoked potentials.[14, 15]

REFERENCES

1. BORG. E.: *On the neuronal organization of the acoustic middle ear reflex. A physiological and anatomical study.* Brain Res. 49:101, 1973.
2. CARHART, R.: *Clinical determination of abnormal auditory adaptation.* Arch. Otolaryngol. 65:32, 1957.
3. DAVIS, H., AND SILVERMAN, S. R. (EDS.): *Hearing and Deafness,* vol. 3. Holt, Rinehart and Winston, New York, 1970.
4. DUBLIN, W. B.: *Fundamentals of Sensorineural Auditory Pathology.* Charles C Thomas, Springfield, Illinois, 1976.
5. JERGER, J.: *A simplified tone decay test.* Arch. Otolaryngol. 102:403, 1975.

6. JERGER, J.: Auditory tests for disorders of the central auditory mechanism. In Fields, W. (ed.): *Neurological Aspects of Auditory and Vestibular Disorders*. Charles C Thomas, Springfield, Illinois, 1964.

7. JERGER, J.: *Diagnostic significance of PB word functions*. Arch. Otolaryngol. 93:573, 1971.

8. JERGER, J. (ED.): *Modern Developments in Audiology*. Academic Press, New York, 1973.

9. JERGER, J.: *Studies in impedance audiometry. I. Normal and sensorineural ears*. Arch. Otolaryngol. 96:513, 1972.

10. KORSAN-BENGTSEN, M.: *Distorted speech audiometry*. Acta Otolaryngol. (Suppl. 310):1, 1973.

11. LUSCHER, E., AND SWISLOCKI, J.: *Comparison of the various methods employed in determination of the recruitment phenomenon*. J. Laryngol. 65:187, 1951.

12. OLSEN, W., NOFFSINGER, D., and KURDZIEL, S.: *Acoustic reflex and reflex decay*. Arch. Otolaryngol. 101:622, 1975.

13. OLSEN, W., AND NOFFSINGER, D.: *Comparison of one new and three old tests of auditory adaptation*. Arch. Otolaryngol. 99:94, 1974.

14. STARR, A. AND ACHOR, L. J.: *Auditory brain stem responses in neurological disease*. Arch. Neurol. 32:761, 1975.

15. STOCKARD, J. J., STOCKHARD, J. E., AND SHARBROUGH, F. W.: *Detection and localization of occult lesions with brain stem auditory responses*. Mayo Clin. Proc. 52:761, 1977.

16. ZAKRISSON, J., BORG, E., AND BLOM, S.: *The acoustic impedance change as a measure of stapedius muscle activity in man*. Acta Otolaryngol. 78:357, 1974.

CHAPTER 7

Differential Diagnosis of Vestibular System Disease

ANATOMIC LOCALIZATION

Lesions of the vestibular system can be conveniently broken down into five anatomic sites: 1) the vestibular end organ and vestibular nerve terminals; 2) the vestibular ganglia and nerve within the internal auditory canal; 3) the cerebellopontine angle; 4) the brain stem and cerebellum; and 5) the vestibular projections to the cerebral cortex. Because of the constellation of associated symptoms and signs, diseases involving these anatomic localizations can usually be identified from the information gained in the history and examination. Although some diseases may affect more than one anatomic site, it is useful to keep each location in mind when formulating a differential diagnosis. Table 10 summarizes the signs associated with pathological changes in each anatomic site.

Labyrinth and Eighth Nerve Terminals

Clinical symptoms and signs associated with lesions of the labyrinth overlap to a considerable extent those produced by disease of the eighth nerve terminals. Single or intermittent episodes of vertigo occur frequently with unilateral disorders, rarely with bilateral disease. Symptoms such as hearing loss, tinnitus, pressure, pain and drainage in the ear are often reported, and examination of the tympanic membrane may reveal evidence of infection, hemorrhage or tumor in the middle ear (see Fig. 49). A positive fistula test suggests a communication between the perilymph and middle ear space.

On clinical vestibular examination (see Chapter 4) the patient past points and falls toward the side of an acute unilateral labyrinthine lesion. Vestibular nystagmus and positional nystagmus, particularly paroxysmal positional nystagmus, commonly occur in all stages. Caloric examination usually reveals a vestibular paresis, or occasionally a directional preponderance, or both. In the case of acute end organ lesions, smooth pursuit and optokinetic nystagmus are transiently impaired when the target moves contralateral to the damaged labyrinth. With bilateral disease, the patient demonstrates ataxia when vision is inhibited, and the caloric and rotatory responses are diminished bilaterally.

Table 10. Findings associated with vestibular involvement at different levels

	End Organ and Nerve Terminals	Ganglia and Intracanal Nerve	Cerebello-pontine Angle	Intrinsic Brain Stem and Cerebellum	Cortical Projections
Ear Exam	Inflamed and/or perforated drum, keratoma, positive fistula test, temporal bone fracture	Zoster vessicles in external canal	—	—	—
Neurologic Exam Other Than Eighth Nerve	—	Ipsilateral seventh nerve	Ipsilateral fifth, sixth and seventh nerve and cerebellar	Multiple cranial nerves, long tracts, cerebellar, ocular	Visual field defects, aphasia, hemiparesis, hemianesthesia
Equilibrium	Ipsilateral past pointing, falling and turning with acute lesions	Ipsilateral past pointing, falling and turning with acute lesions	Ataxia with eyes open increases with eyes closed	Ataxia prominent with eyes open	—
Pathologic Nystagmus	Vestibular, stationary and paroxysmal positional	Vestibular, stationary positional	Vestibular, stationary positional, gaze paretic	All varieties	Gaze paretic
Caloric and Rotatory Testing	Vestibular paresis,* directional preponderance	Vestibular paresis, directional preponderance	Vestibular paresis, directional preponderance	Directional preponderance, hyperactive responses, dysrhythmia, impaired fixation suppression, perverted or disconjugate nystagmus	Directional preponderance

Eye Tracking and OKN	Transient contralateral pursuit and OKN impairment	Transient contralateral pursuit and OKN impairment	Progressive ipsilateral pursuit and OKN impairment	Saccade, pursuit and OKN impairment	Contralateral saccade accuracy and ipsilateral OKN and pursuit impairment
Auditory Exam Pure Tone	Conductive or sensorineural	Sensorineural	Sensorineural	—	—
Speech Discrimination	Relatively preserved	Impaired early	Impaired early	—	—
Impedance Studies	Immobile tympanic membrane	Impaired stapedius reflex	Impaired stapedius reflex	Impaired stapedius reflex	—
Other	Recruitment	Tone decay	Tone decay	Impaired comprehension of competing or distorted messages	Impaired comprehension of competing or distorted messages
Routine X-rays	Sclerosing mastoiditis, malformation, keratoma, erosion of middle or inner ear	Enlarged internal auditory canal, transverse fracture line	Erosion of internal auditory canal opening	Calcification in tumor or cyst	Calcification in tumor or cyst

* Vestibular paresis identified by caloric test only.

171

Auditory testing and routine x-rays are particularly useful in determining a labyrinthine anatomic localization.[174, 330] An air-bone gap on pure tone audiometry and decreased drum mobility on tympanometry indicate a conductive hearing loss and suggest involvement of the middle ear in addition to the inner ear. If a sensorineural hearing loss is present, the finding of good speech discrimination and recruitment favors an end organ rather than a nerve disorder. Routine x-rays of the mastoid bone may provide evidence of chronic infection or erosion from a keratoma (cholesteatoma). Malformations or more subtle changes caused by infection are often identified by laminograms of the middle and inner ear.

Vestibular Ganglia and Nerve Within the Canal

The vestibular ganglia consists of bipolar neurons grouped into two linearly arranged cell masses associated with the superior and inferior divisions of the vestibular nerve trunk. The superior division innervates the cristae of the anterior and lateral canals, the macule of the utricle and the anterosuperior part of the macule of the saccule; the inferior division innervates the crista of the posterior canal and the remainder of the succular macule. Just medial to the ganglia the two divisions of the vestibular nerve merge in the internal auditory canal where they are joined by the cochlear and facial nerves (see Fig. 7). The close approximation of these three nerves in the narrow confines of the internal auditory canal accounts for the characteristic clinical profile of lesions originating in the canal.

Compared to its occurrence in end organ disease, vertigo is less common with vestibular ganglion and nerve lesions, particularly if the pathologic process is slow in developing. Hearing loss and tinnitus are often present, but ear pressure or pain are not. The findings from vestibular examination cannot be distinguished from those of end organ disease. The most useful evidence for anatomic localization is facial weakness from involvement of the seventh nerve. Sensorineural hearing loss is often associated with tone decay, impaired speech discrimination and either a diminished or absent stapedius reflex.[174] X-rays of the internal auditory canal may reveal a fracture line, an erosion or a congenitally narrow canal.[330]

Cerebellopontine (CP) Angle

The CP angle is bounded by the pons, the cerebellum and the temporal bone. The seventh and eighth nerves leave the pons, run through the angle, and enter the temporal bone by way of the internal auditory canal (see Fig. 15). Lesions of the CP angle usually produce a slow, progressive loss of vestibular function and of hearing without episodic vertigo. The fifth and seventh cranial nerves are commonly involved, causing ipsilateral facial numbness and weakness. In later stages of progression, involvement of the sixth, ninth and tenth nerves gives rise to diplopia, dysphonia and dysphagia. Compression of the brain stem and cerebellum results in ipsilateral gaze dysfunction and dysmetria of the extremities.

Caloric examination confirms an ipsilateral loss of vestibular function (a vestibular paresis) in approximately 80 percent of patients with CP angle tumors. Frequently a combination of vestibular nystagmus and asymmetric horizontal gaze paretic nystagmus occurs;[16] the former is caused by vestibular nerve involvement, the latter by brain stem compression on the side of the large amplitude nystagmus. With brain stem compression smooth pursuit and optokinetic nystagmus may be impaired when the target moves either toward the involved CP angle or in both directions.[16] Auditory testing usually reveals a sensorineural hearing loss, impaired speech discrimination, tone decay and loss of the stapedius reflex.[174, 295] Erosion of the medial lip of the internal auditory canal is found on radiologic examination if a tumor has arisen in the canal and grown into the angle.[145, 330] Computerized tomography can regularly identify large CP angle tumors (> 1 cm in diameter)[322] but for detection of most small tumors, particularly those confined to the internal auditory canal, cisternography with air or dye is required.[145, 322]

Brain Stem and Cerebellum

Since vestibular pathways run throughout the brain stem and cerebellum, it is not surprising that vestibular symptoms and signs are common with lesions involving these structures. At the same time, because of the close approximation of other neuronal centers and fiber tracts in the brain stem and cerebellum it is unusual to find lesions that produce isolated vestibular symptoms and signs.

Ataxia associated with cerebellar disease is present whether the patient's eyes are open or closed and, therefore, can usually be distinguished from vestibular ataxia. Ataxia with eyes open can occur after an acute vestibular lesion, but is rapidly compensated for within a few days. Brain stem and cerebellar lesions cause many types of pathologic nystagmus that are discussed in detail in Chapter 4. Rebound nystagmus is specific for cerebellar lesions, dissociated nystagmus suggests involvement of pathways connecting the sixth and third nerve nuclei, and fixation nystagmus is most frequently produced by lesions of the medulla and midline cerebellum. Positional nystagmus that is nonfatigable, not inhibited by fixation and present in multiple positions suggests a brain stem or cerebellar lesion. Vestibular nystagmus can be caused by brain stem lesions particularly if they involve the vestibular nerve root entry zone, but it is accompanied by other brain stem signs and is not effectively inhibited by fixation. Similarly, unilateral caloric hypoexcitability is occasionally produced by brain stem lesions involving the root entry zone, but a directional preponderance more commonly occurs. Saccade, pursuit and optokinetic nystagmus abnormalities are common with brain stem and cerbellar lesions (see Tests of Visual-Ocular Control, Chapter 5).

Hearing loss for pure tones rarely occurs with brain stem lesions unless the lesion is massive or specifically involves the cochlear nerve root entry zone.[174, 175] Routine speech discrimination is normal but abnormalities of central processing of auditory information are identified using simultaneous competing messages or distorted messages.[175] The stapedius reflex may decay abnormally or may be absent because of interruption of the reflex pathways in the brain stem.[134, 175] Routine x-rays seldom identify intrinsic brain stem and cerebellar lesions. If the cerebrospinal fluid circulation is obstructed, skull x-rays may reveal signs of increased pressure caused by obstructive hydrocephalus or calcification in a tumor or cyst. With few exceptions, computerized tomography reliably identifies tumor or hemorrhage in the substance of the brain stem or cerebellum.[227, 235] When computerized tomography is unavailable, one must rely on air contrast or positive contrast encephalography to outline the lesion.

Cortical Vestibular Projections

Although vertigo frequently accompanies supratentorial lesions, it is unclear whether destruction of vestibular cortical projections can cause the symptom. Vertigo may be related to associated brain stem compression or involvement of the labyrinths by the same pathologic process or secondary metabolic changes. Spiegel and Alexander[307] reviewed a large series of patients with supratentorial tumors who complained of vertigo and concluded that even though the majority of instances could be explained on the basis of secondary involvement of the brain stem and/or labyrinths, some cases remained in which the vertigo appeared to be secondary to the supratentorial lesion. Temporal lobe lesions were more frequently associated with vertigo than were lesions in any other lobe. The definition of vertigo was not restricted to an illusion of movement, however, and therefore the patients may have been reporting dizziness associated with damage to other orienting systems.

Although the association between destructive cortical lesions and vertigo is unclear, there is little doubt that excitatory foci of the cortex can produce vertigo. Foerster,[101] Morsier[78] and Penfield and associates[252, 253] were able to induce illusions of rotation by stimulating different cortical areas in patients undergoing brain surgery. The most common locations were the region of the intraparietal sulcus and the posterosuperior gyrus of the temporal lobe. These studies are consistent with the clinical finding of vertigo as part of the aura in patients with well documented focal epilepsy. Although auditory aura phenomena (such as ringing or peculiar sounds) occasionally accompany vertigo with temporal lobe foci, pure tone hearing loss does not occur with supratentorial lesions[171] unless there is bilateral massive involvement of the temporal lobes.[173] Routine speech discrimination is normal with unilateral cortical lesions but special audiometric testing may reveal impaired understanding of spoken phrases, particularly if competing sentences are presented to each ear simultaneously.[172] The message presented to the ear contralateral to the lesion is suppressed. The stapedius reflex is normal since it is a brain stem reflex.

Normal results are usually obtained from caloric examination in patients with supratentorial lesions, although occasionally a directional preponderance will be found (either toward or away from the side of the lesion).[140] The finding is of little localizing value. Frontoparietal lesions produce hypometria of contralateral voluntary saccades while deep parieto-occipital lesions impair smooth pursuit and optokinetic nystagmus when the target moves toward the side of the lesion. With the development of computerized tomography, it is now possible to accurately localize supratentorial lesions without risk to the patient. This should improve our understanding of the pathogenesis of symptoms and signs associated with lesions of the vestibulocortical projections.

ETIOLOGY OF VESTIBULAR SYSTEM DISEASE

Once an anatomic localization has been made, the clinician can formulate a differential diagnosis. The diseases considered in the differential diagnosis depend on the location of pathologic changes, but even more important on the history of the illness. Table 11 lists the most common diseases to be considered with each of the five anatomic sites: the remainder of this chapter will deal with the distinguishing features of those diseases.

Infection

Bacterial Infection

Acute suppurative labyrinthitis has become rare since the introduction of antibiotics, but it produces a clinical syndrome that should be easily recognized.

174

Symptoms include the sudden onset of severe vertigo, nausea, vomiting and unilateral hearing loss. The infection originates either in the middle ear or the cerebrospinal fluid. When labyrinthitis is associated with chronic otitis media, the most common infecting organisms are *Diplococcus pneumoniae, Hemophilus influenza* and *beta-hemolytic streptococcus*.[245,311] *Tuberculosis* should be considered in a patient known to have pulmonary tuberculosis.[169] Bacteria enter the labyrinth from the middle ear through the oval and round windows or after eroding through the bony walls. Patients with bacterial meningitis develop labyrinthitis when bacteria enter the perilymphatic space from the cerebrospinal fluid by way of the cochlear aqueduct or internal auditory canal. The most common invading organisms are *Hemophilus influenza* and *meningococcus*.[103,156]

After an initial accumulation of polymorphs in the perilymphatic space, a fine fibrillar precipitate forms throughout the perilymphatic and endolymphatic spaces.[282] Following blockage of fluid circulation, and perhaps necrosis of the membranous labyrinth, the disease usually produces an irreversible unilateral loss of vestibular and auditory function.

Some otitic bacterial infections, rather than invading the labyrinth, produce irritation and biochemical damage to the membranes by their toxins and endotoxins.[282] This condition is called toxic or *serous labyrinthitis* and is associated with varying degrees of vertigo and hearing loss. In many instances the physician arrives at this diagnosis in retrospect when the patient has recovered and all or part of vestibular and auditory function remain. Because of permanent impairment of fluid resorption some patients go on to develop recurrent episodes of vertigo and hearing loss typical of *endolymphatic hydrops* (see Meniere's syndrome).

Chronic otitic infections produce several types of labyrinthine damage, some of which go on to involve the vestibular nerve and its central connections. Chronic middle ear infections with perforation of the tympanic membrane often lead to an invasion of the middle ear and other pneumatized areas of the temporal bone by keratinizing squamous epithelium from the external canal.[131,282] This *keratoma* (cholesteatoma) either accumulates slowly for years or develops rapidly with recurrent acute infections. A keratoma usually develops in the epitympanic space after penetrating a perforation in Schrapnell's membrane (see Fig. 49). From here it extends posteriorly into the antrum, into the central mastoid tract, or inferiorly into the middle ear where it erodes the ossicles and bony labyrinth. Keratomas incite resorption of adjacent bone by a process of pressure erosion. When infected, the keratomatous mass may erode through the temporal bone into the intracranial cavity, producing central nervous system symptoms and signs.

With chronic labyrinthitis a *fistula* may develop in the bony labyrinth, producing an artificial communication between perilymph and the middle ear.[282] The fistula is caused by either progressive rarefying osteitis or keratomatous erosion. Patients with a perilymph fistula experience incapacitating episodes of vertigo when they sneeze or cough because of the sudden change in middle ear pressure.

Infections involving the perilabyrinthine bone may extend into the apical regions of the petrous bone, producing *petrositis*. Petrositis often presents as Gradenigo's syndrome[127] consisting of: 1) otitis media, 2) paralysis of the ipsilateral external rectus muscle from involvement of the abducens nerve as it crosses the petrous bone, and 3) pain behind the ipsilateral eye from involvement of the trigeminal ganglion at the semilunar fossa. This syndrome is often associated with vertigo and hearing loss from either concomitant erosion of the bony labyrinth or involvement of the eighth nerve in its bony canal. Destruction of the facial nerve,

Table 11. Common disorders affecting the vestibular system

	End Organ and Nerve Terminals	Ganglia and Intracanal Nerve	Cerebello-pontine Angle	Intrinsic Brain Stem and Cerebellum	Cortical Projections
Infection	Labyrinthitis: viral, bacterial, syphilitic, mycotic; keratoma	Herpes zoster, vestibular mononeuritis, petrositis	Basilar meningitis, abscess, petrositis	Focal viral encephalitis, abscess	Focal viral encephalitis, abscess
Vascular	VBI, occlusion: int. aud. artery, ant. vestibular artery; hemorrhage	Occlusion branch of int. aud. artery	Aneurysm, arteriovenous malformation, anomalous arteries	VBI, infarction: lateral medullary, pontomedullary, cerebellum; hemorrhage: brain stem, cerebellum	Temporal-parietal infarction
Neoplastic	Carcinoma: primary and metastatic; sarcoma, glomus body tumors	Vestibular schwannoma, glomus body tumors, carcinoma, sarcoma	Schwannomas, meningioma, epidermoid cyst, metastatic carcinoma	Infiltrating astrocytomas, teratoma, medulloblastoma, ependymoma	Astrocytoma, Oligodendroglioma
Traumatic	Temp. bone fracture, labyrinth concussion, postsurgical, barotrauma, round window rupture	Transverse fractures, penetrating wound	Avulsion of eighth nerve	Contusion: brain stem, cerebellum	Post-traumatic seizure focus

Category				
Metabolic	Diabetes, otosclerosis, Paget's disease, osteogenesis imperfecta, fibrous dysplasia, osteopetrosis, uremia	Diabetes, Paget's disease, osteogenesis imperfecta, fibrous dysplasia, osteopetrosis, familial ataxia syndromes	Diabetes, thiamine deficiency, familial ataxia syndromes	—
Developmental Defects	Genetic and acquired malformations of the inner ear	Atresia int. aud. canal, agenesis of eighth nerve	Basilar impression, Arnold-Chiari malformation, syringobulbia	—
Toxic	Aminoglycosides, salicylates, alcohol	Chemotherapeutic agents, heavy metals	Alcohol, heavy metals	—
Unknown or Multiple Causes	Meniere's disease, Cogan's syndrome, cupulolithiasis, vestibular neuronitis	Vestibular neuronitis, Bell's palsy	Multiple sclerosis, migraine	Psychomotor seizures

obliteration of the carotid artery, thrombosis of the lateral and petrosal sinuses, and involvement of the nerves of the jugular foramen are less frequent accompaniments (for anatomic relationships see Fig. 15).

Otitis externa, usually a benign disorder, produces a debilitating disease called *malignant external otitis* in elderly diabetic patients.[56] Infection with *Pseudomonas aeruginosa* invades the junction of the cartilaginous and osseous portions of the external auditory canal and spreads to the temporo-occipital bones. The most common neurologic sequella is involvement of the facial nerve in the fallopian canal or at the stylomastoid foramen.[89, 291] Occasionally multiple cranial nerves are compressed extradurally and in rare cases the infection spreads across the dura to produce a purulent meningitis. Prolonged treatment with effective antibiotics (carbenicillin disodium, gentamycin sulfate) has improved the previously poor prognosis in this condition.[89]

Extension of infection from the temporal bone into the cranial cavity demands rapid diagnosis and effective therapy to prevent permanent neurologic sequellae or death.[76, 254] Acute or chronic middle ear infection enters the intracranial cavity by breaking through the roof of the epitympanic recess (see Middle Ear, Chapter 2). With chronic otitis media an acute exacerbation of infection usually occurs within a few weeks before the intracranial extension. In a patient with otitic infection who is febrile and continues to complain of severe ear and mastoid pain or headache despite antibiotic therapy, intracranial extension of the infection should be suspected. Localized neurologic signs frequently do not develop until late in the disease process, and the diagnosis should be made before focal signs develop.

The most common intracranial complication of otitic infections is *extradural abscess,* a collection of purulent fluid between the dura mater and bone of the middle or posterior fossa.[282] The dura mater is usually an effective barrier and the infection remains localized outside of the nervous system. Extradural abscesses in the middle fossa may become large and compress the temporal lobe while abscesses in the posterior fossa remain small because of the tight attachments of the dura.[254] The initial symptoms of fever, severe headache and vomiting without focal neurologic signs create a diagnostic and therapeutic problem.[76] Computerized tomography discloses a well defined extradural abscess but misses small collections of extradural pus. Results from cerebrospinal fluid examination are often normal. In some cases an associated subperiosteal abscess can be identified on routine skull x-rays. Surgical exploration to rule out an epidural abscess is necessary in those patients with negative x-ray and cerebrospinal fluid results whose symptoms persist despite adequate medical management.[254]

Spread of the infection across the dura from the epidural space may result in thrombophlebitis of the lateral venous sinus, subdural abscess, meningitis and/or brain abscess. The use of antimicrobial drugs have made all of these conditions rare. *Venous thrombophlebitis* is usually manifested by a clinical syndrome of spiking fevers, shaking chills and profuse sweating (the symptoms of septicemia).[75, 76] The thrombophlebitis may spread backward into the cerebral veins producing recurrent focal epileptic attacks or status epilepticus.[254] Thrombosis of the superior sagittal sinus impairs the resorptive function of the arachnoid granules and leads to so-called otitic hydrocephalus.[75]

Subdural abscess characteristically produces severe generalized headache, vomiting, meningism and eventually focal neurologic signs from compression of the brain.[153] Usually a prodromal period of 24 to 36 hours elapses before focal neurologic signs develop, during which time results from the spinal fluid examination may be within normal limits (the arachnoid membrane acts as an effective barrier between the subdural space and spinal fluid). Computerized tomography can identify subdural abscesses during this prodromal period and should aid in improving the previously poor prognosis of this condition.[182] The clinical picture of *meningitis* is similar to that of subdural abscess except that focal neurologic signs develop only with an associated abscess.[212] The diagnosis rests on the finding of white blood cells, increased protein and decreased glucose in the cerebrospinal fluid.

Brain abscesses from otitic infections are usually localized in the middle third of the temporal lobe or in the anterior part of the lateral lobe of the cerebellum.[254] Neurologic signs associated with a temporal lobe abscess are often subtle, particularly if the patient has received inadequate antibiotic therapy.[151,229] An upper quadrant hemianopia can result from involvement of the optic radiations on either side, and when the abscess is in the dominant hemisphere speech may be abnormal. Usually some weakness of the contralateral face and arm occurs but gross paralysis is rare. The signs of a cerebellar abscess are more prominent. The patient usually complains of severe neck stiffness and holds his head rigid in a tilted position. Neurologic examination reveals ataxia, dysrhythmia and dysmetria of the ipsilateral extremities and the gait is markedly ataxic if the patient is able to walk. Asymmetric gaze paretic nystagmus is usually present with the larger amplitude directed toward the side of the abscess. As the disease progresses the speech becomes thick and slurred and swallowing difficulty develops. Computerized tomography has revolutionized the diagnosis of brain abscesses and should be the initial diagnostic procedure when abscess is suspected.[182,249]

Viral Infection

Viral labyrinthitis is often part of a systemic viral illness such as measles, mumps and infectious mononucleosis, or it may be an isolated infection of the labyrinth without systemic involvement. In the latter case, the infecting agent is rarely identified, but substantial pathologic evidence exists that the sudden onset of hearing loss and vertigo can be caused by an acute isolated viral infection of the labyrinth.[287]

The difficulty involved in identifying the etiologic agent in viral labyrinthitis is illustrated by the experience with mumps infections. *Mumps* is a common cause of unilateral hearing loss, and less frequently vertigo, in school-age children. In preschool children unilateral hearing loss from mumps infection often goes undetected. Several investigators have suggested that subclinical mumps infections produce sudden unilateral hearing loss in adults.[81,198,278] VanDishoeck and Biernan[81] studied 66 patients within three months of the sudden onset of unilateral hearing loss for serologic or culture evidence of mumps infection. Forty-five of the patients complained of dizziness either before or after the onset of hearing loss. In 14, blood serology for mumps was positive, proving contact with mumps virus, but none of the cultures were positive. Since acute and convalescent sera were not obtained, the relationship between the mumps infection and the onset of symptoms was not clear. None of these patients had parotitis and all had a previous history of childhood mumps infection. Of the remaining patients, positive

179

results from serology testing for exposure to influenza viruses were obtained in 7, and for exposure to enteroviruses in 5. An enterovirus was cultured from the feces of 4 patients.

Upper respiratory tract viral illnesses may involve the inner ear, producing the acute onset of hearing loss and vertigo. Because of the large number of viruses that produce upper respiratory infections it is usually impossible to identify the offending agent either serologically or by culture. Lindsay[198] reported 4 patients who developed sudden unilateral deafness, tinnitus and vertigo within one to two weeks after an acute upper respiratory illness. The vertigo was rapidly compensated and each had partial recovery of hearing over the following three months. Schuknecht and coworkers[287] studied the pathologic changes of the labyrinth in 7 patients who experienced *sudden deafness of unknown cause* and died of unrelated illnesses months to years later. Vertigo accompanied the onset of hearing loss in 3 patients, and 5 had respiratory tract illness when the inner ear symptoms began. The pathologic findings of atrophy of the organ of Corti and less frequently atrophy of the vestibular end organs were similar to those seen with labyrinthitis associated with well documented viral illnesses (such as mumps or measles). The vasculature was intact and the cochlear and vestibular neuronal population was unaffected. Schuknecht concluded that isolated viral labyrinthitis is a common cause of unilateral sudden deafness.

The role of viruses in the production of mononeuritis of the seventh and eighth cranial nerves is ill-defined. An example of such a viral syndrome is *herpes zoster oticus* (also known as the Ramsay Hunt syndrome).[159] The patient initially develops a deep burning pain in the ear followed a few days later by a vesicular eruption in the external auditory canal and concha. At some time after the onset of pain, either before or after the vesicular eruption, the patient may develop hearing loss, vertigo and facial weakness. These symptoms may occur singly or collectively. A small percentage of patients with idiopathic facial palsy (Bell's palsy) have a rise in complement fixation antibodies to zoster antigen.[251] The pathologic findings in patients with herpes zoster oticus consist of perivascular, perineural and intraneural round cell infiltration in the seventh and in both divisions of the eighth nerve.[40, 350]

Controversy exists as to whether or not an *isolated viral mononeuritis of the vestibular nerve* is a common cause of episodic vertigo. In any neurotology clinic many patients present with the acute onset of severe vertigo, nausea and vomiting unassociated with auditory or facial nerve symptoms. Most of these patients gradually improve over one to two weeks, but some develop recurrent episodes. Laboratory studies usually reveal pathologic vestibular nystagmus, unilateral caloric hypoexcitability and normal hearing. A large percentage of such patients report an upper respiratory tract illness within one to two weeks prior to the onset of vertigo. This syndrome frequently occurs in epidemics (*epidemic vertigo*), may affect several members of the same family, and erupts more commonly in the spring and early summer.[49, 57, 205, 335, 342] All of these factors suggest a viral origin, but attempts to isolate an agent have been unsuccessful except for occasional findings of a herpes zoster infection.[147, 214]

The main reason for incriminating the vestibular nerve rather than the labyrinth or brain stem in this syndrome is the absence of associated symptoms and signs. Some pathologic studies[225] support a vestibular nerve site and a probable viral etiology, but only a few studies include complete examinations of the labyrinth and eighth nerve. Further virologic and pathologic studies are needed before the importance of viral mononeuritis as a cause of acute and episodic vertigo can be determined.

Viral encephalomyelitis may involve the vestibular nuclei and nerve roots. After studying several epidemics of viral illnesses in Denmark manifested by isolated vertigo in some patients and by clear signs of brain stem encephalitis in others, Pederson[250] suggested that focal brain stem viral encephalitis is a cause of epidemic vertigo. It is not likely a common cause of isolated episodes of vertigo, however, since no anatomic or physiologic reason exists for the virus to be confined to the vestibular nucleus. *Herpes simplex encephalitis* has a particular predilection for the temporal lobes and therefore can involve the cortical vestibular projection. It usually runs a fulminant course. Dizziness is a frequent complaint in the early stages but vertigo is rarely reported.

Syphilitic Infection

Syphilitic labyrinthitis remains an important cause of episodic vertigo and hearing loss despite the general availability and use of penicillin.[226] Morrison calculated that the prevalence of congenital syphilis in England in 1972 was approximately 1 in 700 or 0.14 percent.[226] About one in three patients with congenital syphilis develop otologic manifestations.[71, 181] Although the number of new cases of congenital syphilis progressively declined from 1930 to 1968 the incidence of new cases appears to have stabilized since 1968.[226] New cases of late acquired syphilis are more common than new congenital cases but otologic manifestations occur less frequently with the former (see below).

The natural history of syphilitic labyrinthitis is a slow relentless progression to profound or total bilateral loss of vestibular and auditory function. This progression is marked by episodes of sudden deafness and vertigo and fluctuation in the magnitude of hearing loss and tinnitus. Penicillin, even in massive doses, may not alter the natural course.[226]

Both *congenital* and *acquired* syphilitic infections produce labyrinthitis as a latent manifestation. The congenital variety is approximately three times as common as the acquired variety.[226] The time of onset of congenital syphilitic labyrinthitis is anywhere from the first to seventh decades with a peak incidence in the fourth and fifth decades, while acquired syphilitic labyrinthitis rarely occurs before the fourth decade and has a peak incidence in the fifth and sixth decades. The congenital variety is often associated with other stigmata of congenital syphilis, such as interstitial keratitis, Hutchinson's teeth, saddle nose, frontal bossing and rhagades. Of these associated signs interstitial keratitis is by far the most common, occurring in approximately 90 percent of patients.[71, 226] The pathologic changes in the labyrinth are similar in the congenital and acquired variety, consisting of inflammatory infiltration of the membranous labyrinth and osteitis of all three layers of the otic capsule.[120, 181] A combination of hydrops of the membranous labyrinth and atrophy of cochlear and vestibular end organs resembles the pathologic findings in idiopathic Meniere's syndrome.[257]

A positive serum fluorescent treponemal antibody absorption (FTA-ABS) test is present in nearly 100 percent of patients with the typical clinical syndrome of congenital and acquired syphilitic labyrinthitis.[226] The serum Venereal Disease Research Laboratory test (VDRL) is positive in only 75 percent of cases, making it an unreliable test for syphilitic labyrinthitis. Cerebrospinal fluid serology is usually negative in both the congenital and acquired varieties.

In a minority of patients syphilitic labyrinthitis, especially the acquired type, is associated with neurosyphilis.[224, 318] The CSF reaction is usually mild and a full-blown neurosyphilitic syndrome seldom occurs. In rare cases, acute meningovascular syphilis accompanies the acquired variety of labyrinthine syphilis, the symptoms and signs of the former frequently overshadowing the labyrinthine findings.

Mycotic Infections

Mycotic infections can involve the vestibular system either in the mastoid bone or in the CP angle. Although the mucorales group of fungi are of low virulence, *mucormycosis* of the mastoid bone has become an increasingly common clinical problem.[133, 234] It occurs in patients who are chronically ill (particularly with diabetes or malignancy) and are receiving chemotherapy or broad-spectrum antibiotic therapy. The organism enters the sinuses from the nose and penetrates the muscular walls of arteries inciting thrombosis and infarction of tissue. The infection may then spread to the petrous apices, the middle and inner ears and into the intracranial cavity. Thrombosis of the major cerebral arteries often develops despite therapy with Amphotericin.

Cryptococcosis and *coccidioidomycosis* produce basilar meningitis with involvement of multiple cranial nerves including the eighth nerve. The clinical picture of an insidious febrile illness is often indistinguishable from that of basilar meningitis caused by *tuberculosis* and *sarcoidosis*. A cerebrospinal fluid profile of lymphocytic pleocytosis, elevated protein and decreased glucose occurs with all four conditions, as does obstruction of cerebrospinal fluid circulation and associated pulmonary lesions. The diagnosis of fungal meningitis is most reliably made by identifying the cryptococcal or coccidioidal antigen in the cerebrospinal fluid using compliment fixation, latex agglutination or immunoflourescent techniques.[50, 122]

Vascular Disease

Ischemia

As discussed in Chapter 2, the vascular supply to the labyrinth, eighth nerve and brain stem arises from a common source, the vertebrobasilar circulation. The vestibular system is subject to two general categories of vascular ischemia: 1) hypoperfusion in the vertebrobasilar system, in which case multiple areas (both peripheral and central) become simultaneously ischemic, or 2) hypoperfusion in the distribution of a single smaller feeding vessel, in which case a circumscribed area of infarction results. In the former case the site of origin of hypoperfusion can be anywhere from the heart and major vessels in the chest and neck to the basilar artery, while in the latter case an occlusion is usually situated near the origin or, less frequently, in the smaller feeding vessel itself. These two categories of ischemia are not mutually exclusive, however; a patient with small vessel disease may be asymptomatic because of collateral circulation but an added hypoperfusion in the vertebrobasilar system can lead to focal ischemia and/or infarction.

VERTEBROBASILAR INSUFFICIENCY (VBI). VBI is a common cause of vertigo in patients over the age of 50.[43, 93, 96, 341] Whether the vertigo originates from ischemia of the labyrinth, brain stem or both structures is not always clear. It is

Table 12. Initial symptoms of vertebrobasilar insufficiency in 65 patients[341]

Symptom	Number	Percentage
Vertigo	32	48
Visual hallucinations	7	10
Drop attacks or weakness	7	10
Visceral sensations	5	8
Visual field defects	4	6
Diplopia	3	5
Headaches	2	3
Other	5	8

abrupt in onset, usually lasting several minutes, and is frequently associated with nausea and vomiting. In a series of 65 patients with VBI reported by Williams and Wilson, vertigo was the initial symptom in 48 percent (Table 12).[341] The key to the diagnosis of VBI is to find associated symptoms resulting from ischemia in the remaining territory supplied by the posterior circulation (those listed in Table 12). These symptoms occur in episodes either in combination with the vertigo or in isolation. Vertigo may be an isolated initial symptom of VBI but repeated episodes of vertigo without other symptoms suggest a disorder other than VBI.[96]

The cause of VBI is usually atherosclerosis of the subclavian, vertebral and basilar arteries.[94, 341] Other less common causes of arterial occlusion include arteritis, emboli, polycythemia, thromboangitis obliterans and hypercoagulation syndromes. In rare cases occlusion or stenosis of the subclavian or innominate arteries just proximal to the origin of the vertebral artery results in the so-called subclavian steal syndrome.[248] In this syndrome, VBI results from a siphoning of blood down the vertebral artery from the basilar system to supply the upper extremities. Vertigo and other symptoms of VBI are precipitated by exercise of the upper extremities. Occasionally episodes of VBI are precipitated by postural hypotension, Stokes-Adams attacks or mechanical compression from cervical spondylosis. Angiography is helpful in localizing the site of lesion with VBI but often a poor correlation exists between the angiographic and clinical findings. Angiography should not be undertaken unless it is required for diagnosis or it is expected to lead to definitive treatment such as removal or bypass of a focal atherosclerotic lesion.

FOCAL VASCULAR SYNDROMES. *Cochlear Infarction.* The role of vascular occlusion in the production of sudden unilateral deafness is disputed.[197, 260] There is little reason to suspect that sudden deafness in young healthy individuals is secondary to vascular disease. As already suggested most of these cases are probably due to viral infections. However, sudden deafness without associated vertigo or brain stem signs in patients with known vascular disease or hypercoagulation syndromes suggests the possibility of occlusion of the common cochlear artery or one of its branches (see Fig. 22). Sudden deafness has been reported in patients with fat emboli,[166] thromboangitis obliterans[186] and macroglobulinemia.[272] Atherosclerotic disease is also associated with sudden deafness but pathologic confirmation of the site of vascular occlusion is often lacking. Pathologic examination of the cochlea in such patients reveals loss of the organ of Corti, and degenerative changes in the stria vascularis, spiral ligament and distal cochlear nerve

183

fibers.[139] A similar picture is produced in animals after occlusion of the internal auditory artery.[258]

Infarction of the Vestibular Labyrinth. Ischemia confined to the anterior vestibular artery distribution results in infarction of the utricular macule and the cristae of the horizontal and anterior semicircular canals (see Fig. 22). The clinical picture is that of a sudden destruction of one vestibular labyrinth, i.e. sudden onset of severe vertigo without hearing loss or brain stem signs. The patient, recovering from the acute manifestations, often develops episodes of paroxysmal positional nystagmus lasting for several months. Schuknecht[283] postulated that the cause of this paroxysmal positional nystagmus is ischemic necrosis of the utricular macule causing a release of otoconia that settles on the intact cupula of the posterior semiciruclar canal (see Cupulolithiasis). Lindsay and Hemenway[201] reported 7 cases of this syndrome, with examination of the temporal bone in 1 case. All were elderly patients with atherosclerotic vascular disease. The lesion consisted of degeneration of part of Scarpa's ganglion and nerves to the utricle and the anterior and horizontal semicircular canals with a mass of convoluted vessels in the internal auditory meatus, indicating a vascular occlusion as the cause.

Lateral Medullary Syndrome (Wallenberg's Syndrome). The zone of infarction producing the lateral medullary syndrome consists of a wedge of the dorsolateral medulla just posterior to the olive. Although the syndrome is commonly known as that of the posteroinferior cerebellar artery, Fisher and coworkers[97] demonstrated that it usually occurs from occlusion of the ipsilateral vertebral artery, and only rarely with occlusion of the posteroinferior cerebellar artery. Major symptoms include vertigo, nausea, vomiting, intractable hiccupping, ipsilateral facial pain, diplopia, dysphagia and dysphonia.[119]

On examination the following abnormalities may be found: 1) ipsilateral Horner's syndrome from involvement of the preganglionic sympathetic fibers originating in the hypothalamus, 2) ipsilateral loss of pain and temperature sensation on the face due to involvement of the nucleus and descending tract of the fifth nerve, 3) ipsilateral paralyses of the palate, pharynx and larynx from involvement of the nucleus ambiguus and the exiting fibers of the ninth and tenth nerves, 4) ipsilateral facial and lateral rectus weakness from involvement of the sixth and seventh nerves, 5) ipsilateral dysmetria, dysrhythmia and dysdiadokinesia from involvement of the cerebellum, and 6) contralateral loss of pain and temperature sensation on the body from involvement of the crossed spinothalamic fibers. Hearing loss does not occur because the lesion is caudal to the cochlear nerve entry zone and cochlear nuclei.

Patients with Wallenberg's syndrome suffer a prominent motor disturbance that causes their body and extremities to deviate toward the lesion side as if being pulled by a strong external force.[23, 38] This so-called lateropulsion also affects the oculomotor system, causing excessively large voluntary and involuntary saccades directed toward the side of the lesion while saccades away from the lesion side are abnormally small.[188] Spontaneous vestibular nystagmus toward the side of the lesion is usually present with eyes closed[28, 221] while fixation nystagmus in the opposite direction occurs with eyes open and fixating.[188, 221] This results in the unusual occurrence of a spontaneous nystagmus that changes direction with opening and closing of the eyes. If one performs caloric examination with the patient's eyes closed a directional preponderance toward the side of the lesion occurs, whereas with the eyes open a directional preponderance away from the side of the lesion is found.[221] Patients with Wallenberg's syndrome also demonstrate instability of fixation,[221] impaired smooth pursuit[221] and skew deviation.[296]

Lateral Pontomedullary Syndrome. Ischemia in the distribution of the anteroinferior cerebellar artery usually results in infarction of the dorsolateral pontomedullary region and the inferolateral cerebellum.[2, 119] Since the labyrinthine artery arises from the anteroinferior cerebellar artery approximately 80 percent of the time, infarction of the membranous labyrinth is a common accompaniment. Severe vertigo, nausea and vomiting are the initial and most prominent symptoms. Other associated symptoms include unilateral hearing loss, tinnitus, facial paralysis, and cerebellar asynergy. In addition to the signs of ipsilateral hearing loss, facial weakness and cerebellar dysfunction, examination discloses ipsilateral loss of pain and temperature sensation on the face from involvement of the trigeminal nucleus and tract and contralateral decreased pain and temperature sensation on the body from involvement of the crossed spinothalamic tract. Vestibular examination reveals spontaneous vestibular nystagmus away from the side of the lesion and a caloric vestibular paresis on the side of the lesion from involvement of the labyrinth and vestibular nerve. The clinical course is that of an acute onset followed by gradual improvement over a variable period. Vertigo may persist for several weeks to months because of damage to the central compensation mechanisms.

Cerebellar Infarction. In some instances occlusion of the vertebral artery, the posteroinferior cerebellar artery or the anteroinferior cerebellar artery results in infarction confined to the posteroinferior cerebellar hemisphere without accompanying brain stem involvement.[85, 193, 314] The initial symptoms are severe vertigo, vomiting and ataxia and since typical lateral medullary signs do not occur, the mistaken diagnosis of an acute peripheral labyrinthine disorder might be made. The key differential point is the finding on examination of prominent ipsilateral cerebellar signs including asymmetric gaze paretic nystagmus (larger amplitude directed toward the side of the lesion). After a latent interval of 24 to 96 hours, some patients develop progressive brain stem dysfunction due to compression by a swollen cerebellum. A relentless progression to quadriplegia, coma, and death follows unless the compression is surgically relieved.[193, 314]

Hemorrhage

INTRALABYRINTHINE. Spontaneous hemorrhage into the inner ear mainly occurs in patients with an underlying bleeding diathesis. Leukemia is the most common bleeding disorder associated with labyrinthine hemorrhage.[246, 286] Such patients experience sudden onset of unilateral deafness and severe vertigo. Pathologic examination of the inner ear reveals hemorrhage into the perilymphatic space with smaller focal hemorrhages in the endolymphatic space. The vestibular and cochlear end organs, although morphologically intact, are rendered nonfunctional apparently from altered fluid chemistry. A similar condition may follow from blows to the head without the occurrence of bony fracture. Schuknecht and coworkers[288] produced labyrinthine hemorrhage in 5 of 9 cats given experimental head blows that did not produce fractures. The hemorrhage was confined to the perilymph in 4 of 5 animals but in 1 cat blood was also found in the endolymph. The red blood cells that remain in the labyrinthine fluids for extended periods of time might, the authors speculated, interfere with the chemical balance of the fluids leading to degenerative changes in the sensory and neural structures.

185

SUBARACHNOID.   Vertigo is not an infrequent early symptom in acute subarachnoid hemorrhage. Subarachnoid blood enters the ear via two routes—the
cochlear aqueduct and the internal auditory canal.[157, 255] The cochlear aqueduct is
sufficiently large in approximately 50 percent of patients to allow free access of
blood cells to the perilymphatic space. Blood usually cannot enter the perilymphatic or endolymphatic space via the internal auditory canal but it can interfere with
the inner ear function by entering the area of the modiolus and dissecting along the
perineural space of the vestibular nerve as far as the subepithelial layers of the
macules and cristae. The facial nerve may also be affected by blood dissecting in
the perineural spaces of the fallopian canal.

Unruptured *aneurysms* can compress the eighth nerve in the CP angle, producing hearing loss and vertigo.[236, 262] The clinical picture is indistinguishable from
other CP angle mass lesions and angiography is required to identify the nature of
the mass. Minor bleeding may indicate involvement of other nearby cranial nerves
in which case red blood cells would be found on CSF examination. A similar
picture is produced by *arteriovenous malformations* and anomalous or *tortuous
arteries in the CP angle*.

INTRAPARENCHYMAL.   Spontaneous intraparenchymal hemorrhages into the
brain stem and cerebellum produce dramatic clinical syndromes frequently pro-
gressing to loss of consciousness and death.[80] The cause of hemorrhage is *hyper-
tensive vascular disease* in approximately two-thirds of the patients. *Anticoag-
ulation therapy, cryptic arteriovenous malformations* and *bleeding diathesis* are
also important etiologic factors whether alone or in combination with hyperten-
sion.

Because of its potential reversibility, *cerebellar hemorrhage* deserves particular
emphasis. The initial symptoms of acute cerebellar hemorrhage are vertigo,
nausea, vomiting, headache and inability to stand or walk.[80, 104, 243] Examination in
this initial period usually reveals nuchal rigidity, prominent cerebellar signs, ipsilateral facial paralysis and ipsilateral gaze paralysis. The pupils are bilaterally
small but reactive. Approximately 50 percent of patients lose consciousness
within 24 hours of the initial symptoms and 75 percent become comatose within
one week of onset. The condition is often fatal unless surgical decompression is
performed. The earlier the syndrome is recognized the more likely that surgery
will be successful. Once the patient is comatose almost none survive.[44] Midline
cerebellar hemorrhage is particularly difficult to diagnose because it produces
bilateral signs and generally runs a more fulminant course than lateralized hemorrhage.

In contrast to cerebellar hemorrhage, spontaneous hemorrhage into the brain
stem is associated with rapid loss of consciousness usually without prodromal
symptoms. *Intrapontine hemorrhage* results in rapid onset of coma, flaccid quadriplegia, loss of horizontal eye movements, pinpoint reactive pupils, and ocular
bobbing.[80, 98] *Hemorrhage into the medulla* is associated with rapid cardiorespiratory failure and death. Computerized axial tomography has proved to be remarkably effective in identifying hemorrhage in the brain stem and cerebellum.[227]

Neoplasia

Primary Carcinoma

Epidermoid carcinomas arise from epidermal cells of the auricle, external auditory canal or the middle ear and mastoid. The prognosis is good for tumors

confined to the auricle and external canal but not for those invading the middle ear and mastoid. The latter are frequently associated with prominent labyrinthine symptoms which typically include vertigo, hearing loss, pain, otorrhea, mastoid swelling and facial paralysis.[195, 304] The tumor is frequently visible in the external canal and erosion of the temporal bone is apparent on x-ray examination. To treat invasion of the middle ear and mastoid a subtotal resection of the temporal bone is required if the enitre tumor is to be removed. Other less common tumors originating in the external auditory canal and middle ear include *adenoid cystic carcinoma, basal cell carcinoma, mucoepidermoid carcinoma* and *ceruminoma*. These tumors in general are less malignant but occasionally will be locally invasive. Adenoid cystic carcinoma arising from glandular tissue of the external canal and middle ear is often associated with distant metastasis.

Sarcoma

Osteogenic sarcoma and *chondrosarcoma* both occur as rare primary tumors of the temporal bone,[67, 70] running fulminant courses in young adults. Osteolytic lesions with irregular borders indicate the malignant nature of the tumor on x-ray. *Rhabdomyosarcoma* of the middle ear usually occurs in children under the age of five.[167] The initial symptom is often facial paralysis which is misdiagnosed as idiopathic Bell's palsy. In later stages the tumor extends beyond the middle ear to involve the petrous apex and may invade the posterior or middle cranial fossae. Radiologic studies should be obtained on any infant presenting with idiopathic facial paralysis to rule out a rhabdomyosarcoma.

Glomus Body Tumors

Glomus tumors are the most common tumor of the middle ear and next to schwannomas are the most common tumor of the temporal bone. Glomus tumors arise in the glomera of the chemoreceptor system which may be found along the vagus nerve, glossopharyngeal nerve, Jacobson's nerve (tympanic branch of the ninth nerve) and the nerve of Arnold (postauricular branch of the tenth nerve).[138] The most common tumor sites are the glomus jugulare (jugular bulb), glomus tympanicum (middle ear) and the glomus vagale (along the course of the vagus nerve). Glomus vagale and jugulare tumors often involve the labyrinth and cranial nerves while glomus tympanicum tumors usually produce only local symptoms such as conductive hearing loss, pulsatile tinitus and rhinorrhea because of the tumor bulk in the middle ear. Invasion of the labyrinth is an uncommon but serious prognostic sign and is often associated with extension to the petrous apex and into the middle and posterior fossa. The jugular foramen syndrome consisting of ninth, tenth and eleventh nerve involvement occurs with glomus jugulare and vagale tumors.[306] Involvement of the twelfth nerve is an ominous sign indicating destruction of the jugular foramen with tumor extension into the hypoglossal canal and usually into the posterior fossa.

The diagnosis of glomus tumor is often made when routine examination discloses a reddish-blue pulsating mass behind the tympanic membrane (see Fig. 49). Occasionally tumor tissue can be seen in the floor of the external auditory canal. Polytomography is critical for demonstrating the extent of bone destruction. Intracranial invasion is suggested by destruction of the floor of the middle fossa and the posteromedial surface of the petrous apex. With glomus jugulare tumors a jugular venogram reveals a filling defect in the jugular bulb with destruction of the upper end of the internal jugular vein.[111, 112] Angiography usually demonstrates a highly vascular tumor whose blood supply is derived predominantly from a branch of the external carotid artery or less frequently from the vertebral artery.

Schwann Cell Tumors

Tumors arising from the sheaths of the cranial and peripheral nerves have been called neuromas, neurilemmomas and neurofibromas, but convincing evidence that they represent a proliferation of the sheath-producing Schwann cells makes schwannoma a more appropriate term.[204, 267, 282] These tumors are the most common of those arising in the temporal bone and are nearly always associated with neurotologic symptoms and signs. They arise from the vestibular nerve in the internal auditory canal in well over 90 percent of cases and rarely originate from the cochlear nerve.[282] The term acoustic neuroma, therefore, is inappropriate on two accounts. Infrequently the tumor arises from the vestibular nerve terminals near the end organ, in which case end organ destruction occurs, or it may arise from the nerve after it leaves the canal in the CP angle, in which case it can be relatively large before producing symptoms and signs. Schwannomas are usually small, firm encapsulated tumors that grow very slowly. Occasionally hemorrhage into the tumor, cyst formation or associated edema produces clinical evidence of more rapid growth.

Vestibular schwannomas beginning in the internal auditory canal produce symptoms by compressing the nerves in the narrow confines of the canal. As the tumor enlarges it protrudes through the internal auditory meatus, producing a funnel-shaped erosion of the bone surrounding the canal, stretching adjacent nerve roots over the surface of the mass and deforming the brain stem and cerebellum. Vestibular schwannomas account for approximately 10 percent of intracranial tumors and over 75 percent of CP angle tumors.[118] By far the most common symptoms associated with vestibular schwannomas are slowly progressive hearing loss and tinnitus from compression of the cochlear nerve. These symptoms occurred in 90 to 100 percent of patients in several large series.[87, 118] Rarely an acute hearing loss occurs apparently from compression of the labyrinthine vasculature. Vertigo occurs in less than 20 percent of patients but approximately 50 percent complain of imbalance or dysequilibrium. Next to the auditory nerve, the most commonly involved cranial nerves (by compression) are the seventh and fifth, producing facial weakness and numbness, respectively. Involvement of sixth, ninth, tenth, eleventh and twelfth nerves occurs only in the late stages of disease with massive tumors.[69] Large vestibular schwannomas may also produce increased intracranial pressure from obstruction of cerebrospinal fluid outflow resulting in severe headaches and vomiting.

Any patient with a slowly progressive hearing loss should be suspected of having a vestibular schwannoma. The diagnosis is supported by audiometric findings of a sensorineural loss, poor speech discrimination, tone decay and an absent stapedius reflex.[16, 176, 295] Caloric testing shows an ipsilateral vestibular paresis in over 90 percent of cases.[16, 87] Laminography of the internal auditory canal usually reveals erosion of the internal acoustic meatus.[145, 330] Computerized tomograpy identifies large tumors extending in the CP angle but posterior fossa myelography is the most useful procedure for identifying small tumors confined to the meatus.[145, 322] Cerebrospinal fluid protein is often elevated with large tumors but usually normal with small tumors confined to the internal auditory meatus.[143] The importance of early diagnosis of these tumors has been repeatedly stressed since their close association with cranial nerves, brain stem, cerebellum, and the basilar vascular system makes them difficult to manage when large but surgically treatable with low morbidity and mortality when small.[261]

Bilateral vestibular schwannomas occur in approximately 5 percent of patients with *von Recklinghausen's disease* and often they are the sole manifestation of the disease.[349] A young patient with a unilateral vestibular schwannoma and a family history of von Recklinghausen's disease has a high probability of developing a second vestibular schwannoma. Schwannomas arising from the seventh and fifth nerves usually produce slowly progressive facial weakness and numbness, respectively. *Facial nerve schwannomas* often begin in the internal auditory canal and are associated with slowly progressive hearing loss, making it difficult to distinguish them from vestibular schwannomas.[265, 301] Early involvement of the facial nerve is the key distinguishing feature. *Trigeminal nerve schwannomas* develop in the anterior CP angle and usually grow into the middle fossa.[125] They are rarely associated with eighth nerve symptoms and signs.

Other CP Angle Tumors

After schwannomas the most common primary tumors of the CP angle are meningiomas and epidermoid cysts.[118] *Meningiomas* arise from arachnoid fibroblasts usually in the posterior aspect of the petrous pyramid near the sigmoid and petrosal sinuses.[162, 232] They displace cranial nerves and compress the brain stem and cerebellum but do not invade brain tissue. In the posterior fossa the lobulated variety is more common than the flat (en-plaque) type. Meningiomas in the CP angle are frequently calcified and induce osteoblastic reaction in adjacent bone. Both of these features are identified by routine x-ray studies. Angiography usually reveals a vascular tumor with major feeding vessels from the external carotid circulation.

Epidermoid cysts arise from congenital epithelial inclusion rests in the area of the petrous apex.[184] They slowly emerge to fill the CP angle, stretching nearby cranial nerves and compressing the brain stem. Symptoms usually begin before the age of 20. In addition to the usual symptoms and signs of CP angle tumors, hemifacial spasm is a frequent early symptom. Erosion of the petrous apex is found on routine x-rays and posterior fossa myelography often reveals a characteristic scalloped surface contour.[154]

Metastatic Neoplasms

Metastatic involvement of the temporal bone is common with several different tumor types but, apparently because of the enchondral layer's resistance, neoplasms rarely invade the bony labyrinth.[231] The most common site of origin for metastatic tumors in order of frequency are: breast, kidney, lung, stomach, larynx, prostate and thyroid gland.[284] The internal auditory canal is a frequent site of metastatic tumor growth.[264] From this site tumor cells destroy the seventh and eighth nerves, and extend into the inner ear or into the CP angle. Irregular destruction of bone by the rapidly growing tumor is usually apparent on x-ray examination. Metastatic tumors from the breast and prostate commonly incite new bone formation.

Tumors of the Brain Stem and Cerebellum

Gliomas arising in the brain stem usually grow slowly and infiltrate the brain stem nuclei and fiber tracts, producing multiple symptoms and signs.[19, 69] Although these tumors are five to ten times more common in children than adults, they still

189

make up approximately 1 percent of adult intracranial tumors.[339] The neurologic symptoms and signs of childhood brain stem gliomas do not differ in essence from those of adults. The typical history is that of relentless, progressive involvement of one brain stem center after another, often ending with destruction of the vital cardiorespiratory centers of the medulla. Vestibular and cochlear symptoms and signs are common (occurring in approximately 50 percent of cases), the brain stem origin of which is usually obvious because of the multiple associated findings.[19] Acquired fixation, gaze paretic and dissociated nystagmus are frequently present and impairment of saccade and pursuit eye movements further suggests an intrinsic brain stem disorder (see Test of Visual-Ocular Control, Chapter 5).

In contrast to brain stem gliomas, *gliomas of the cerebellum* are relatively silent until they become large enough to obstruct CSF circulation or compress the brain stem.[47, 68, 110] The most common symptoms are headache, vomiting and gait imbalance. Approximately 90 percent of patients have papilledema from increased intracranial pressure.[110] Positional vertigo is occasionally the initial symptom of a cerebellar glioma.[132] Paroxysmal positional nystagmus, when present, is atypical since it can be induced in several different positions and is usually nonfatigable. Caloric examination reveals impaired fixation suppression of vestibular nystagmus. Computer tomography and pneumoencephalography are most useful in establishing the diagnosis of both brain stem and cerebellar gliomas but occasionally a low grade infiltrating glioma will not be identified prior to death. Other tumors that produce identical symptoms and signs include teratomas, hemangiomas and hemangioblastomas.[69]

Tumors arising in the fourth ventricle, compressing the vestibular nuclei in its floor, commonly produce vestibular symptoms. *Medulloblastomas,* occurring primarily in children and adolescents, are rapidly growing, highly cellular tumors that arise in the posterior midline or vermis of the cerebellum and invade the fourth ventricle and adjacent cerebellar hemispheres.[164] Vertigo and dysequilibrium are common initial complaints. Headaches and vomiting also occur early from obstructive hydrocephalus and associated increased intracranial pressure. An attack of headache, vertigo, vomiting and visual loss may result from a change in head position producing transient CSF obstruction (Bruns' symptom). As with cerebellar gliomas, positional vertigo and nystagmus may be the presenting symptom and sign. In Nylen's study of nystagmus in patients with subtentorial tumors,[239] 17 of 27 patients with medulloblastoma demonstrated positional nystagmus, and in 2 cases it was the only focal neurologic sign. Grand reported 2 cases of medulloblastoma in which paroxysmal positional nystagmus was the initial abnormal neurologic sign.[129]

Other fourth ventricle tumors that produce similar clinical pictures include *ependymomas, papillomas, teratomas, epidermoid cysts*[102, 163, 269] and in endemic areas *cysticercosis.*[240] The diagnosis of a fourth ventricular mass is made with computerized tomography and pneumonencephalography, but frequently the exact nature of the tumor cannot be determined prior to surgical exploration and biopsy.

Trauma—Blunt Head Trauma

Temporal Bone Fractures

Fractures of the temporal bone are commonly divided into two types: longitudinal and transverse.[183, 282] *Longitudinal fractures* are approximately four times as common as transverse fractures.[95] They pass parallel to the anterior margin of the petrous pyramid and usually extend medially from the region of the gasserian ganglion to the middle ear and laterally to the mastoid air cells. Typically the fracture line transverses the tympanic annulus, lacerating the tympanic membrane and producing a steplike deformity in the external auditory canal (see Fig. 49).[183] Cerebrospinal and hemorrhagic otorrhea are common and the combination of laceration of the tympanic membrane, ossicular damage and hemotympanum produces a conductive hearing loss. Sensorineural hearing loss and vertigo characteristic of inner ear concussion frequently accompany a longitudinal temporal bone fracture but the bony labyrinth is rarely fractured.[285] Damage to the seventh and eighth cranial nerves is infrequent.

Transverse fractures of the temporal bone run orthogonal to the long axis of the petrous pyramid. In contrast to longitudinal fractures, they usually pass through the vestibule of the inner ear, tearing the membranous labyrinth and lacerating the vestibular and cochlear nerves, producing complete loss of vestibular and cochlear function.[95, 310] Vertigo, nausea, and vomiting are prominent for several days after the fracture, typical of acute unilateral vestibular loss. The facial nerve is lacerated in approximately 50 percent of cases and the loss of function may be permanent unless surgical repair is instituted.[136] Examination of the ear reveals hemotympanum but bleeding from the ear occurs infrequently since the tympanic membrane usually remains intact. CSF often fills the middle ear and drains through the eustachian tube into the nasopharynx. Meningitis is a late complication of both types of temporal bone fractures and therefore a CSF fistula must be identified early and surgically repaired.[10]

Labyrinthine Trauma without Skull Fracture

Auditory and vestibular symptoms (either isolated or in combination) frequently follow blows to the head that do not result in a temporal bone fracture.[73, 148, 168] Voss suggested the name labyrinthine concussion for these symptoms.[168] The absence of associated brain stem symptoms and signs and the usual rapid improvement in symptoms following injury support a peripheral localization for the lesion.[184] Although protected by a bony capsule, the delicate labyrinthine membranes are susceptible to blunt trauma.[288] Of 57 cases of labyrinthine concussion reported by Davey,[73] 51 percent resulted from blows to the occipital region, 26 percent to the frontal and 23 percent to other areas. In the majority of cases the blow resulted in loss of consciousness.

By far the most common symptom of labyrinthine concussion is *positional vertigo*.[18, 73, 82, 124] The patient develops sudden brief attacks of vertigo and nystagmus precipitated by changing head position (see Paroxysmal Positional Nystagmus, Chapter 4). Barber[18] reported positional vertigo with 47 percent of head injuries associated with longitudinal temporal bone fractures and with 21 percent of head injuries of a comparable severity without skull fracture. In over 90 percent of the patients, fatigable paroxysmal positional nystagmus was induced with rapid positional testing (see Fig. 51). Convincing evidence exists that post-traumatic positional vertigo and nystagmus are caused by damage to the labyrinth and a possible mechanism is presented later (see Cupulolithiasis). The prognosis for patients with post-traumatic positional vertigo is good, with spontaneous remission occurring in most patients within six weeks and almost always within two years of the head injury.[18, 73, 124, 285]

Sudden deafness following a blow to the head without associated vestibular symptoms is often partially or completely reversible.[88, 273] It is probably caused by intense acoustic stimulation from pressure waves created by the blow that are transmitted through the bone to the cochlea, just as pressure waves are transmitted from air through the conduction mechanism.[161] Supporting this suggestion, the pathologic changes in the cochlea produced by experimental head blows in animals are similar to those produced by intense airborne sound stimuli.[256, 288] These changes consist of degeneration of hair cells and cochlear neurons in the middle turns of the cochlea. Pure tone hearing loss is usually most pronounced at 4000 and 8000 Hz.

Brain Stem Trauma

Although contrary opinions have been expressed,[48, 105] brain stem injury from blunt head trauma is not likely a common cause of isolated auditory and vestibular symptoms.[54, 73] Severe head blows produce petechial hemorrhages and focal infarction in the brain stem but these pathologic changes are invariably associated with alteration in the level of consciousness and multiple neurologic signs. Mitchell and Adams[219] studied serial sections of the brain stem in 100 cases of fatal blunt head injury. Only 18 patients showed no evidence of increased intracranial pressure and of these only 7 had abnormalities in the brain stem attributable to the primary impact. In these 7, other areas of the brain were damaged, suggesting to the authors that so-called "primary brain stem injury" does not exist but rather is one aspect of diffuse brain damage.

Caloric examination is particularly useful in evaluating the brain stem status in patients who are comatose from blunt head injuries.[41, 218, 263] These patients do not produce saccades so that a "normal" response is a conjugate tonic deviation of the eyes toward the side of a cold stimulus or away from the side of a warm stimulus. Absence of this tonic deviation affirms that the brain stem vestibulo-ocular reflex pathways have been damaged, assuming the eighth nerve and end organs are intact. Unilateral loss of tonic deviation or nonconjugate deviation indicates focal involvement of the reflex pathways. The absence of caloric responses after an acute head injury is a poor prognostic sign.[218, 263]

Postconcussion Syndrome

The postconcussion syndrome has long been the center of medicolegal controversy.[66, 217 313] Symptoms include dizziness, headache (usually diffuse), increased irritability, insomnia, forgetfulness, mental obtuseness and loss of initiative, all of which may arise after a severe head injury with loss of consciousness or may follow what seems to have been a trivial blow to the head. Because of the ill-defined nature of these symptoms, it is difficult to localize the site of lesion and the patient is frequently diagnosed as being psychoneurotic (compensation neurosis).[217] The dizziness associated with the postconcussion syndrome is usually a nonspecific lightheadedness. If vertigo is present an additional labyrinthine lesion should be suspected.

Rutherford and coworkers[274] followed 145 patients with concussion from minor head injuries to assess the type and frequency of symptoms and to evaluate whether the symptoms correlated with the severity of injury, associated neurologic signs, or other circumstances related to the injury. Concussion was defined as a period of amnesia, no matter how brief, caused by a blow to the head. All of the patients were released from the hospital after brief observation. Table 13 lists the symptoms and their frequency of occurrence reported by the 145 patients six weeks after the concussion. Approximately one-half were symptom-free while

Table 13. Symptoms reported six weeks after a concussion in 165 patients[274]

Symptom	Number	Percentage
Headache	36	24.8
Anxiety	28	19.3
Insomnia	22	15.2
Dizziness	21	14.5
Irritability	13	9.0
Fatigue	13	9.0
Loss of concentration	12	8.3
Loss of memory	12	8.3
Hearing defect	10	6.9
Sensitivity to alcohol	9	6.2
Depression	8	5.5
Visual defect	7	4.8
Anosmia	4	2.8
Epilepsy	3	2.1
Diplopia	2	1.4
Other	16	11.0
No symptoms	71	49.0

the other half complained of one or more symptoms. In those patients with multiple symptoms no consistent pattern was found to support the concept of a postconcussion syndrome. A significant correlation existed between the presence of multiple symptoms at six weeks and the occurrence of positive neurologic signs and symptoms within 24 hours of the concussion. Postconcussion symptoms were more frequent in women, and in patients who blamed their employers or large impersonal organizations for their accidents. The authors concluded that both organic and psychosomatic factors were involved in the pathogenesis of postconcussion symptoms.

Surgical Trauma

Patients who have undergone surgery near the inner ear frequently develop vestibular and auditory symptoms during the postoperative period.[6, 282] Most commonly implicated are 1) mastoidectomy for infection and/or keratoma and 2) stapedectomy for otosclerosis. With *mastoid surgery,* the lateral semicircular canal may be inadvertently opened because of its prominent position in the floor of the mastoid antrum. A perilymph fistual results and if the membranous labyrinth is torn the resulting communication between endolymph and perilymph leads to profound unilateral loss of auditory and vestibular function.[6] The bony fistula usually requires surgical exploration and repair.

Stapedectomy provides amelioration of severe conductive hearing loss in patients with fixed immobile stapes, but several complications result in disabling vestibular and auditory symptoms. The most important complication, a fistula of the oval window, manifests itself anytime from a few days to months after surgery.[150, 152, 158] Its characteristic symptoms are dysequilibrium, episodic vertigo, and a sensorineural hearing loss that fluctuates in severity. Vestibular examination frequently reveals vestibular nystagmus, positional nystagmus, and decreased caloric response. Other complications of stapedectomy include reparative granuloma, foreign bodies in the vestibule and adhesions in the vestibule.[108,202] Dysequilibrium, episodic vertigo and fatigable paroxysmal positional nystagmus may be associated with each of these complications.

Rupture of the Oval and Round Windows

Fistulae of the oval and round windows result from impact noise, deep water diving, severe physical exertion or blunt head injury without skull fracture.[91,121,266,319] The mechanism of the rupture is a sudden negative or positive pressure change in the middle ear or possibly a sudden increase in CSF pressure transmitted to the inner ear via the cochlear aqueduct. Clinically, the rupture leads to the sudden onset of vertigo and/or hearing loss. Goodhill and coworkers[121] explored the middle ear in 21 cases of sudden deafness and found evidence of fistulae of the oval window in 9, round window in 1, and both windows in 5 ears. Ten of the fifteen patients with fistulae had a definite history of severe exertion or head trauma prior to the onset of symptoms. Most patients complained of vertigo and had vestibular nystagmus and/or caloric hypoexcitability. It is unlikely that labyrinthine window rupture is a common cause of sudden deafness, however, and surgical exploration is only indicated when a clear cut association exists between the onset of symptoms and either exertion, barometric change, head injury or impact noise.[282]

Metabolic Disorders

Diabetes Mellitus

Vestibular symptoms and signs are common in patients with diabetes mellitus but convincing evidence does not exist for a specific vestibular lesion.[180] In those diabetic patients with vestibular dysfunction whose temporal bones and nervous systems have been studied at necropsy, pathologic changes can be explained on the basis of associated vascular disease.[179,206,282] Three types of vascular changes occur with diabetes mellitus: 1) endothelial proliferation narrowing the lumens of arterioles, capillaries and venules, 2) arteriosclerotic narrowing of small arteries and arterioles, and 3) atherosclerotic narrowing of large arteries. These vascular changes may damage the vestibular system from the peripheral end organ and vestibular nerve to its diffuse CNS connections.

The most common finding in the labyrinth of patients with diabetes mellitus is a PAS-positive thickening of the capillary walls,[179] most prominent in the vascular stria of the cochlea where it probably accounts for the progressive bilateral high frequency hearing loss characteristic of the disease. Similar changes are found in the vestibular end organs which, along with degeneration of the vestibular nerve and ganglion, could explain the frequent complaints of chronic dysequilibrium and dizziness in diabetic patients.

Sudden onset of hearing loss and/or vertigo in patients with diabetes mellitus results from occlusion of the vessels to the labyrinth or the eighth nerve.[180] Cranial nerve mononeuropathy is a well known clinical phenomenon associated with diabetes mellitus and is most likely due to arteriosclerotic occlusion of arterioles supplying the cranial nerves. Atherosclerosis of larger vessels predisposes the patient to transient vertebrobasilar insufficiency and to specific occlusive syndromes such as the anterior vestibular artery syndrome and the lateral medullary

194

syndrome. Gladney and Shepherd[115] suggested that auditory and vestibular dysfunction occur in the prediabetic state similar to the retinal and renal changes that develop before the onset of clinical diabetes mellitus. This supposition was based on the finding of abnormal glucose tolerance in 19 patients with auditory and vestibular symptoms of unknown cause. These findings may have represented a sampling deviation, however, and better controlled studies are needed before such symptoms are ascribed to the prediabetic state.

Uremia

Multiple causes of auditory and vestibular symptoms can be identified in patients with chronic renal disease.[30] The same pathologic process can affect both the kidneys and the labyrinths, as seen in Alport's syndrome (hereditary nephritis and deafness), diabetes mellitus and Fabry's disease. Immunosuppressive treatment either of the primary renal disorder or to avoid transplant rejection predisposes the patient to otologic infections, often with exotic or saprophytic organisms. Patients with renal disease are particularly vulnerable to the ototoxic effects of aminoglycoside antibiotics and ototoxic diuretics because of their inability to clear these substances from the blood—probably the most common cause of auditory and vestibular symptoms in uremic patients.[30]

Hyponatremia causes reversible hearing loss and tinnitus in patients undergoing chronic hemodialysis. Yassin and coworkers[348] found a high degree of correlation between hearing loss and serum sodium levels irrespective of the blood urea level. The hearing loss could be corrected by returning the serum sodium level to normal in 80 percent of patients with acute renal failure and in 52 percent of those with chronic renal failure. Patients undergoing chronic hemodialysis and those receiving kidney transplants often experience ill-defined fluctuating auditory and vestibular symptoms. Oda and coworkers[241] performed necropsy studies on the temporal bones of 8 patients with chronic uremia who had undergone long term hemodialysis therapy (24 to 546 treatments). At least one kidney transplant was performed in 7 of the 8 patients. Vestibular symptoms occurred in 5 patients and auditory symptoms in 3; all symptoms began after the start of hemodialysis. Abnormal concretions were found in the vascular stria of the cochlea and in the subepithelial connective tissue of the macules and cristae in 7 of the 8 patients. The source of these abnormal deposits is unknown.

Metabolic Disorders of the Temporal Bone

Otosclerosis is a disease of the bony labyrinth that usually manifests itself by immobilizing the stapes and thereby producing a conductive hearing loss.[53, 191] Seventy percent of patients with clinical otosclerosis notice hearing loss between the ages of 11 and 30. A positive family history for otosclerosis is reported in approximately 50 percent of cases. Although this disease is primarily considered a disorder of the cochlea, vestibular symptoms and signs are more common than is generally appreciated. Approximately 25 percent of patients with proven otosclerosis complain of episodic vertigo and unsteadiness when walking. Virolainen[332] compared the results of vestibular function testing in 60 patients with otosclerosis and 20 normal controls. Over 50 percent of the patients had abnormalities in the following order of frequency: caloric vestibular paresis, heightened threshold of angular acceleration, caloric directional preponderance and positional nystagmus.

The basic pathologic process of otosclerosis is a resorption of normal bone, often around blood vessels, and its replacement by cellular fibrous connective tissue.[282] With time, immature basophilic bone is produced in the resorption space; after several cycles of resorption and new bone formation a mature acidophilic bone with a laminated matrix is produced. Areas of predilection for otosclerotic foci include the oval window region, the round window niche, the anterior wall of the internal auditory canal and within the stapedial footplate. Sando and coworkers[277] studied 4 temporal bones of 2 patients with otosclerosis who complained of prominent vestibular symptoms and found otosclerotic foci in opposition to the superior vestibular nerve in each. Vestibular nerve degeneration distal to these foci was also present and 3 of the 4 temporal bones exhibited a marked degeneration of the sensory epithelium of the cristae of the lateral semicircular canals. The authors speculated that these pathologic changes could explain the frequent clinical vestibular disorders occurring with otosclerosis. Although conductive hearing loss is the hallmark of otosclerosis, a combined conductive sensorineural hearing loss pattern is frequent.[135] The sensorineural component is perhaps caused by foci of otosclerosis next to the spiral ligament of the cochlea producing atrophy of the spiral ligament.

Paget's disease is a metabolic disorder of bone marked by pronounced osteoclastic resorption of old fully-calcified bone and deposition of new osteoid layers that calcify normally. The clinical picture varies from the classic one of an enlarged skull, progressive kyphosis and short stature to the more common restricted forms confined to the skull, spine, pelvis and femur.[74] Hearing loss is a common symptom initially described by Paget in his early reports and subsequently studied in detail by numerous investigators.[58, 74, 244, 317] A progressive combined sensorineural and conductive hearing loss is usually found. The vestibular labyrinth may also be progressively destroyed resulting in unsteadiness of gait and, in rare cases, episodic vertigo. In the late stages complete destruction of the bony labyrinth may occur with invasion of the inner ears, fractures and degeneration of the membranous labyrinth.[200] The diagnosis rests on the characteristic roentgenographic findings of areas of increased density of bone with loss of the normal architecture, mingled with areas of decreased bone density. The skull is enlarged with indistinct margins giving a "cotton wool" appearance.

Other less common temporal bone disorders that are associated with hearing loss include *osteogenesis imperfecta*,[242, 294] *fibrous dysplasia*[293, 321] and *osteopetrosis*.[144, 177] Because the clinical picture is often indistinguishable from that of otosclerosis the diagnosis depends on finding the characteristic roentgenographic features of each disease.

Thiamine Deficiency

Wernicke's encephalopathy is a common clinical syndrome caused by thiamine deficiency (usually secondary to malnutrition from chronic alcoholism).[331] It is characterized by the subacute onset of confusion, ophthalmoplegia, and ataxia of stance and gait. Vertigo and hearing loss are not common complaints. The truncal ataxia is often dramatic, with the patient being unable to take even a few steps without support, and yet standard cerebellar function testing with finger-to-nose and heel-to-shin is usually normal or minimally impaired. The ataxia is increased with eye closure or darkness. These findings suggest a combination of midline cerebellar and either proprioceptive or vestibular impairment. Two recent reports[113, 123] have documented impaired bithermal caloric responses in 56 patients with acute Wernicke's encephalopathy. The majority of patients did not respond to caloric stimulation, even with ice water. Symmetrical gaze paretic nystagmus was also a frequent finding in the acute stages.

Although the ophthalmoplegia, confusion and ataxia rapidly respond to thiamine replacement, the patient is frequently left with a memory disorder (Korsakoff's syndrome) and mild ataxia. In patients receiving thiamine replacement, the vestibular function as measured by serial caloric testing slowly returns toward normal over several weeks, although in some cases the recovery is asymmetric and incomplete.

The main pathologic changes involving the vestibular system in Wernicke's encephalopathy take place in the vestibular nuclei. In the studies by Victor and coworkers,[331] the medial vestibular nucleus was involved in 71 percent of cases, with the lateral, superior and descending nuclei being involved in 50, 36 and 30 percent of cases, respectively. The changes in the vestibular nuclei were relatively mild, however, compared to the frank necrosis and demyelination occurring in other areas. Experimental studies in thiamine deficient rats[320] reveal that the earliest pathologic changes originate in the vestibular nuclei, particularly the lateral nucleus. The nerve terminals and axons degenerate without evidence of damage to the neuronal parikaria. Neurologic signs appear even before these early pathologic changes. Loss of transketolase activity (a thiamine dependent enzyme) in the lateral pontine tegmentum including the lateral vestibular nuclei correlates better with the onset of clinical signs. Injection of thiamine promptly restores transketolase activity and improves clinical signs. Apparently the majority of clinical findings (including the impaired vestibular function) are secondary to thiamine dependent enzyme loss in the brain stem and only after prolonged and/or repeated episodes of deficiency do irreversible structural changes occur.

Familial Ataxia Syndromes

Auditory and vestibular disturbances are common in the hereditary ataxia syndromes although in many instances the site of pathologic involvement has not been adequately investigated.[15, 42, 271] Of the well defined syndromes, *Friedreich's ataxia, olivopontocerebellar degeneration, Roussy-Lévy syndrome* and *Refsum's disease* are all associated with loss of vestibular and auditory function. In addition, several isolated families with atypical ataxia syndromes associated with hearing loss and absent vestibular function have been reported.[42] Clinically the loss of vestibular function may be overshadowed by the cerebellar findings and only after performing caloric or rotatory testing is the impaired vestibular function recognized. Because of the progressive bilateral symmetrical loss of vestibular function, vertigo is rarely experienced. Pathologic nystagmus commonly occurs including gaze paretic, vestibular, positional and rebound nystagmus.[15]

Only a few pathologic studies of the audiovestibular end organs and nervous pathways have been reported in patients with hereditary ataxia. Spoendlin[309] studied the temporal bones in 2 sisters with Friedreich's ataxia and found extensive degeneration of the neurons of the eighth nerve (both auditory and vestibular) with preservation of the peripheral receptor organs. These changes correlated with the clinical findings of progressive bilateral deafness and caloric hypoexcitability for several years prior to death. Involvement of the vestibular nuclear complex has been well documented in several familial ataxia syndromes but the vestibular nerves and labyrinths have not been examined in the patients.[42] The vestibular dysfunction associated with familial ataxia syndromes is probably due to a

197

combination of vestibular nuclei and nerve degeneration without involvement of the vestibular end organs.

Developmental Defects

Malformations of the Inner Ear

Although congenital deafness is usually recognized during infancy, congenital vestibular impairment is not because the manifestations are more subtle. Children learn to use other sensory information to compensate for vestibular loss and appear normal on standard developmental tests. Congenital deafness has therefore received extensive study while congenital vestibular loss has been relatively neglected. Congenital deformities of the inner ear are divided into two major categories: hereditary and acquired. Hereditary disorders result from abnormal genes and acquired disorders result from abnormal development of a normal fertilized egg.

HEREDITARY. Several hereditary syndromes produce sensorineural deafness and bilateral vestibular loss. *Alport's syndrome* is manifested by a sex-linked dominantly inherited sensorineural deafness and interstitial nephritis. Miller and coworkers[216] found decreased vestibular responses in several patients with Alport's syndrome and suggested an associated vestibular system disorder. The inner ear histology is normal and tomographic x-ray studies are negative, which is consistent with the absence of bony defects.[107, 216] Abnormalities of lipid and amino acid metabolism have been reported but the exact enzyme defect or defects are yet to be identified.[282]

Waardenburg's syndrome is a dominantly inherited sensorineural deafness associated with: 1) lateral displacement of the medial canthae and lacrimal punctae, 2) hyperplastic high nasal root, 3) hyperplasia of the medial portions of the eyebrows, 4) partial or total heterochromia iridis and 5) circumscribed albinism of the frontal head hair (white forelock).[333] Vestibular function is usually impaired bilaterally[208] and tomographic x-ray studies of the temporal bone reveal bony anomalies of the inner ear. Ophthalmologic evaluation can be helpful in defining the characteristic eye signs. Of particular importance, Marcus[208] studied a large family with Waardenburg's syndrome and found several children who had vestibular malfunction despite normal hearing with minimal or no other signs of the syndrome.

A combination of recessively inherited retinitis pigmentosa and sensorineural deafness is known as *Usher's syndrome*.[141, 329] The hearing loss is present at birth but the retinitis pigmentosa is not recognized until about the age of 10 when the patient develops night blindness and/or contraction of the visual fields. Caloric responses are usually diminished bilaterally.[334]

Extra or transposed chromosomes result in multiple congenital defects. *Trisomy 13* and *trisomy 18* are both associated with malformations of the inner ear and decreased auditory and vestibular function.[39, 190] The more common trisomy 21 (Down's syndrome) does not produce ear deformities.[282]

ACQUIRED. The most common cause of acquired congenital malformations of the inner ear is maternal *rubella* infection during the critical developmental period (first 9 weeks of gestation for vestibular development and first 25 weeks for auditory development). Infants born to mothers who acquire rubella in the first trimester of pregnancy may have multiple congenital defects including cataracts, patent ductus arteriosus, microcephaly, dental defects, and generally impaired growth and development.[19, 339] Hearing loss is more common than vestibular function loss (apparently because of the longer critical developmental period). Although less common, the infant's fully developed inner ear can be damaged by a maternal rubella infection in the last two trimesters.[223] Other important causes of acquired congenital inner ear defects include: maternal drug or toxin ingestion, hyperbilirubinemia, anoxia associated with a difficult birth, and cretinism.[282]

PATHOLOGY. The first pathologic study of an inner ear congenital malformation was reported by Mundini in 1791.[228] The *Mundini malformation* consists of subtotal development of the osseous and membranous labyrinth with only the basal turn of the cochlea being completely formed.[25] The endolymphatic duct system is dilated and the vestibular labyrinth is underdeveloped. This deformity occurs with many different syndromes, both hereditary and acquired, and is invariably associated with some (and often complete) loss of auditory and vestibular function. Cochleosaccular dysgenesis initially described by Scheibe consists of dysplasia of the pars inferior (cochlea and saccule) with a fully developed bony labyrinth and normal pars superior (semicircular canals and utricle).[279] The *Scheibe deformity* is frequently produced by congenital rubella accounting for the relative sparing of vestibular function in many of these children. A rare deformity characterized by complete failure of development of the inner ear (*Michel deformity*) is associated with total loss of auditory and vestibular function. This deformity has been found in several patients with Thalidomide anomalies of the ear.[315] X-ray tomography of the inner ear is particularly helpful in identifying malformations but it can only identify bony malformations[170] and not those of the sensory epithelium. Because of its bony changes the Mundini malformation is most consistently identified by tomography.

Malformations of the Foramen Magnum Region

BONY. Bony malformations of the craniovertebral junction occur frequently and may bear no relation to clinical findings.[215, 308] Two of the more common defects, fusion of the cervical vertebrae and basilar impression, are associated with the clinical complaint of dizziness and with other bony defects and malformations of the brain stem and cerebellum. *Basilar impression* is a deformity of the base of the skull in which the bony rim of the foramen magnum is elevated into the cranial cavity. Cerebellar ataxia and damage to the lower cranial nerves result from cerebellar and brain stem compression. The diagnosis is confirmed when lateral x-rays of the skull demonstrate that the odontoid process extends well above Chamberlain's line (line drawn from the posterior edge of the hard palate to the posterior lip of the foramen magnum).[55]

Many different varieties of *cervical vertebral fusion* have been reported. Klippel and Feil initially described a patient with only 4 cervical vertebrae that were fused into a single column of bone.[187] These anatomic features were associated with a clinical triad of short neck, low hairline and limitation of neck movements. Although partial coalescence of two or more cervical vertebrae occurs in many patients, few develop the syndrome originally described by Klippel and Feil. Spillane and coworkers[308] suggested that fusion of cervical vertebrae should be called congenital cervical synostosis and that the term *Klippel-Feil* should be used to describe only typical clinical syndromes associated with either complete fusion of the cervical spine or reduction in the number of cervical vertebrae. Patients with the classic Klippel-Feil syndrome have a high incidence of deafness. McLay and Maran[213] studied the temporal bone of one such patient and found a vestigial inner ear having a rudimentary cystic cavity for a cochlea and only one semicircular canal, incompletely formed. The inner ear abnormalities with Klippel-Feil syndrome may be unilateral or bilateral and may be appreciated on tomographic study of the temporal bone.

SOFT TISSUE. Of the cervicomedullary developmental defects *syringobulbia* and *Arnold-Chiari malformations* commonly produce vestibular symptoms. Either may be associated with bony defects of the craniovertebral region and frequently the two deformities occur together in the same patient. Both may be associated with cervical *syringomyelia*. Syrinx formation in the medulla (syringobulbia) damages any of the lower cranial nerve nuclei, but most often involves the twelfth nuclei and the descending tract and nucleus of the fifth nerve, producing atrophy, and fasciculations of the tongue and loss of pain and temperature sensation on one or both sides of the face. Dysphonia and dysphagia are also prevalent because of damage to the ninth and tenth nuclei.[20] Pathologic nystagmus is a common finding in all reported series and occasionally it is the only abnormal neurologic sign.[323] Fixation nystagmus (either horizontal or vertical), periodic alternating nystagmus and dissociated nystagmus may occur when eyes are open and fixating, vestibular nystagmus when fixation is inhibited. Patients with fixation nystagmus and periodic alternating nystagmus complain of oscillopsia and in some reported cases this is the initial symptom of syringobulbia.

Arnold in 1894 and Chiari in 1895 described a congenital malformation of the hindbrain in which the brain stem and cerebellum were elongated downward into the cervical canal. Most frequently the deformity manifests itself in the first few months of life and is associated with hydrocephalus and other nervous system malformations. Less frequent but more important to the neurotologist are those cases in which the onset of symptoms and signs is delayed until adult life. These cases often present with subtle neurologic symptoms and signs and are usually unassociated with other developmental defects.[17] The most common neurologic symptom is slowly progressive unsteadiness of gait which the patient frequently describes as dizziness. Vertigo and hearing loss occur in less than 10 percent of patients.[276] On neurologic examination the patient is ataxic with eyes open, suggesting midline cerebellar involvement. Pathologic nystagmus is nearly always present.[24, 308] Downbeat fixation nystagmus in particular occurs frequently with Arnold-Chiari malformation[64] but other forms of fixation nystagmus (upbeat and horizontal), periodic alternating nystagmus and rebound nystagmus also occur. As with syringobulbia, oscillopsia is a common complaint. Any adult presenting with oscillopsia and fixation nystagmus should be suspected of having syringobulbia and/or an Arnold-Chiari malformation. Dysphagia, hoarseness and dysarthria result from stretching of the lower cranial nerves and obstructive hydrocephalus results from occlusion of the basal cisterns. The diagnosis is made with contrast studies (air and oil) of the cervicomedullary junction region.

Toxic Disorders

Aminoglycosides

The common ototoxic aminoglycosides are *streptomycin, kanamycin, neomycin* and *gentamycin*. Although each of these drugs produce both auditory and vestibular loss, streptomycin and gentamycin are relatively specific for the vestibular end organ while kanamycin and neomycin primarily damage the auditory end organ.

Streptomycin was the first antibiotic found to be effective against tuberculosis. Many of the early clinical reports documented that parenteral streptomycin in a dose of 2 to 3 gms per day usually resulted in complete loss of vestibular function in two to four weeks.[45, 90] More prolonged treatment results in progressive auditory impairment. The patient rarely complains of vertigo but consistently reports unsteadiness of gait, particularly at night or in a darkened room. Serial caloric examinations document a progressive bilateral loss of vestibular responsiveness. Some patients develop spontaneous vestibular nystagmus with the fast component directed away from that ear which shows a more rapidly decreasing caloric response. Because of this highly selective effect on the vestibular end organ streptomycin has been used to produce a chemical vestibulectomy in patients with episodic vertigo from Meniere's syndrome.[299]

The sensorineural hearing loss caused by aminoglycosides usually begins at the high frequencies and progresses to a flat 60 to 70 db loss across all frequencies. Neomycin has the undesirable effect of producing delayed ototoxic effects that may occur weeks to months following administration.[292] Serial audiograms are mandatory for any patient receiving aminoglycosides, but because of these delayed effects it is difficult to monitor neomycin toxicity. In patients with renal failure all of the aminoglycosides should be used with great caution and neomycin should rarely be used.

The ototoxicity of the aminoglycosides has been convincingly shown to be due to hair cell damage in the inner ear. Unlike penicillin and other common antibiotics, aminoglycosides are concentrated in the perilymph and endolymph.[312] Streptomycin primarily damages the hair cells of the cristae with relative sparing of the hair cells of the macules and cochlea. When streptomycin is given to animals hair cell damage is most pronounced in the central part of the crista, type I hair cells being more vulnerable than type II hair cells.[196, 338] According to histologic studies the loss of hair cells is not associated with changes in the supporting elements or the vestibular nerves. Lundquist and Wersäll[203] found gentamycin to be more toxic than streptomycin when given in equal doses to guinea pigs. Their histologic studies of the vestibular hair cells in the gentamycin treated guinea pigs revealed a ballooning of the cell surface and mitochondrial degeneration beginning in the type I cell. Loss of cochlear hair cells has been documented with each of the aminoglycosides. The external hair cells of the basal turn of the cochlea appear to be particularly vulnerable.

Salicylates

Patients receiving high dose salicylate therapy frequently complain of hearing loss, tinnitus, dizziness, loss of balance and, occasionally, vertigo. Sensorineural hearing loss involves all frequencies and is associated with recruitment, suggesting a cochlear rather than a nervous system etiology.[128, 211, 230] The tinnitus is high pitched and frequently precedes the onset of hearing loss. Both hearing loss and tinnitus invariably occur when the plasma salicylate level approaches 0.35 mg per milliliter.[128] Caloric testing often reveals bilaterally depressed responses consistent with bilateral vestibular end organ damage.[32] All symptoms and signs are rapidly reversible after the cessation of salicylate ingestion (usually within 24 hours). As with aminoglycosides, salicylates are highly concentrated in the perilymph and preliminary evidence suggests that they interfere with enzymatic activity of the hair cells and/or the cochlear neurons.[298]

Heavy Metals

Both lead and mercury intoxication are known to produce auditory and vestibular symptoms, but the pathophysiologic mechanism of these symptoms is poorly understood. Gozdzik-Zolnierkiewicz and Moszynski[126] found segmental demyelination and axonal degeneration of the eighth nerve in 23 of 32 young guinea pigs given weekly intraperitoneal injections of 1 percent *lead* acetate solution for seven weeks. The end organs and ganglion cells showed no visible morphologic changes. Wilpizeski[343] performed similar experiments in adult squirrel monkeys and found minimal changes in the auditory and vestibular systems both on chemical and histologic examination. The difference in findings may be due to the well known decreased susceptibility of the adult nervous system to lead toxicity. Hearing loss and vertigo have occasionally been reported in isolated cases of childhood and adult lead poisoning, but no detailed study has been undertaken of auditory and vestibular function in a large population of lead poisoned patients.

In contrast to lead, two large patient populations with organic *mercury poisoning* have undergone detailed neurotologic testing in Japan. Mizukoshi and coworkers[220] studied 144 patients with organic mercury poisoning acquired from eating contaminated fish caught in the Aganagawa River in Niigata. Impaired hearing was found in 50 percent of the patients and 67 percent complained of dizziness and unsteadiness of gait. Episodes of vertigo were reported in 10 percent. Audiologic examination revealed sensorineural hearing loss, usually consistent with a cochlear origin in the early stages and a retrocochlear origin in later stages. Spontaneous vestibular nystagmus was present in 27 percent, 17 percent had gaze paretic nystagmus and 65 percent positional nystagmus. Results of caloric testing were reported to be abnormal in 46 percent of cases with a directional preponderance being the most consistent finding. Unfortunately, normative data were not included for comparison and therefore the frequent occurrence of a caloric directional preponderance must be interpreted with caution. Similar findings on neurotologic examination were reported in patients who acquired mercury poisoning from eating seafood caught in Minamata Bay.[238]

The site of vestibular and auditory dysfunction in mercury poisoned patients is unknown. Anniko and Sarkady[9] produced chronic mercury intoxication in guinea pigs and found distortion of the endothelial cells of labyrinthine blood vessels. They speculated that these morphologic changes cause altered vascular permeability and impaired labyrinthine function. Necropsy studies have not been performed on the temporal bones and eighth nerves from patients dying of mercury intoxication. Examination of the CNS in such patients reveals a selective sensitivity of the granule-cell layer of the neocerebellum but cases of demyelination of the subcortical and brain stem white matter and peripheral nerves have also been reported.[160, 316]

Alcohol

Acute alcohol intoxication is regularly associated with unsteadiness of gait, slurring of speech and, occasionally, vertigo. The gait unsteadiness with eyes open and slurring of speech are suggestive of cerebellar dysfunction but an additional vestibular dysfunction must also be considered. Vestibular function testing with rotatory stimulation in patients with alcohol intoxication has revealed normal vestibulo-ocular reflex gain in the dark but impaired fixation suppression of vestibular nystagmus consistent with cerebellar dysfunction.[114, 137] Wilkinson and coworkers[340] showed that vestibulo-ocular (doll's eye) movements were normal in alcohol intoxicated subjects when equal-velocity smooth pursuit movements were markedly impaired.

Positional nystagmus is a well documented effect of alcohol on the vestibular system.[11] Within 30 minutes after ingesting a moderate amount of alcohol (for example, 100 ml of whiskey) the subject develops a direction-changing stationary positional nystagmus (SPN) often associated with vertigo. The SPN beats to the right in the right lateral position and to the left in the left lateral position. Nystagmus is not present in the supine position and the SPN is inhibited by fixation. The primary phase SPN reaches its peak in about two hours at approximately the time of peak blood alcohol level (0.1 percent for the above example). Four to five hours after alcohol ingestion, when the blood alcohol level is below 0.01 percent, SPN is still present, but now is right-beating in the left lateral position and left-beating in the right lateral position (secondary phase). The SPN can last up to 12 hours at which time alcohol cannot be detected in the blood.

The studies of Money and Myles[222] provide a reasonable explanation for alcohol positional nystagmus. These investigators produced a direction-changing SPN in the reverse direction of primary alcohol SPN by giving the subjects heavy water, H_3O. When subjects with alcohol direction-changing SPN (primary phase) were given H_3O the nystagmus disappeared. The authors interpreted these findings to indicate that alcohol and heavy water direction-changing SPN were due to a variable rate of diffusion of alcohol and heavy water into the cupula and the surrounding endolymph. In the primary phase of alcohol SPN, alcohol rapidly diffuses into the base of the cupula because of the latter's proximity to blood capillaries while it slowly diffuses into the endolymph. The cupula then has a lower specific gravity than the endolymph and acts as a gravity sensing organ, maintaining a slight deflection as long as the position is held. After approximately three hours, the endolymph and cupula have approximately the same alcohol concentration and the SPN disappears. As the blood alcohol level falls the reverse situation occurs with the cupula being heavier than the surrounding endolymph, and the secondary phase of SPN occurs.

Syndromes of Unknown or Multiple Causes

Meniere's Syndrome

CLINICAL PICTURE. Meniere's syndrome is characterized by fluctuating hearing loss and tinnitus, episodic vertigo and a sensation of fullness or pressure in the ear. The clinical syndrome was first described by Prosper Meniere in 1861 but Hallpike and Cairns made the first clinicopathologic correlation with hydrops of the labyrinth.[14, 142] Subsequently numerous pathologic studies have been reported and the pathologic findings of endolymphatic hydrops are remarkably consistent in patients with the syndrome originally described by Meniere.

Typically the patient with Meniere's syndrome develops a sensation of fullness and pressure along with decreased hearing and tinnitus in one ear. Vertigo rapidly follows reaching a maximum intensity within minutes and then slowly subsiding over the next several hours. The patient is usually left with a sense of unsteadiness and dizziness for days after the acute vertiginous episode. In the early stages the hearing loss is completely reversible but in later stages a residual hearing loss remains. Tinnitus may persist between episodes but usually increases in intensity during the acute episode. Nausea and vomiting often occur and the patient prefers to lie in bed without eating until the acute symptoms pass. Such episodes occur at irregular intervals for years with long periods of remission unpredictably inter-mixed. Eventually severe permanent hearing loss develops and the episodic na-ture spontaneously disappears ("burnt-out phase"). In approximately 20 percent of patients bilateral involvement will occur.[60]

Variations from this classic picture occur, particularly in the early stages of the disease process, but the diagnosis remains uncertain unless the combination of fluctuating hearing loss and vertigo occurs. Although so-called vestibular Meniere's and cochlear Meniere's have been proposed as variations of the classic syndrome, clinicopathologic correlation of isolated vestibular and auditory disor-ders with selective endolymphatic hydrops of the vestibular and auditory labyrinth is lacking. Some patients with well documented Meniere's syndrome experience abrupt episodes of falling to the ground without loss of consciousness or associated neurologic signs. These episodes have been called otolithic catas-trophes by Tumarkin[327] because of his suspicion that they represented acute stimulation of the otoliths from the hydrops.

DIAGNOSIS. The key to the diagnosis of Meniere's syndrome is to document fluctuation in the pure tone audiometric thresholds.[5] In the early stages the pure tone hearing loss is usually greater in the lower frequencies but this finding cannot be absolutely relied upon. Speech discrimination is relatively preserved and re-cruitment usually occurs consistent with the cochlear site of dysfunction. Vestibu-lar examination may reveal spontaneous vestibular nystagmus and either a ves-tibular paresis or directional preponderance on caloric examination. During the acute episode vestibular nystagmus may be directed toward the involved ear, suggesting an excitatory rather than a destructive effect. Complete loss of either auditory or vestibular function is unusual with Meniere's syndrome.

PATHOPHYSIOLOGY. The principle pathologic finding in patients with Meniere's syndrome is an increase in the volume of endolymph associated with a distention of the entire endolymphatic system.[7] The membranous labyrinth pro-gressively dilates until the saccular wall makes contact with the stapes footplate and the cochlear duct occupies the entire vestibular scala. The cochlear and vestibular end organs and nerves show minimal pathologic changes. Membranous labyrinth herniations and ruptures are common, the latter frequently involving Reissner's membrane and the walls of the saccule, utricle and ampullae. Occa-sionally a rupture is followed by complete collapse of the membranous labyrinth.

Although the pathologic changes in Meniere's syndrome have been well de-scribed, the mechanism for its fluctuating symptoms and signs are not well under-stood. Perfusing the perilymph space of animals with a potassium solution inhibits the bioelectric activity of the cochlea and produces prominent vestibular nystag-mus.[282, 297] When the artificial perfusate is stopped the potassium is slowly cleared from the perilymph and labyrinthine function returns to normal in two to three hours. These observations led to the theory that the episodes of hearing loss and vertigo that occur with Meniere's syndrome are caused by ruptures in the mem-branes separating endolymph from perilymph, producing a sudden increase in potassium concentration in the latter.[192] Another possible explanation for the fluctuating symptoms is mechanical deformation of the end organ that is reversible as the endolymphatic pressure decreases.[8, 199] The dramatic sudden falling attacks initially described by Tumarkin are likely due to sudden deformation or displace-ment of one of the vestibular sense organs.

ETIOLOGY. Several diseases are known to produce Meniere's syndrome but in the majority of cases the cause is unknown. Bacterial, viral and syphilitic labyrinthitis (see Infection) can all lead to endolymphatic hydrops and typical symptoms and signs of Meniere's syndrome. The hydrops apparently results from damage to fluid resorptive mechanisms due to inflammation and scarring. Several authors have suggested that the term Meniere's disease should apply to the idiopathic variety and secondary syndromes should be referred to as Meniere's syndrome or endolymphatic hydrops. This can lead to confusion. A simpler approach is to refer to those cases with unknown cause as idiopathic Meniere's syndrome and to those when a specific disorder is known as Meniere's syndrome secondary to that specific disorder, such as Meniere's syndrome secondary to syphilitic labyrinthitis.

Multiple etiologic possibilities have been proposed for idiopathic Meniere's syndrome including allergy,[79, 344] endocrine disturbances,[116, 117] infection,[194, 347] sympathetic vasomotor disturbances,[247] and psychosomatic factors.[305, 336] Patients with idiopathic Meniere's syndrome frequently have a positive family history (in some reports as high as 50 percent), suggesting genetic predisposing factors.[31, 46] Several investigators have produced endolymphatic hydrops in animals by either blocking the endolymphatic duct or destroying the endolymphatic sac.[26, 185, 233, 289] This led to a series of surgical procedures designed to open the endolymphatic duct in patients with idiopathic Meniere's syndrome. The results of such surgical procedures have been reported with varying degrees of enthusiasm; further controlled studies are needed to assess their usefulness. At the present time no compelling evidence exists to choose one cause over another for Meniere's syndrome.

Cogan's Syndrome

In 1945, Cogan described 4 patients who presented with a clinical syndrome of interstitial keratitis, episodic vertigo, tinnitus and profound deafness.[63] These patients had no clinical or laboratory evidence of syphilis or any other specific disease. Since this original report approximately 50 clinical studies have been reported and a few cases have been studied pathologically.[59, 302, 345] The onset of symptoms is abrupt with severe vertigo, nausea, vomiting and hearing loss. The hearing loss may initially be unilateral but within a few weeks to months both sides are involved. The eye and ear manifestations may occur simultaneously or the onset of one may be delayed for several months. The only other nervous system sign reported has been bilateral facial weakness in 2 patients.

Audiologic examination reveals a sensorineural pure tone hearing loss, which is often complete. Caloric responses are diminished or absent. Visual acuity is usually normal but slit lamp examination of the cornea reveals a granular infiltrate, patchy in distribution, situated predominantly in the posterior half of the cornea.

Cogan's syndrome is often part of a general systemic illness.[61, 100] Five reported cases occurred in patients with well documented polyarteritis nodosa; one patient had proven sarcoidosis. In many other cases described in the literature clinical manifestations suggested collagen vascular disease. One of us (RB) has followed a patient who developed biopsy-proven polyarteritis nodosa three years after presenting with symptoms and signs of Cogan's syndrome. Pathologic studies of the temporal bone are sparse and have not shown localized vasculitis even in patients with prominent vasculitis in other organs. The most consistent finding has been diffuse degeneration of all neural elements in the inner ear. Endolymphatic hydrops was found in 1 case. In accord with speculation that Cogan's syndrome is an immunological disorder, patients have responded transiently to steroid treatment. The usual course, however, is that of progression to bilateral deafness with or without steroid treatment.

Cupulolithiasis

The term cupulolithiasis was introduced by Schuknecht when he proposed a new theory on the pathophysiology of positional vertigo of the "benign" paroxysmal type (see Chapter 4, Positional Nystagmus).[281] Schuknecht studied the temporal bones of 2 patients who had manifested typical fatigable paroxysmal positional nystagmus in the left head-hanging position and found basophilic deposits on the cupulae of the posterior canals of the left ear in each patient. The posterior canal cupulae of the right ears were normal in appearance. Schuknecht and Ruby[290] subsequently reported another identical case, then examined 391 temporal bones from 245 individuals to assess the incidence in the general population of cupular deposits. They found small deposits in 125, medium deposits in 20 and large deposits in 4; in none did the deposits exceed the size of those found in the 3 patients with paroxysmal positional nystagmus.

Schuknecht postulated that the cupular basophilic deposits were otoconia released from a degenerating utricular macula. The otoconia settles on the cupula of the posterior canal (situated directly under the utricular macule) causing it to become heavier than the surrounding endolymph and thus sensitive to changes in the gravity vector. When the patient moves from the sitting to head-hanging position (provocative test for paroxysmal positional nystagmus) the posterior canal moves from an inferior to superior position, a utriculofugal displacement of the cupula occurs, and a burst of nystagmus is produced. Schuknecht further speculated that the latency before nystagmus onset is due to the period of time required for the otoconial mass to be displaced and that fatigability is caused by dispersement of particles in the endolymph. Consistent with this theory, the burst of rotatory paroxysmal positional nystagmus is in the plane of the posterior canal of the "down" ear with the fast component directed upward, as would be predicted from ampullofugal stimulation of the posterior canal (unpublished observation). Additional support for this concept has come from a report showing disappearance of fatigable paroxysmal positional nystagmus after the ampullary nerve has been sectioned from the posterior canal on the diseased side.[109] This mechanism cannot explain all cases of fatigable paroxysmal positional nystagmus, however, which may occur with lesions of the cerebellum in animals[92] and with CNS lesions in humans.[149]

Vestibular Neuronitis

The term vestibular neuronitis was introduced by Dix and Hallpike[82] to describe a clinical syndrome manifested by vestibular symptoms and signs (either acute or chronic) that were not associated with auditory or other neurologic findings. Of the initial 100 patients described, some complained of acute episodes of vertigo while others reported a persistent feeling of dysequilibrium when walking or standing. A prior history of febrile illness or ear, nose and throat infection was frequently elicited. Abnormal caloric responses were found in all 100 cases—bilateral in 47 and unilateral in 53. Caloric vestibular paresis occurred most commonly, followed by a combined vestibular paresis and directional preponderance and, in a few cases, the latter alone. Because of the absence of cochlear signs and because of impaired galvanic responses in 13 of 16 patients tested, Dix and Hallpike hypothesized that the vestibular lesion was localized to the peripheral nervous pathways up to and including the vestibular nuclei in the brain stem. The term vestibular neuronitis they felt would "encompass this uncertainty" of pathologic localization.

On reviewing the case material reported by Dix and Hallpike, one may reach the conclusion that they were dealing with a group of patients manifesting vestibular disorders of multiple causes. It is likely that infectious, postinfectious, vascular and toxic disorders were all represented in their sample. The only common finding in all the patients was abnormal caloric responses, which documents a vestibular impairment but provides little information about cause. Therefore, the use of the term vestibular neuronitis as a specific disease entity may suggest that the pathologic process is known when in fact it is not. Drachman and Hart[84] proposed that the term vestibulopathy of unknown cause was more appropriate for describing isolated vestibular disorders for which a specific diagnosis could not be made. As an understanding of vestibular disease pathophysiology improves this category should become smaller.

Bell's Palsy

Bell's palsy has been considered a cranial mononeuropathy of unknown cause limited to the facial nerve. Some patients complain of dizziness, however, and vestibular testing may reveal evidence of vestibular impairment.[259, 268, 270] The dizziness is usually described as a sense of unsteadiness but vertigo occurs in a small percentage of patients. Caloric testing reveals a vestibular paresis on the side of the facial paralysis in approximately 20 percent of the cases and occasionally responses are decreased bilaterally. Two likely possibilities to explain the associated vestibular findings in patients with Bell's palsy are: 1) the same disease process involves the seventh and eighth nerves or 2) the swollen facial nerve compresses the superior vestibular nerve which it closely accompanies in the internal auditory canal. Support for the first possibility derives from the similar picture of combined seventh and eighth nerve involvement with herpes zoster oticus and the frequent finding of serologic evidence of viral infection in patients with Bell's palsy.[4, 326] Support for the second possibility can be found in the report by Adour and coworkers[3] in which 2 patients being treated for Bell's palsy with large doses of steroids experienced vertigo when the steroids were abruptly stopped. They postulated the vertigo was due to rebound edema of the facial nerve resulting in compression of the vestibular nerve.

Multiple Sclerosis

Multiple sclerosis is a CNS demyelinating disease of unknown cause with onset usually in the third and fourth decades of life.[52, 210] The key to the diagnosis is the finding of disseminated signs of CNS dysfunction manifested in an alternately remitting and exacerbating course. No specific laboratory test for multiple sclerosis exists but spinal fluid gamma globulin is elevated in 80 to 90 percent of patients at some time in the course of the disease. The symptoms of multiple sclerosis are too diverse to enumerate, emanating from lesions anywhere in the CNS from the spinal roots and spinal cord to the subcortical white matter. Certain symptoms do deserve comment, however, because of the consistency of their occurrence. Blurring and/or loss of vision due to demyelination of the optic nerve (retrobulbar neuritis) is the initial symptom of multiple sclerosis in approximately 20 percent of cases. Diplopia, weakness, numbness, and ataxia also occur early in the disease process. Vertigo is the initial symptom in approximately 5 percent of cases and is reported at some time during the course of the disease in as many as 50 percent of patients.[29, 210] Hearing loss rarely occurs initially but approximately 10 percent of patients will eventually develop some detectable hearing loss (usually in the later stages).[237]

The findings on examination are as diverse as the symptoms.[210] In most longstanding cases there are signs of involvement of the pyramidal tracts (hyperreflexia, extensor plantar responses), cerebellum (intention tremor, ataxia, scanning speech), sensory tracts (impaired vibratory and postural sensitivity) and visual pathways (decreased visual acuity and pallor of the optic discs). Pathologic nystagmus is found in approximately 90 percent of multiple sclerosis patients during the course of their disease. Multiple sclerosis produces every variety of pathologic nystagmus described in Chapter 4. The finding of dissociated nystagmus on lateral gaze or acquired pendular fixation nystagmus is particularly helpful in diagnosing multiple sclerosis since these two varieties are common with multiple sclerosis and relatively unusual with other disease processes. [12, 62] All varieties of positional nystagmus including fatigable paroxysmal positional nystagmus occur in patients with multiple sclerosis and caloric examination is abnormal in approximately 25 percent of patients.[1, 72] Vestibular paresis (either unilateral or bilateral) and directional preponderance can each occur. In addition to documenting pathologic nystagmus and quantifying caloric responses, ENG recordings are particularly useful in evaluating patients with suspected multiple sclerosis since they detect smooth pursuit, saccade and optokinetic nystagmus abnormalities that are not apparent on visual inspection of eye movements.[209, 237, 303]

The demyelination in multiple sclerosis is confined to CNS myelin; the myelin produced by oligodendrogliocytes. Peripheral nerve myelin produced by Schwann cells is not affected. Since both peripheral and cranial nerves contain CNS myelin at their root entry zones, a demyelinated plaque involving the root entry zone may produce signs of peripheral nerve dysfunction. Plaques involving the vestibular and auditory root entry zones can explain the findings of unilateral caloric hypoexcitability and hearing loss in patients with multiple sclerosis. In a typical demyelinated plaque the majority of myelin sheaths are destroyed and those that remain become swollen and fragmented. The axis cylinders and neurons are relatively spared so that conduction of nerve impulses still occurs although at a decreased frequency and rate. Whether the remissions and exacerbations of symptoms and signs are related to repair of demyelinated regions or changes in the physiology of nerve conduction unrelated to demyelination is currently unknown. It has been repeatedly shown, however, that there is a poor correlation between the clinical symptoms experienced during life and pathologic findings at necropsy.

Migraine

Migraine is a syndrome characterized by periodic headaches.[346] It is often familial and occurs in many complex patterns and settings.[106] Two types of migraine headaches are commonly encountered—classic and common. *Classic migraine* begins with an aura (usually visual although other neurologic symptoms, including vertigo, are not uncommon) before the onset of a severe unilateral throbbing headache. The aura usually lasts 10 to 20 minutes and the headache begins as the aura diminishes. The headache reaches a peak in approximately one hour and then gradually subsides, disappearing in four to eight hours. Nausea and vomiting usually accompany the onset of head pain. The visual phenomena (most commonly a scintillating scotoma) and other focal neurologic symptoms usually occur on the side opposite to that in which the headache subsequently occurs.

Common migraine can best be described as a "sick" headache. It is preceded by vague prodromal symptoms but aura phenomena are absent. The headache (usually unilateral but occasionally bilateral) builds slowly in intensity and may go on for several days in a row. Nausea, vomiting, diarrhea, chills and prostration often occur. The mechanism of migraine (common and classic) is incompletely understood but the most likely explanation is that the headache is due to dilatation of extracranial and dural arteries and the aura phenomena are due to constriction of intracranial arteries resulting in transient ischemia in the territory of the constricted vessel.[346]

Dizziness is a common complaint with both classic and common migraine and patients frequently report a sense of unsteadiness during the entire period of headache. Vertigo is less common and usually occurs only during the aura of classic migraine. Bickerstaff[33] reported an unusual variety of migraine in which the aura consisted of posterior fossa symptoms such as vertigo, ataxia, dysarthria and tinnitus along with positive visual phenomena in both visual fields. These aura symptoms lasted from 2 to 45 minutes and were followed by a throbbing unilateral occipital headache. Between attacks many of the patients experienced classic migraine episodes and over the years the atypical episodes were replaced with more typical ones. Adolescent girls comprised 26 of the 34 reported cases and the attacks were strikingly related to their menstrual periods. Bickerstaff postulated that the aura phenomena were secondary to vasoconstriction in the vertebrobasilar system and called the syndrome *basilar artery migraine*. He further postulated that patients with vertigo as part of a more usual migraine aura (such as visual scotoma) develop ischemia simultaneously in the distribution of several vessels including the basilar artery.

The possibility of an association between *migraine and Meniere's syndrome* was initially suggested by Meniere in his original paper on the syndrome. Since then numerous cases have been reported in which migraine and Meniere's attacks occurred in the same patient. Most commonly, the patient has classic migraine episodes for many years before developing symptoms and signs of Meniere's syndrome. Atkinson[13] reported 4 such patients and postulated a common vascular abnormality for the two disorders, in one case affecting the CNS and in the other the labyrinth. He reported that treatment successful in relieving the vertigo of Meniere's syndrome also relieved the migraine headaches. This interesting hypothesis deserves further attention but no well controlled studies have been conducted demonstrating an increased incidence of the combined occurrence of migraine and Meniere's syndrome.

Patients with migraine demonstrate more vestibular abnormalities on neurotologic examination than age-matched control subjects. Dursteler[86] studied 30 patients with migraine, 13 percent of whom complained of vertigo during their attacks. Pathologic vestibular nystagmus was found in 17 percent and 33 percent had abnormal caloric responses. Both of these findings were significantly different from the control population at the 0.025 level. Audiologic testing by comparison was normal. Dursteler also proposed a common vascular cause for the migraine and vestibular impairment.

Focal Seizure Disorders

Since well documented cortical projections from the vestibular nuclei exist it could be predicted that focal epileptic discharge from some areas of the cortex would result in sensations of altered orientation and vertigo (see Chapter 3, Subjective Sensation). In Penfield and Kristansen's[252] series of 222 patients with focal seizures in which the irritable focus was identified at the time of surgery, 9 reported an ictal sensory experience of vertigo. In 8 of these patients the causal lesion was found in the posterior half of the superior temporal gyrus or at the parietotemporal junction. Electric stimulation of these areas produced vertiginous experiences similar to those experienced during a spontaneous seizure. Other investigators reported vertiginous auras with lesions in other parts of the temporal and parietal lobe, suggesting that corticovestibular projections were more diffuse than suggested by Penfield and Kristansen's studies.

Smith[300] studied 120 patients with focal seizures who experienced vestibular symptoms as part of their aura. He attempted to define the cortical focus of origin on the basis of associated symptoms. The most common vestibular symptom was a sense of spinning (occurring in 55 percent of cases) followed by a sense of linear movement occurring in 30 percent of cases. Common associated symptoms and their frequency of occurrence were: visceral and autonomic in 62 percent, visual in 45 percent, auditory in 28 percent and somatosensory in 22 percent. Of the visceral and autonomic complaints an abnormal epigastric sensation was most frequently followed by nausea, mastication and salivation. Visual illusions and hallucinations occurred frequently suggesting a close functional relationship between cortical visual and vestibular projections. Auditory symptoms included tinnitus, auditory hallucinations and auditory illusions. Mapping the suspected cortical foci on the basis of these associated symptoms suggested that lesions of the frontal, parietal and temporal cortex can result in vestibular symptoms as part of the aura phenomena. It must be emphasized, however, that episodic vertigo as an isolated manifestation of a focal seizure disorder is a rarity if it occurs at all.

Behrman and Wyke[27] reported an unusual case in which caloric stimulation induced a complex seizure beginning with vertigo followed by right-sided clonic motor activity. EEG recordings made at the time of the seizure registered bitemporal theta activity. The authors postulated that these seizures represented a form of reflex epilepsy and proposed the term vestibulogenic seizure to emphasize the vestibular role in seizure induction. Several subsequent reports of vestibulogenic seizures have been published; the most complete being that of Cantor.[51] Cantor's patient developed typical temporal lobe seizures after a cold caloric stimulus in the right ear only. EEG recording suggested that a focus in the contralateral temporal lobe was activated by the caloric stimulus. Cantor postulated that the caloric stimulus induced a seizure because of the excessive responsiveness of a damaged, deafferented cortex.

Cervical Vertigo

Although the term cervical vertigo has been used as a specific diagnosis, several different mechanisms exist by which lesions in the cervical region might produce vertigo.

VASCULAR LESIONS. Because of their long course through the bony canal of the cervical vertebrae, the vertebral arteries are vulnerable to compression by cervical osteoarthritic spurs.[146] Frequently compression results from a particular head movement such as lateral rotation or hyperextension. Extreme hyperextension of the neck can occlude the vertebral arteries even in normal subjects but collateral circulation via the carotid arteries is usually adequate to prevent symptoms.[94] In patients with atherosclerotic vascular disease the already compromised cerebral circulation may be further impaired by vertebral occlusion and symptoms of VBI result (see section on vascular disease). Typical histories in such patients are those of: 1) a housewife who develops VBI when reaching for an item from a high overhead shelf and 2) a truck driver who develops VBI when backing his vehicle from a loading dock.

As discussed previously, vertigo is a prominent symptom with VBI but is invariably associated with other brain stem symptoms and signs and rarely, if ever, occurs as an isolated recurrent symptom.[96] Vertebral angiography with the head and neck in the provocative position may demonstrate the site of vertebral artery blockage. Surgical removal of the osteoarthritic spurs has been accomplished in a small number of patients.[337]

The so-called posterior cervical sympathetic syndrome of Barre is a disputed cause of vertigo arising from cervical lesions. Barre proposed that cervical lesions might irritate the sympathetic vertebral plexus and result in a decreased blood flow to the labyrinth due to constriction of the internal auditory artery.[22] Although numerous clinical reports of Barre's syndrome have been published, few objective data exist to support an association between episodic vertigo and cervical sympathetic dysfunction. Since intracranial circulation is autoregulated independently of cervical sympathetic control it is unlikely that lesions of the vertebral sympathetic plexus could produce focal constriction of the vasculature to the inner ear.

ALTERED PROPRIOCEPTIVE INPUT.   The role of lesions involving the deep neck proprioceptive afferents in the production of vertigo and dyseqilibrium is disputed (see Neck-Vestibular Interaction, Chapter 3). Some investigators feel that cervical lesions are a common cause of vertigo[37, 130, 178, 275] while others feel they are a rare cause.[189] Interruption of unilateral neck afferent input in normal human subjects by injection of a local anesthetic near the upper cervical joints results in vertigo and ataxia.[77] The subjects report a sensation of falling or tilting toward the side of injection and when walking they deviate toward the injected side. Although animals consistently develop spontaneous nystagmus after unilateral cervical anesthesia, human subjects have not done so despite prominent vertigo and ataxia. This may be due either to a species specificity or to some difficulty with injecting local anesthetics near the upper cervical vertebrae in humans.[77]

Biemond[34, 35] described 5 patients with unilateral cervicobrachial radiculoneuritis who developed vertigo and positional nystagmus when assuming a particular position. The positional nystagmus beat toward the side of the diseased brachial plexus. In 4 of these patients the vertigo and nystagmus cleared as the radiculoneuritis cleared. The same author[36] reported a patient who developed positional vertigo and nystagmus after unilateral section of the third and fourth cervical sensory roots in the course of removal of multiple neurinomas. For several days after the operation the patient developed nystagmus when rotating the head with respect to the trunk and on turning the entire body about its longitudinal axis. In these and other reports of vestibular symptoms and signs associated with neck lesions a concomitant vestibular lesion cannot be ruled out. For example, the same etiologic factor might produce a radiculoneuritis and a labyrinthitis and surgical procedures involving cervicodorsal roots often result in the loss of large quantitites of CSF that might in turn affect labyrinthine function.[280] Despite these reservations, however, convincing reports suggest that certain acute lesions of the high cervicodorsal roots may lead to symptoms indistinguishable from those produced by labyrinthine disease.

A more perplexing problem because of the frequency of occurrence and the medicolegal ramifications is the role of the soft tissue injuries of the neck (whiplash injuries) in producing vertigo and dysequilibrium.[155, 165, 324, 328] The type of dizziness is often ill-defined but vertigo is occasionally described. In many instances the dizziness lasts for months or years after the injury although it usually disappears as the swelling and pain subside. Several reports indicate a high incidence of positional and spontaneous nystagmus on electronystagmographic examination in such patients.[65, 325] Unfortunately, matched control subjects have not been studied and the findings must be interpreted with caution since normal subjects frequently have both spontaneous and positional nystagmus when tested with eyes closed (see Recording Pathologic Nystagmus, Chapter 5).

From the known anatomic substrate for neck-vestibular interaction (see Chapter 3) it is unlikely that lesions involving only soft tissues of the neck could produce vertigo and dysequilibrium. The major neck afferent input to the vestibular nuclei arises in the paravertebral joints and capsules with a relatively minor input from the paravertebral muscles. The skin and superficial muscles do not appear to provide any input to the vestibular nuclei. In addition, the relative contribution of neck afferent input to the vestibular nuclei is small compared to direct labyrinthine and visual signals transmitted via the cerebellum. Lesions involving the neck afferents in primates are rapidly compensated and therefore prolonged dizziness after neck injuries of any type would be difficult to explain on the basis of damage to the neck afferent input to the vestibular nuclei.[77]

REFERENCES

1. AANTAA, E., RIEKKINEN, P. J., AND FREY, H. J.: *Electronystagmographic findings in multiple sclerosis.* Acta Otolaryngol. 75:1, 1973.

2. ADAMS, R.: *Occlusion of the anterior inferior cerebellar artery.* Arch Neurol. Psychiat. 49:765, 1943.

3. ADOUR, K., ET AL.: *Prednisone treatment for idiopathic facial paralyses (Bell's palsy).* New Eng. J. Med. 287:1268, 1972.

4. ADOUR, K. K., AND DOTY, H. E.: *Electronystagmographic comparison of acute idiopathic and Herpes zoster facial paralysis.* Laryngoscope 83:2029, 1973.

5. ALFORD, B.: *Menieres disease: criteria for diagnosis and evaluation of therapy for reporting. Report of Subcommittee on Equilibrium and its Measurement.* Trans. Amer. Acad. Ophthalmol. Otolaryngol. 76:1462, 1972.

6. ALTMAN, F.: *Healing of fistulas of the human labyrinth: Histopathologic studies.* Arch. Otolaryngol. 43:409, 1946.

7. ALTMAN, F., AND KORNFELD, M.: *Histological studies of Menieres disease.* Ann. Otol. Rhinol. Laryngol. 74:915, 1965.

8. ALTMAN, F., AND ZECHNER, G.: *The pathology and pathogenesis of endolymphatic hydrops. New investigations.* Arch. Klin. Exper. Ohr-Nas-Kehlkheilk 192:1, 1968.

9. ANNIKO, M., AND SARKADY, L.: *Morphological changes of labyrinthine blood vessels following metal poisoning.* Acta Otolaryngol. 83:441, 1977.

10. APPLEBAUM, E.: *Meningitis following trauma to the head and face.* JAMA 173:1818, 1960.

11. ASCHAN, G., AND BERGSTEDT, M.: *Positional alcoholic nystagmus (PAN) in man following repeated alcohol doses.* Acta Otolaryngol. (Suppl. 330):15, 1975.

12. ASCHOFF, J. C., CONRAD, B., AND KORNHUBER, H. H.: *Acquired pendular nystagmus with oscillopsia in multiple sclerosis: a sign of cerebellar nuclei disease.* J. Neurol. Neurosurg. Psychiat. 37:570, 1974.

13. ATKINSON, M.: *Meniere's syndrome and migraine; observations on a common causal relationship.* Ann. Intern. Med. 18:797, 1943.

14. ATKINSON, M.: *Menieres original papers: Reprinted with an English translation together with commentaries and biographical sketch.* Acta Otolaryngol. (Suppl. 162):14, 1961.

15. BALOH, R. W., KONRAD, H. R., AND HONRUBIA, V.: *Vestibulo-ocular function in patients with cerebellar atrophy.* Neurology 25:160, 1975.

16. BALOH, R. W., ET AL.: *Cerebellar-pontine angle tumors: Results of quantitative vestibulo-ocular testing.* Arch. Neurol. 33:507, 1976.

17. BANERJI, N. K., AND MILLAR, J. H. D.: *Chiari malformation presenting in adult life.* Brain 97:157, 1974.

18. BARBER, H.: *Positional nystagmus especially after head injury.* Laryngoscope 74:891, 1964.

19. BARNETT, H. J., AND HYLAND, H. H.: *Tumours involving the brain stem.* Quant. J. Med. 21:265, 1952.

20. BARNETT, H. J. M., FOSTER, J. B., AND HUDGSON, P.: *Syringomyelia.* Saunders, London, 1973.

21. BARR, B., AND LUNDSTRÖM, R.: *Deafness following maternal rubella.* Acta Otolaryngol. 53:413, 1961.

22. BARRÉ, M. J. A.: *Sur un syndrome sympathique cervical postérieur et sa cause fréquente: l'árthrite cervicale.* Rev. Neurol. 1:1246, 1926.

23. BARRÉ, M. J. A.: Le nystagmus et le syndrome vestibulaire dans plusiers cas personnels de syndrome de Babinski-Negeotte et de Wallenberg. Rev. Otoneurooptalmol. 5:945, 1927.

24. BARROWS, L. J., AND COGAN, D. G.: *Ocular manifestations of the Arnold-Chiari malformation.* AMA Arch. Neurol. Psychiat. 72:116, 1954.

25. BEAL, D., DAVEY, P., AND LINDSAY, J.: *Inner ear pathology of congenital deafness.* Arch. Otolaryngol. 85:134, 1967.

26. BEAL, D.: *Effect of endolymphatic sac ablation in the rabbit and cat.* Acta Otolaryngol. 66:333, 1968.

27. BEHRMAN, S., AND WYKE, B. D.: *Vestibulogenic seizures. A consideration of vertiginous seizures, with particular reference to convulsions produced by stimulation of labyrinthine receptors.* Brain 81:529, 1958.

28. BENDER, M. B.: Disorders of eye movements. In: *Handbook of Clinical Neurology.* North-Holland Publishing Company, Amsterdam, 1969.

29. BENTZEN, O., JELNES, K., AND THYGESEN, P.: *Acoustic and vestibular function in multiple sclerosis.* Acta Psychiat. Scand. 26:265, 1951.

30. BERGSTROM, L., ET AL.: *Hearing loss in renal disease: clinical and pathological studies.* Ann. Otol. Rhinol. Laryngol. 82:555, 1973.

31. BERNSTEIN, J.: *Occurrence of episodic vertigo and hearing loss in families.* Ann. Otol. Rhinol. Laryngol. 74:1011, 1965.

32. BERNSTEIN, J. M., AND WEISS, A. D.: *Further observations on salicylate ototoxicity.* J. Laryngol. Otol. 81:915, 1967.

33. BICKERSTAFF, E. R.: *Basilar artery migraine.* Lancet 1:15, 1961.

34. BIEMOND, A.: *On a new form of experimental position-nystagmus with the rabbit and its clinical value.* Proc. K. Ned. Akad. Wet. 42:370, 1939.

35. BIEMOND, A.: *Further observations about the cervical form of positional nystagmus and its anatomical base.* Proc. K. Ned. Akad. Wet. 43:901, 1940.

36. BIEMOND, A.: *Nystagmus de position d'origine cervicale.* Psychiat. Neurol. Neuroclin. 64:149, 1961.

37. BIEMOND, A., AND DEJONG, J. M. B. V.: *On cervical nystagmus and related disorders.* Brain 92:437, 1969.

38. BJERNER, K., AND SILFVERSKIÖLD, B. P.: *Lateropulsion and imbalance in Wallenberg's syndrome.* Acta Neurol. Scand. 44:91, 1968.

39. BLACK, F., ET AL.: *Middle and inner ear abnormalities, 13–15 (D_1) trisomy.* Arch. Otolaryngol. 93:615, 1971.

40. BLACKLEY, B., FRIEDMANN, I., AND WRIGHT, I.: *Herpes zoster auires associated with facial nerve palsy and auditory nerve symptoms.* Acta Otolaryngol. 63:533, 1967.

213

41. BLEGVAD, B.: *Caloric vestibular reaction in unconscious patients.* Arch. Otolaryngol. 75:36, 1962.

42. BOGAERT, L. VAN, AND MARTIN, L.: *Optic and cochleovestibular degenerations in the hereditary ataxias. I. Clinico-pathological and genetic aspects.* Brain 97:15, 1974.

43. BRADSHAW, P., AND MCQUAID, P.: *The syndrome of vertebrobasilar insufficiency.* Quart. J. Med. 32:279, 1963.

44. BRENNEN, R. W., AND BERGLAND, R. M.: *Acute cerebellar hemorrhage. Analysis of clinical findings and outcome in 12 cases.* Neurology 27:527, 1977.

45. BROWN, H., AND HINSHAW, H.: *Toxic reaction of streptomycin on the eighth nerve apparatus.* Proc. Staff Meeting, Mayo Clinic 21:347, 1946.

46. BROWN, M.: *The factor of heredity in labyrinthine deafness and paroxysmal vertigo (Meniere's syndrome).* Ann. Otol. Rhinol. Laryngol. 58:665, 1949.

47. BUCY, P. C., AND THIEMAN, P. W.: *Astrocytomas of the cerebellum.* Arch. Neurol. 24:125, 1971.

48. BRUNNER, H.: *Disturbances of the function of the ear after concussion of brain.* Laryngoscope 50:921, 1940.

49. BURROWES, W.: *Acute labyrinthitis.* Brit. Med. J. 2:408, 1952.

50. CANDILL, R. G., SMITH, C. E., AND REINARZ, J. A.: *Coccidioidal meningitis: A diagnostic challenge.* Am. J. Med. 49:360, 1970.

51. CANTOR, F. K.: *Vestibular-temporal lobe connections demonstrated by induced seizures.* Neurology 21:507, 1971.

52. CARTER, S. D., SCIARRA, D., AND MERRITT, H. H.: *The course of multiple sclerosis as determined by autopsy-proven cases.* Res. Publ. Assn. Nerv. Ment. Dis. 28:471, 1950.

53. CAWTHORNE, T.: *Otosclerosis.* J. Laryngol. 69:437, 1955.

54. CAWTHORNE, T.: Discussion of Chapters XII and XIII. In Fields, W. S., and Alford, B. R. (eds.): *Neurologic Aspects of Auditory and Vestibular Disorders.* Charles C Thomas, Springfield, Illnois, 1964.

55. CHAMBERLAIN, W. E.: *Basilar impression (platybasia).* Yale J. Biol. Med. 11:847, 1939.

56. CHANDLER, J.: *Malignant external otitis.* Laryngoscope 78:1257, 1968.

57. CHARTERS, A.: *Epidemic vertigo in Kenya.* E. African Med. J. 34:7, 1957.

58. CLEMIS, J., ET AL.: *The clinical diagnosis of Paget's disease of the temporal bone.* Ann. Otol. Rhinol. Laryngol. 76:611, 1967.

59. CODY, D., AND WILLIAMS, N.: *Cogan's syndrome.* Laryngoscope 70:447, 1960.

60. CODY, D.: Rehabilitation for sensorineural hearing loss. In Paparella, M., Hohmann, A., and Huff, J. (eds.): *Clinical Otology—An International Symposium.* C. V. Mosby Co., St. Louis, Missouri, 1971.

61. COGAN, D., AND DICKERSIN, G.: *Non-syphilitic interstitial keratitis with vestibuloauditory symptoms.* Arch. Ophthalmol. 71:172, 1964.

62. COGAN, D. G.: *Internuclear ophthalmoplegia typical and atypical.* Arch. Ophthalmol. 84:583, 1970.

63. COGAN, D. G.: *Syndrome of nonsyphilitic interstitial keratitis and vestibuloauditory symptoms.* Arch. Ophthalmol. 33:144, 1945.

64. COGAN, D. G.: *Down-beat nystagmus.* Arch. Ophthalmol. 80:757, 1968.

65. COMPERE, W. E. Jr.: *Electronystagmographic findings in patients with "whiplash" injuries.* Laryngoscope 78:1226, 1968.

66. COURVILLE, C. B.: *Commotio Cerebri. Cerebral Concussion and the Postconcussion Syndrome in Their Medical and Legal Aspects.* San Lucas Press, Los Angeles, 1953.

67. COVENTRY, M., AND DAHLIN, D.: *Osteogenic sarcoma, a critical analysis of 430 cases.* J. Bone Jt. Surg. 39-A:741, 1957.

68. CUSHING, H.: *Experiences with cerebellar astrocytomas. A critical review of 26 cases.* Surg. Gynec. Obstet. 52:129, 1931.

69. CUSHING, H.: *Intracranial Tumors.* Charles C Thomas, Springfield, Illinois, 1935.

70. DAHLIN, D.: *Bone Tumors.* Charles C Thomas, Springfield, Illinois, 1957.

71. DALSGAARD-NEILSON, E.: *Correlation between syphilitic interstitial keratitis and deafness.* Acta Ophthalmol. 16:635, 1938.

72. DAM, M., ET AL.: *Vestibular aberrations in multiple sclerosis.* Acta Neurol. Scand. 52:407, 1975.

73. DAVEY, L. M.: *Labyrinthine trauma in head injury.* Conn. Med. 29:250, 1965.

74. DAVIES, D.: *Paget's disease of the temporal bone: A clinical and histopathological survey.* Acta Otolaryngol. (Suppl 242):7, 1968.

75. DAWES, J.: Complications of infections of the middle ear. In Scott-Brown, W., Ballantyne, J., and Groves, J. (eds.): *Diseases of the Ear, Nose and Throat.* Butterworth and Company, London, 1965.

76. DAWES, J. D. K.: *Discussion on intracranial complications of otogenic origin.* Proc. Roy. Soc. Med. 54:315, 1961.

77. DE JONG, P. T. V. M., ET AL.: *Ataxia and nystagmus induced by injection of local anesthetics in the neck.* Ann. Neurol. 1:240, 1977.

78. DE MORSIER, J.: *Contribution a l'étude des centres vestibulaires corticaux et des hallucinations lilliputiennes.* Encéphale 33:57, 1938.

79. DERLACKI, E.: *Medical management of endolymphatic hydrops.* Laryngoscope 75:1518, 1965.

80. DINSDALE, H. B.: *Spontaneous hemorrhage in the posterior fossa: A study of primary cerebellar and pontine hemorrhage with observations on the pathogenesis.* Arch. Neurol. 10:200, 1964.

81. DISHOECK, H. VAN, AND BIERMAN, T.: *Sudden perceptive deafness and viral infection (report of the first one hundred patients).* Ann. Otol. Rhinol. Laryngol. 66:963, 1957.

82. DIX, M., AND HALLPIKE, C.: *The pathology, symptomatology and diagnosis of certain common disorders of the vestibular systems.* Ann. Otol. Rhinol. Laryngol. 61:987, 1952.

83. DOHLMAN, G.: *The mechanism of secretion and absorption of endolymph in the vestibular apparatus.* Acta Otolaryngol. 59:275, 1965.

84. DRACHMAN, D. A., AND HART, C. W.: *An approach to the dizzy patient.* Neurology 22:323, 1972.

85. DUNCAN, G. W., PARKER, S. W., AND FISHER, C. M.: *Acute cerebellar infarction in the PICA territory.* Arch. Neurol. 32:364, 1975.

86. DÜRSTELER, M. R.: *Migräne und Vestibularapparat.* J. Neurol. 210:253, 1975.

87. ERICKSON, L., SORENSON, G., AND MCGAVRAN, M.: *A review of 140 acoustic neurinomas (neurilemmomas).* Laryngoscope 75:601, 1965.

88. ESCHER, F.: *Die Otologische Beurteilung des Schädeltraumatikers.* Pract. Oto-Rhino-Laryngol. 10(Suppl. I):4, 1948.

89. FADAN, A.: *Neurological sequella of malignant external otitis.* Arch. Neurol. 32:204, 1975.

90. FARRINGTON, R., ET AL.: *Streptomycin toxicity. Reactions to highly purified drug on long-continued administration to human subjects.* JAMA 134:679, 1947.

91. FEE, G.: *Traumatic perilymphatic fistulas.* Arch. Otolaryngol. 88:477, 1968.

92. FERNANDEZ, C. A. R., AND LINDSAY, J. R.: *Experimental observations on postural nystagmus in the cat.* Ann. Otol. Rhinol. Laryngol. 68:816, 1959.

93. FIELDS, W.: Vertigo related to alteration in arterial blood flow. In Wolfson, R. (ed.): *The Vestibular System and Its Diseases.* University of Pennsylvania Press, Philadelphia, 1966.

94. FIELDS, W. S.: *Arteriography in the differential diagnosis of vertigo.* Arch. Otolaryngol. 85:111, 1967.

95. FISCHER, J., AND WOLFSEN, L.: *The Inner Ear.* Grune and Stratton, New York, 1943.

96. FISHER, C. M.: *Vertigo in cerebrovascular disease.* Arch. Otolaryngol. 85:855, 1960.

97. FISHER, C. M., KARNES, W. E., AND KUBIK, C. S.: *Lateral medullary infarction—the pattern of vascular occlusion.* J. Neuropath. Exp. Neurol. 20:323, 1961.

98. FISHER, C. M.: *Ocular bobbing.* Arch. Neurol. 11:543, 1964.

99. FISHER, C. M., ET AL.: *Atherosclerosis of the carotid and vertebral arteries. Extracranial and intracranial.* J. Neuropath. Exp. Neurol. 24:455, 1965.

100. FISHER, E., AND HELLSTROM, H.: *Cogan's syndrome and systemic vascular disease: Analysis of pathologic features with reference to its relationship to thromboangitis obliterans (Buerger).* Arch. Path. 75:572, 1961.

101. FOERSTER, O.: Sensible corticale Felder. In Bumke, O., and Foerster, O. (eds.): *Hrsg. Handbuch der Neurologie 6.* Springer, Berlin, 1936.

102. FOKES, E. C., AND EARLE, K. M.: *Ependymomas: Clinical and pathological aspects.* J. Neurosurg. 30:585, 1969.

103. FRASER, J., AND DICKIE, J.: *Meningetic neuro-labyrinthitis.* Proc. Roy. Soc. Med. 13:23, 1920.

104. FREEMAN, R. E., ET AL.: *Spontaneous intracerebellar hemorrhage. Diagnosis and surgical treatment.* Neurology 23:84, 1973.

105. FRIEDMAN, A. P., BRENNER, C., AND DENNY-BROWN, D.: *Post-traumatic vertigo and dizziness.* J. Neurosurg. 2:36, 1945.

106. FRIEDMAN, A. P.: The infinite variety of migraine. In Smith, R. (ed.): *Background to Migraine.* William Heinemann, Ltd., London, 1970.

107. FUJITA, S., and HAYDEN, R. C.: *Alport's syndrome.* Arch. Otolaryngol. 90:453, 1969.

108. GACEK, R.: *The diagnosis and treatment of poststapedectomy granuloma.* Ann. Otol. Rhinol. Laryngol. 79:970, 1970.

109. GACEK, R.: *Transection of the posterior ampullary nerve for relief of benign paroxysmal positional vertigo.* Ann. Otol. Rhinol. Laryngol. 83:569, 1974.

110. GEISSINGER, J. D., AND BUCY, P. C.: *Astrocytomas of the cerebellum in children. Long-term study.* Arch. Neurol. 24:125, 1971.

111. GEJROT, T., and LAURÉN, T.: *Retrograde venography of the internal jugular veins and transverse sinuses: Techniques and roentgen anatomy.* Acta Otolaryngol. 57:556, 1964.

112. GEJROT, T., and LAURÉN, T.: *Retrograde jugularography in diagnosis of glomus tumors in the jugular region.* Acta Otolaryngol. 58:191, 1964.

113. GHEZ, C.: *Vestibular paresis: A clinical feature of Wernicke's disease.* J. Neurol. Neurosurg. Psychiat. 33:134, 1969.

114. GILSON, R. D., ET AL.: *Effects of different alcohol dosages and display illumination on tracking performance during vestibular stimulation.* Aerospace Med. 43:656, 1972.

115. GLADNEY, J. H., AND SHEPHERD, D. C.: *Labyrinthine dysfunction in latent and early manifest diabetes.* Ann. Otol. Rhinol. Laryngol. 79:984, 1970.

116. GODLOWSKI, Z.: *Endocrine management of selected cases of allergy based on enzymatic mechanism of sensitization.* Arch. Otolaryngol. 71:513, 1960.

117. GOLDMAN, H.: *Hypoadrenocorticism and endocrinologic treatment of Meniere's disease.* N.Y. J. Med. 62:377, 1962.

118. GONZALEZ-REVILLA, A.: *Differential diagnoses of tumors at the cerebellopontine recess.* Bull. Johns Hopkins Hosp. 83:187, 1948.

119. GOODHART, S. P., AND DAVISON, C.: *Syndrome of the posterior inferior and anterior inferior cerebellar arteries and their branches.* Arch. Neurol. Psychiat. 35:501, 1936.

120. GOODHILL, V.: *Syphilis of the ear: a histopathological study.* Ann. Otol. Rhinol. Laryngol. 48:676, 1939.

121. GOODHILL, V., ET AL.: *Sudden deafness and labyrinthine window ruptures: Audio-vestibular observations.* Ann. Otol. Rhinol. Laryngol. 82:2, 1973.

122. GOODMAN, J. S., KAUFMAN, L., AND KOENIG, M. G.: *Diagnosis of cryptococcal meningitis. Value of immunologic detection of cryptococcal antigen.* New Eng. J. Med. 285:434, 1971.

123. GOOR, C., ENDTZ, L. J., AND MULLER KOBOLD, M. J. P.: *Electronystagmography for the diagnosis of vestibular dysfunction in Wernicke-Korsakoff syndrome.* Clin. Neurol. Neurosurg. 78:112, 1975.

124. GORDON, N.: *Post-traumatic vertigo, with special reference to positional nystagmus.* Lancet 1:1216, 1954.

125. GORDY, P. D.: *Neurinoma of the gasserian ganglion.* J. Neurosurg. 22:90, 1965.

126. GOZDZIK-ZOLNIERKIEWICZ, T., AND MOSZYNSKI, B.: *VIIIth nerve in experimental lead poisoning.* Acta Otolaryngol. 68:85, 1969.

127. GRADENIGO, G.: *Sulla leptomeningite circoscritta e sulla paralisi dell'abducente di origine otitica.* G. Accad. Med. Torino 10:59, 1904.

128. GRAHAM, J., AND PARKER, W.: *The toxic manifestations of sodium salicylate therapy.* Quart J. Med. 18:153, 1948.

129. GRAND, W.: *Positional nystagmus: An early sign of medullablastoma.* Neurology 21:1157, 1971.

130. GRAY, L. P.: *Extra-labyrinthine vertigo due to cervical muscle lesions.* J. Laryngol. 70:352, 1956.

131. GRAY, J.: *The treatment of cholesteatoma in children.* Proc. Roy. Soc. Med. 57:769, 1964.

132. GREGORIUS, F. K., CRANDALL, P. H., AND BALOH, R. W.: *Positional vertigo in cerebellar astrocytoma. Report of two cases.* Surgical Neurol. 6:283, 1976.

216

133. GREGORY, J., GOLDEN, A., AND HAYMAKER, W.: *Mucormycoses of central nervous system: report of three cases.* Bull. Johns Hopkins Hosp. 73:405, 1943.

134. GREISEN, O., AND RASMUSSEN, P.: *Stapedius muscle reflexes and otosurgical examinations in brain stem tumors.* Acta Otolaryngol. 70:366, 1970.

135. GROSS, C.: *Sensori-neural hearing loss in clinical and histologic otosclerosis.* Laryngoscope 79:104, 1969.

136. GROVE, W. E.: *Skull fractures involving the ear: a clinical study of 211 cases.* Laryngoscope 49:678, 1939.

137. GUEDRY, F. E., ET AL.: *Some effects of alcohol on various aspects of oculomotor control.* Aviat. Space Environ. Med. 46:1008, 1975.

138. GUILD, S.: *The glomus jugulare, a nonchromaffin paraganglion, in man.* Ann. Otol. Rhinol. Laryngol. 62:1045, 1953.

139. GUSSEN, R.: *Sudden deafness of vascular origin: A human temporal bone study.* Ann. Otol. Rhinol. Laryngol. 85:94, 1976.

140. HAKAS, P., AND KORNHUBER, H. H.: *Der vestibuläre Nystagmus bei grobhirnläsionen des Menchen.* Arch. Psychiat. Nervenkr. 200:19, 1959.

141. HALLGREN, B.: *Retinitis pigmentosa combined with congenital deafness with vestibulo-cerebellar ataxia and mental abnormality in a proportion of cases. A clinical and genetico-statistical study.* Acta Psychiat. Scand. (Suppl. 138):9, 1959.

142. HALLPIKE, C., AND CAIRNS, H.: *Observations on the pathology of Meniere's syndrome.* J. Laryngol. 53:625, 1938.

143. HAMBLEY, W., GORSHENIN, A., AND HOUSE, W.: *The differential diagnosis of acoustic neuroma (neurilemmomas).* Laryngoscope 75:601, 1965.

144. HAMERSMA, H.: *Osteopetrosis (marble bone disease) of the temporal bone.* Laryngoscope 80:1518, 1970.

145. HANAFEE, W., AND WILSON, G.: *Pontocerebellar angle tumors: Newer diagnostic methods.* Arch. Otolaryngol. 92:236, 1970.

146. HARDIN, C. A., WILLIAMSON, W. P., and STEEGMAN, A. T.: *Vertebral artery insufficiency produced by cervical osteoarthritis spurs.* Neurology 10:855, 1960.

147. HART, C.: *Vestibular paralysis of sudden onset and probable viral etiology.* Ann. Otol. Rhinol. Laryngol. 74:33, 1965.

148. HART, C. W.: Traumatic vestibular impairment in the nervous system. In: *Human Communication and Its Disorders, 3.* Raven Press, New York, 1975.

149. HARRISON, M. S., AND OZSAHINOGLU, C.: *Positional vertigo.* Arch. Otolaryngol. 101:675, 1975.

150. HARRISON, W., ET AL.: *The perilymph fistula problem.* Laryngoscope 80:1000, 1970.

151. HEINEMAN, H. S., BRAUDE, A. I., AND OSTERHOLM, J. L.: *Intra cranial suppurative disease. Early presumptive diagnosis and successful treatment without surgery.* JAMA 218:1542, 1971.

152. HEMENWAY, W., HILDYARD, V., AND BLACK, F.: *Post stapedectomy perilymph fistulas in the Rocky Mountain area: The importance of nystagmography and audiometry in diagnosis and early tympanotomy in prognoses.* Laryngoscope 78:1687, 1968.

153. HITCHCOCK, E., AND ANDREADIS, A.: *Subdural empyema: A review of 29 cases.* J. Neurol. Neurosurg. Psychiat. 27:422, 1964.

154. HITSELBERGER, W., and GARDNER, G. JR.: *Other tumors of the cerebellopontine angle.* Arch. Otolaryngol. 88:712, 1968.

155. HINOKI, M.: *Clinical aspects of traumatic cervical vertigo.* J. Jap. Med. Assoc. 60:745, 1968.

156. HOF, E.: *Meningitis und Labyrinthitis im Kindesalter.* ORL 38 (Suppl. 1):25, 1976.

157. HOLDEN, H., AND SCHUKNECHT, H.: *Distribution pattern of blood in the inner ear following spontaneous subarchnoid hemorrhage.* J. Laryngol. 82:321, 1968.

158. HOUSE, H.: *The fistula problem in otosclerosis surgery.* Laryngoscope 77:1410, 1967.

159. HUNT, J.: *On herpetic inflammations of the geniculate ganglion. A new syndrome and its complications.* J. Nerv. Ment. Dis. 34:73, 1907.

160. HUNTER, D., AND RUSSELL, D. S.: *Focal cerebral and cerebellar atrophy in a human subject due to organic mercury compounds.* J. Neurol. Neurosurg. Psychiat. 17:235, 1954.

161. IGARASHI, M., SCHUKNECHT, H., AND MYERS, E.: *Cochlear pathology in humans with stimulation deafness.* J. Laryngol. 78:115, 1964.

217

162. IGARASHI, M., ET AL.: *Cerebellopontine meningiomas and the temporal bone.* Arch. Otolaryngol. 94:224, 1971.

163. INGRAHAM, F. D., AND BAILEY, O. T.: *Cystic teratomas and teratoid tumors of the central nervous system in infancy and childhood.* J. Neurosurg. 3:511, 1946.

164. INGRAHAM, F. D., BAILEY, O. T., AND BARKER, W. F.: *Medullablastoma cerebelli.* New Eng. J. Med. 238:171, 1948.

165. ISHII, S.: Significance of soft tissue neck injuries in the post-traumatic syndrome. In Walker, A. E., Caveness, W. F., and Critchley M., (eds.): *The Late Effects of Head Injury.* Charles C Thomas, Springfield, Illinois, 1964.

166. JAFFE, B.: *Sudden deafness—a local manifestation of systemic disorders: Fat emboli, hypercoagulation and infections.* Laryngoscope 80:788, 1970.

167. JAFFE, B., FOX, J., AND BATSAKIS, J.: *Rhabdomyosarcoma of the middle ear and mastoid.* Cancer 27:29, 1971.

168. JAMA: *Is there a labyrinthine concussion?* In Foreign Letters, 103:1721, 1934.

169. JEANES, A., AND FRIEDMANN, I.: *Tuberculosis of the middle ear.* Tubercle, The Journal of the British Tuberculosis Association 41:109, 1960.

170. JENSEN, J.: *Congenital anomalies of the inner ear.* Radiologic Clinics of North America 12:473, 1974.

171. JERGER, J.: *Observations in auditory behavior in lesions of the central auditory pathways.* Arch. Otolaryngol. 71:797, 1960.

172. JERGER, J.: Auditory tests for disorders of the central auditory mechanism. In Fields, W. (ed.): *Neurological Aspects of Auditory and Vestibular Disorders.* Charles C Thomas, Springfield, Illinois, 1964.

173. JERGER, J., ET AL.: *Bilateral lesions of the temporal lobe: A case study.* Acta Otolaryngol. (Suppl. 258):7, 1969.

174. JERGER, J. (ed.): *Modern Developments in Audiology.* Academic Press, New York, 1973.

175. JERGER, J., AND JERGER, S.: *Auditory findings in brain stem disorders.* Arch. Otolaryngol. 99:342, 1974.

176. JOHNSON, E. W.: *Auditory test results in 500 cases of acoustic neuromas.* Arch. Otolaryngol. 103:152, 1977.

177. JONES, M., AND MULCAHY, N.: *Osteopathia striata, osteopetrosis, and impaired hearing.* Arch. Otolaryngol. 87:116, 1968.

178. JONGKEES, L. B. W.: *Cervical vertigo.* Laryngoscope 79:1473, 1969.

179. JORGENSEN, M.: *The inner ear in diabetes mellitus.* Arch. Otolaryngol. 74:373, 1961.

180. JORGENSEN, M., AND BUCH, N.: *Studies on inner-ear function and cranial nerves in diabetics.* Acta Otolaryngol. 53:350, 1961.

181. KARMODY, C., AND SCHUKNECHT, H.: *Deafness in congenital syphilis.* Arch. Otolaryngol. 83:18, 1966.

182. KAUFMAN, D. M., AND LEEDS, N. E.: *Computed tomography (CT) in the diagnosis of intracranial abscesses. Brain abscess, subdural empyema, and epidural empyema.* Neurology 27:1069, 1977.

183. KELEMEN, G.: *Fractures of the temporal bone.* Arch. Otolaryngol. 40:333, 1944.

184. KEVILLE, F. J., AND WISE, B. L.: *Intracranial epidermoid and dermoid tumors.* J. Neurosurg. 16:564, 1959.

185. KIMURA, R., AND SCHUKNECHT, H.: *Membranous hydrops in the inner ear of the guinea pig after obliteration of the endolymphatic sac.* Pract. Oto-Rhino-Laryngol. 27:343, 1965.

186. KIRIKAE, I., ET AL.: *Sudden deafness due to Buerger's disease.* Arch. Otolaryngol. 75:502, 1962.

187. KLIPPEL, M., AND FEIL, A.: *Un cas d'absence des vertebres cervicales.* Nouv. Iconogr. Salpet. 25:223, 1912.

188. KOMMERELL, G., and HOYT, W. F.: *Lateropulsion of saccadic eye movements. Electrooculographic studies in a patient with Wallenberg's syndrome.* Arch. Neurol. 28:313, 1973.

189. KORNHUBER, H. H.: Nystagmus and related phenomena in man: an outline of otoneurology. In Kornhuber, H. H. (ed.): *Handbook of Sensory Physiology,* vol. VI, part 2. Springer-Verlag, Berlin, 1974.

190. KOS, A., SCHUKNECHT, H., AND SINGER, J.: *Temporal bone studies in 13—15 and 18 trisomy syndromes.* Arch. Otolaryngol. 83:439, 1966.

191. LARSSON, A.: *Otosclerosis: A genetic and clinical study.* Acta Otolaryngol. (Suppl. 154):6, 1960.

192. LAWRENCE, M., AND MCCABE, B.: *Inner ear mechanics and deafness. Special considerations of Meniere's syndrome.* JAMA 171:1927, 1959.

193. LEHRICH, J. R., WINKLER, G. F., AND OJEMANN, R. G.: *Cerebellar infarction with brain stem compression.* Arch. Neurol. 22:490, 1970.

194. LEMPERT, J., ET AL.: *New theory for the correlation of the pathology and the symptomatology of Meniere's disease.* Ann. Otol. Rhinol. Laryngol. 61:717, 1952.

195. LEWIS, J.: *Cancer of the ear: A report of 150 cases.* Laryngoscope 70:551, 1960.

196. LINDEMAN, H.: *Regional differences in sensitivity of the vestibular sensory epithelia to ototoxic antibiotics.* Acta Otolaryngol. 67:177, 1969.

197. LINDSAY, J., AND ZURDEMA, J.: *Inner ear deafness of sudden onset.* Laryngoscope 60:238, 1950.

198. LINDSAY, J.: *Sudden deafness due to virus infection.* AMA Arch. Otolaryngol. 69:13, 1959.

199. LINDSAY, J., KOHUT, R., AND SCIARRA, P.: *Meniere's disease: Pathology and manifestations.* Ann. Otol. Rhinol. Laryngol. 76:1, 1967.

200. LINDSAY, J., AND LEHMAN, R.: *Histopathology of the temporal bone in advanced Paget's disease.* Laryngoscope 79:213, 1969.

201. LINDSAY, J. R., AND HEMENWAY, W. G.: *Postural vertigo due to unilateral sudden partial loss of vestibular function.* Ann. Otol. Rhinol. Laryngol. 65:692, 1956.

202. LINTHICUM, F. JR.: *Histological evidence of the causes of failure in stapes surgery.* Ann. Otol. Rhinol. Laryngol. 80:67, 1971.

203. LUNDQUIST, P., AND WERSÄLL, J.: *The ototoxic effect of gentamicin: An electron microscopical study.* In: *Gentamicin First International Symposium,* Paris, 1967.

204. LUSE, S.: *Electron microscopic studies of brain tumors.* Neurology 10:881, 1960.

205. MACKIEWICZ, J.: *Vertigo epidemic.* Pol. Tyg. Lek. 18:48, 1963.

206. MAKISHIMA, K., AND TANAKA, K.: *Pathological changes of the inner ear and central auditory pathways in diabetics.* Ann. Otol. Rhinol. Laryngol. 80:218, 1971.

207. MAKISHIMA, K., SOBEL, S. F., AND SNOW, J. B.: *Histopathologic correlates of otoneurologic manifestations following head trauma.* Laryngoscope 86:1303, 1976.

208. MARCUS, R.: *Vestibular function and additional findings in Waardenburg's syndrome.* Acta Otolaryngol. (Suppl. 229):7, 1968.

209. MASTAGLIA, F. L., ET AL.: *Evoked potentials, saccadic velocities, and computerized tomography in diagnosis of multiple sclerosis.* Brit. Med. J. 1:1315, 1977.

210. MCALPINE, D., LUMSDEN, C. E., AND ACHESON, E. D.: *Multiple sclerosis. A reappraisal.* Churchill Livingstone, Edinburgh and London, 1972.

211. MCCABE, P., AND DEY, F.: *The effect of aspirin upon auditory sensitivity.* Ann. Otol. Rhinol. Laryngol. 74:312, 1965.

212. MCLAY, K.: *Otogenic meningitis.* J. Laryngol. 68:140, 1954.

213. MCLAY, K., AND MARAN, A.: *Deafness and Klippel-Feil syndrome.* J. Laryngol. 83:175, 1969.

214. MERIFIELD, D.: *Self-limited idiopathic vertigo (epidemic vertigo).* Arch. Otolaryngol. 81:355, 1965.

215. MICHIE, I., AND CLARK, M.: *Neurological syndromes associated with cervical and craniocervical anomalies.* Arch. Neurol. 18:241, 1968.

216. MILLER, G. W., ET AL.: *Alport's syndrome.* Arch. Otolaryngol. 92:419, 1970.

217. MILLER, H.: *Mental sequelae of head injury.* Proc. Roy. Soc. Med. 59:257, 1966.

218. MINDERHOUD, J. M., VAN WOERKOM, T. C. AND VAN WEERDEN, T. W.: *On the nature of brain stem disorders in severe head injured patients. II. A study on caloric vestibular reactions and neurotransmitter treatment.* Acta Neurochirugica 34:23, 1976.

219. MITCHELL, D. E., AND ADAMS, J. H.: *Primary focal impact damage to the brainstem in blunt head injuries. Does it exist?* Lancet 2:215, 1973.

220. MIZUKOSHI, K., ET AL.: *Neurotological studies upon intoxication by organic mercury compounds.* ORL 37:74, 1975.

219

221. MOBERG, A., ET AL.: *Imbalance nystagmus and diplopia in Wallenberg's syndrome.* Acta Otolaryngol. 55:269, 1962.

222. MONEY, K. E., AND MYLES, W. S.: *Heavy water nystagmus and effects of alcohol.* Nature 247:404, 1974.

223. MONIF, G., HARDY, J., AND SEVER, J.: *Studies in congenital rubella, Baltimore 1964—1965. I. Epidemiologic and virologic.* Bull. Johns. Hopkins Hosp. 118:85, 1966.

224. MOORE, J. E.: *The Modern Treatment of Syphilis.* Bailiere, London, 1973.

225. MORGENSTEIN, K., AND SEUNG, H.: *Vestibular neuronitis.* Laryngoscope 81:131, 1971.

226. MORRISON, A. W.: Late syphilis. In: *Management of Sensorineural Deafness.* Butterworths, Boston, 1975.

227. MÜLLER, H. R., ET AL.: *The contribution of computerized axial tomography to the diagnosis of cerebellar and pontine hemorrhages.* Stroke 6:467, 1975.

228. MUNDINI, C.: *Anatomia surdi nedi sectio.* De Bononiensi Scientiarum et Artium Instituto Atque Academia Commentarii, Boniensi 7:28, 419, 1791.

229. MYERS, E., AND BALLANTINE, H.: *The management of otogenic brain abscess.* Laryngoscope 75: 273, 1965.

230. MYERS, E., BERNSTEIN, J., AND FOSTIROPOLOUS, G.: *Salicylate ototoxicity. A clinical study.* New Eng. J. Med. 273:587, 1965.

231. NAGER, F.: *Ueber die Knochenopathologie der Labyrinthkapsel.* Acta Otolaryngol. 26:127, 1968.

232. NAGER, G.: *Meningiomas Involving the Temporal Bone: Clinical and Pathological Aspects.* Charles C Thomas, Springfield, Illinois, 1964.

233. NAITO, T.: *Clinical and pathological studies of Meniere's disease.* Sixtieth Annual Meeting of the Oto-Rhino-Laryngol. Soc. of Japan, Tokyo, March, 1959.

234. New England Journal of Medicine: *Case records of the Massachusetts General Hospital.* 279:1220, 1968.

235. NEW, P. F. J., ET AL.: *Computed tomography with the EMI scanner in the diagnosis of primary and metastatic ultracranial neoplasms.* Radiology 114:75, 1975.

236. NIJENSOHN, D. E., SAEZ, R. J., AND REAGAN, T. J.: *Clinical significance of basilar artery aneurysms.* Neurology 24:301, 1974.

237. NOFFSINGER, D., ET AL.: *Auditory and vestibular aberrations in multiple sclerosis.* Acta Otolaryngol. (Suppl. 303):7, 1972.

238. NOSAKA, Y., SETOGUTI, A., AND SUKO, H.: *Auditory and vestibular disturbances in Minamata disease.* Kumamoto Med. J. 32:1465, 1958 (in Japanese).

239. NYLEN, C. O.: *The oto-neurological diagnoses of tumors of the brain.* Acta Otolaryngol. (Suppl. 33):81, 1939.

240. OBRADOR, S.: *Cysticercosis cerebri.* Acta Neurochir. 10:320, 1962.

241. ODA, M., ET AL.: *Labyrinthine pathology of chronic renal failure patients treated with hemodialysis and kidney transplantation.* Laryngoscope 84:1489, 1974.

242. OPHEIM, O.: *Loss of hearing following the syndrome of Van der Hoeve-de Kleyn.* Acta Otolaryngol. 65:337, 1968.

243. OTT, K. H., ET AL.: *Cerebellar hemorrhage. Diagnosis and treatment.* Arch. Neurol. 31:160, 1974.

244. PAGET, J.: *On a form of chronic inflammation of bones (osteitis deformans).* Medico-Chirurgical Trans. 60:37, 1877.

245. PALVA, T., FRIEDMANN, I., AND PALVA, A.: *Mastoiditis in children.* J. Laryngol. 78:977, 1964.

246. PAPARELLA, M., ET AL.: *Otological manifestations of leukemia.* Laryngoscope 83:1510, 1973.

247. PASSE, E., AND SEYMOUR, J.: *Meniere's syndrome: successful treatment by surgery on the sympathetic.* Brit. Med. J. 2:812, 1948.

248. PATEL, A., AND TOOLE, J. F.: *Subclavian steal syndrome—reversal of cephalic blood flow.* Medicine 44:289, 1965.

249. PAXTON, R., AND AMBROSE, J.: *The EMI-scanner. A brief review of the first 650 patients.* Br. J. Radiol. 47:530, 1974.

250. PEDERSEN, E.: *Epidemic vertigo. Clinical picture and relation to encephalitis.* Brain 83:566, 1959.

251. Peitersen, E., and Anderson, P.: *Spontaneous course of 220 peripheral nontraumatic facial palsies.* Acta Otolaryngol. (Suppl. 224):296, 1967.

252. Penfield, W., and Kristiansen, K.: *Epileptic seizure patterns: A study of the localizing value of initial phenomena in focal cortical seizures.* Charles C Thomas, Springfield, Illinois, 1951.

253. Penfield, W., and Jasper, H.: *Epilepsy and the Functional Anatomy of the Human Brain.* Little, Brown and Co., Boston, 1954.

254. Pennybacker, J.: *Discussion on intracranial complications of otogenic origin.* Proc. Roy. Soc. Med. 54:309, 1961.

255. Perlman, H., and Lindsay, J.: *Relation of the internal ear spaces to the meninges.* Arch. Otolaryngol. 29:12, 1939.

256. Perlman, H.: *Minimal shock pulse trauma to the cochlea: Acute and chronic.* Laryngoscope 58:466, 1948.

257. Perlman, H., and Leek, J.: *Late congenital syphilis of the ear.* Laryngoscope 62:1175, 1952.

258. Perlman, H., Kimura, R., and Fernández, C.: *Experiments on temporary obstruction of the internal auditory artery.* Laryngoscope 69:591, 1959.

259. Philipszoon, A.: *Nystagmus and Bell's palsy.* Pract. Oto-Rhino-Laryngol. 24:233, 1962.

260. Polus, K.: *The problem of vascular deafness.* Laryngoscope 82:24, 1972.

261. Pool, J., and Pava, A.: *The Early Diagnosis and Treatment of Acoustic Nerve Tumors.* Charles C Thomas, Springfield, Illinois, 1957.

262. Pool, J. L., and Potts, D. G.: *Aneurysms and Arteriovenous Anomalies of the Brain: Diagnosis and Treatment.* Hoeber Medical Division, New York, 1965.

263. Poulsen, J., and Zilstrorff, K.: *Prognostic value of the caloric vestibular test in the unconscious patients with cranial trauma.* Acta Neurol. Scand. 48:282, 1972.

264. Proctor, B., and Lindsay, J.: *Tumors involving the petrous pyramid of the temporal bone.* Arch. Otolaryngol. 46:180, 1947.

265. Pulec, J.: *Facial nerve tumors.* Ann. Otol. Rhinol Laryngol. 78:962, 1969.

266. Pullen, F. II: *Round window membrane rupture: a cause of sudden deafness.* Trans. Amer. Acad. Ophthalmol. Otolaryngol. 76:1444, 1972.

267. Ramondi, A., Mullan, S., and Eraus, J.: *Human brain tumors: An electromicroscopic study.* J. Neurosurg. 19:731, 1962.

268. Rauchbach, E., and Stroud, M. H.: *Vestibular involvement in Bell's palsy.* Laryngoscope 85:1396, 1975.

269. Ringertz, N., and Reymond, A.: *Ependymomas and choroid plexus papillomas.* J. Neuropathol. Exp. Neurol. 8:355, 1949.

270. Robert, F., and Pfaltz, C.: *Vestibuläre Funklionsstörungen bei idiopathischer Faciallisparese (Lokalisations-und Kompensationsprobleme).* Arch. Ohr. Nas.-Kehlk-Heilk. 197:183, 1970.

271. Roger, H., and Cain, J.: *Les symptomes vestibulaires et oculaires dans les Lérédo-dégénérations spino-cérébelleuses.* Revue Oto-Neuro-Ophtal. 20:406, 1948.

272. Ruben, R., et al.: *Sudden sequential deafness as the presenting symptom of macroglobulinemia.* JAMA 209:1364, 1969.

273. Rüedi, L., and Furrer, W.: *Das akustische trauma.* Pract. Oto-Rhino-Laryngol. 8:177, 1946.

274. Rutherford, W. H., Merrett, J. D., and McDonald, J. R.: *Sequelae of concussion caused by minor head injuries.* Lancet 1:1, 1977.

275. Ryan, G. M. S., and Cope, S.: *Cervical vertigo.* Lancet 2:1355, 1955.

276. Saez, R. J., Onofrio, B. M., and Yanagihara, T.: *Experience with Arnold-Chiari malformation, 1960 to 1970.* J. Neurosurg. 45:416, 1976.

277. Sando, I., et al.: *Vestibular pathology in otosclerosis temporal bone histopathological report.* Laryngoscope 84:593, 1974.

278. Saunders, W., and Lippy, W.: *Sudden deafness and Bell's palsy: a common cause.* Ann. Otol. Rhinol. Laryngol. 68:830, 1959.

279. Scheibe, A.: *A case of deaf-mutism with auditory atrophy and anomalies of development in the membranous labyrinth of both ears.* Arch. Otolaryngol. 11:12, 1892.

221

280. SCHMIDT, W.: *Über den Einfluss der Liquorentnahme auf das Ergebnis der Vestibularisprüfung.* Mschr. Ohrenheilk. Lar.-Rhinol. 76:299, 1942.

281. SCHUKNECHT, H.: *Cupulolithiasis.* Arch. Otolaryngol. 90:765, 1969.

282. SCHUKNECHT, H. F.: *Pathology of the Ear.* Harvard Univ. Press, Cambridge, Mass. 1974.

283. SCHUKNECHT, H.: *Positional vertigo: clinical and experimental observations.* Trans. Amer. Acad. Ophthalmol. Otolaryngol. 66:319, 1962.

284. SCHUKNECHT, H., ALLAM, A., AND MURAKAMI, Y.: *Pathology of secondary malignant tumors of the temporal bone.* Ann. Otol. Rhinol. Laryngol. 77:5, 1968.

285. SCHUKNECHT, H., AND DAVISON, R.: *Deafness and vertigo from head injury.* Arch. Otolaryngol. 63:513, 1956.

286. SCHUKNECHT, H., IGARASHI, M., AND CHASIN, W.: *Inner ear hemorrhage in leukemia.* Laryngoscope 75:662, 1965.

287. SCHUKNECHT, H., KIMURA, R., AND NAUFAL, P.: *The pathology of sudden deafness.* Acta Otolaryngol. 76:75, 1973.

288. SCHUKNECHT, H., NEFF, W., AND PERLMAN, H.: *An experimental study of auditory damage following blows to the head.* Ann. Otol. Rhinol. Laryngol. 60:273, 1951.

289. SCHUKNECHT, H., NORTHROP, C., AND IGARASHI, M.: *Cochlear pathology after destruction of the endolymphatic sac in the cat.* Acta Otolaryngol. 65:479, 1968.

290. SCHUKNECHT, H., AND RUBY, R.: *Cupulolithiasis.* Adv. Oto-Rhino-Laryngol. 20:434, 1973.

291. SCHWARZ, G. A., BLUMENKRANTZ, M. J., AND SUNDMAKER, W. L.: *Neurologic complications of malignant external otitis.* Neurology 21:1077, 1971.

292. SHAMBAUGH, G., JR., ET AL.: *Dihydrostreptomycin deafness.* JAMA 170:1657, 1959.

293. SHARP, M.: *Monostotic fibrous dysplasia of the temporal bone.* J. Laryngol. 84:697, 1970.

294. SHEA, J., SMYTH, G., AND ALTMANN, F.: *Surgical treatment of the hearing loss associated with osteogenesis imperfecta tarda.* J. Laryngol. 77:679, 1963.

295. SHEEHY, J. L., AND INZER, B. E.: *Acoustic reflex test in neuro-otologic diagnosis. A review of 24 cases of acoustic tumors.* Arch. Otolaryngol. 102:647, 1976.

296. SILFVERSKIÖLD, B. P.: *Skew deviation in Wallenberg's syndrome.* Acta Neurol. Scand. 41:381, 1965.

297. SILVERSTEIN, H.: *The effects of perfusing the perilymphate space with artificial endolymph.* Ann. Otol. Rhinol. Laryngol. 79:754, 1970.

298. SILVERSTEIN, H., BERNSTEIN, J., AND DAVIES, D.: *Salicylate ototoxicity. A biochemical and electrophysiological study.* Ann. Otol. Rhinol. Laryngol. 76:118, 1967.

299. SINGLETON, E., AND SCHUKNECHT, H.: *Streptomycin sulfate in the management of Meniere's disease.* Otolaryngol. Clin. North Amer. October:531, 1968.

300. SMITH, B. H.: *Vestibular disturbances in epilepsy.* Neurology 10:465, 1960.

301. SMITH, C., ET AL.: *Facial palsy caused by facial nerve tumor.* Laryngoscope 81:1542, 1971.

302. SMITH, J. L.: *Cogan's syndrome.* Laryngoscope 80:121, 1970.

303. SOLINGEN, L. D., ET AL.: *Subclinical eye movement disorders in patients with multiple sclerosis.* Neurology 27:614, 1977.

304. SORENSEN, H.: *Cancer of the middle ear and mastoid.* Acta Radiol. 54:460, 1960.

305. SORENSEN, L. K., ET AL.: *Meniere's disease. A neuropsychological study.* Acta Otolaryngol. 83:266, 1977.

306. SPECTOR, G. J., ET AL.: *Neurologic implications of glomus tumors in the head and neck.* Laryngoscope 85:1387, 1975.

307. SPIEGEL, E. A., AND ALEXANDER, A.: *Vertigo in brain tumors with special reference to results of labyrinth examination.* Ann. Otol. Rhinol. Laryngol. 45:979, 1936.

308. SPILLANE, J. D., PALLIS, C., AND JONES, A. M.: *Developmental abnormalities in the region of the foramen magnum.* Brain 80:11, 1957.

309. SPOENDLIN, H.: *Optic and cochleovestibular degenerations in the hereditary ataxias. II. Temporal bone pathology in two cases of Friedreich's ataxia with vestibulo-cochlear disorders.* Brain 97:41, 1974.

310. STENGER, P.: *Bertrag zur Kenntnis der nach Kopfverletzungen auftretenden Veränderungen in Inneren Ohr.* Arch. Ohrenheilk. 79:43, 1909.

311. STEWART, J.: *Histopathology of mastoiditis*. J. Laryngol. 43:689, 1928.

312. STUPP, H.: *Untersuchung der Antibiotikaspiegel in deu Innenohrflussigkeiten und ihre Bedeutung für die Spezi-fische Ototoxizität der Ammoglykosidantibiotika*. Acta Otolaryngol. (Suppl. 262):8, 1970.

313. SYMONDS, C.: *Concussion and its sequelae*. Lancet 1:1, 1962.

314. SYPERT, G. W., AND ALVORD, E. C.: *Cerebellar infarction*. Arch. Neurol. 32:357, 1975.

315. TAKEMORI, S., TANAKA, Y., AND SUZUKI, J.: *Thalidomide anomalies of the ear*. Arch. Otolaryngol. 10:425, 1976.

316. TAKEUCHI, T., ET AL.: *A pathological study of Minamata disease in Japan*. Acta Neuropath. 2:40, 1962.

317. TAMARI, M.: *Histopathologic changes in the temporal bone in Paget's disease*. Ann. Otol. Rhinol. Laryngol. 51:170, 1942.

318. TAMARI, M., AND ITKIN, P.: *Penicillin and syphilis of the ear*. Eye, Ear, Nose, Throat Monthly 30:252, 1951.

319. TAYLOR, P. H., AND BICKNELL, P. G.: *Rupture of the round window membrane*. Ann. Otol. Rhinol. Laryngol. 85:105, 1976.

320. TELLEZ, I., AND TERRY, R. D.: *Fine structure of the early changes in the vestibular nuclei of the thiamine-deficient rat*. Amer. J. Path. 52:777, 1968.

321. TEMBE, D.: *Fibro-osseous dysplasia of the temporal bone*. J. Laryngol. 84:107, 1970.

322. THOMSEN, J., GYLDENSTED, C., AND LESTER, J.: *Computer tomography of cerebellopontine angle lesions*. Arch. Otolaryngol. 103:65, 1977.

323. THRUSH, D. C., AND FOSTER, J. B.: *An analysis of nystagmus in 100 consecutive patients with communicating syringomyelia*. J. Neurol. Sci. 20:381, 1973.

324. TOGLIA, J. U.: Dizziness after whiplash injury of the neck and closed head injury. In Walker, A. E., Caveness, W. F., Critchley M., (eds.): *The Late Effects of Head Injury*. Charles C Thomas, Springfield, Illinois, 1964.

325. TOGLIA, J. U.: *Acute flexion-extension injury of the neck: electronystagmographic study of 309 patients*. Neurology 26:808, 1976.

326. TOMITA, H., HAYAKAWA, W., AND HONDO, R.: *Varicella-zoster virus in idiopathic facial palsy*. Arch. Otolaryngol. 95:364, 1972.

327. TUMARKIN, I.: *Otolithic catastrophe; a new syndrome*. Brit. Med. J. 2:175, 1936.

328. UEKE, T.: *Signs of whiplash injury*. Surg. Ther. (Osaka) 22:633, 1970.

329. USHER, C.: *On the inheritance of retinitis pigmentosa, with notes of case*. Roy. London Ophth. Hosp. Rep. 19:130, 1914.

330. VALVASSORI, G. E.: Neuro-otological radiology. In Naunton, R. F. (ed.): *The Vestibular System*. Academic Press Inc., New York, 1975.

331. VICTOR, M., ADAMS, R. D., AND COLLINS, C. H.: *The Wernicke-Korsakoff Syndrome*. Davis, Philadelphia, 1971.

332. VIROLAINEN, E.: *Vestibular disturbances in clinical otosclerosis*. Acta Otolaryngol. (Suppl. 306):7, 1972.

333. WAARDENBURG, P.: *A new syndrome combining developmental anomalies of the eyelids, eyebrows, and nose root with pigmentary defects of the iris and head hair and with congenital deafness*. Amer. J. Hum. Genet. 3:195, 1951.

334. WAGEMANN, W.: *Zur Kenntnis des Usher-Syndroms, einer Sonderferm recessiver Labyrinthschädigungen*. Hals.-Nas.-Ohrenarzt. 9:151, 1960-1961.

335. WALFORD, P.: *An unusual epidemic*. Letter to the Editor. Lancet 1:415, 1952.

336. WATSON, C., ET AL.: *Psychosomatic aspects of Meniere's disease*. Arch. Otolaryngol. 86:543, 1967.

337. WEIBEL, J., AND FIELDS, W. S.: *Angiography of the posterior cervicocranial circulation*. Amer. J. Roentgen. 98:660, 1966.

338. WERSÄLL, J., AND HAWKINS, J. JR.: *The vestibular sensory epithelia in the cat labyrinth and their reactions in chronic streptomycin intoxication*. Acta Otolaryngol. 54:1, 1962.

339. WHITE, H. H.: *Brain stem tumors occurring in adults*. Neurology 13:292, 1963.

340. WILKINSON, I. M. S., KIME, R., AND PURNELL, M.: *Alcohol and human eye movement*. Brain 97:785, 1974.

341. WILLIAMS, D., AND WILSON, T. G.: *The diagnosis of the major and minor syndromes of basilar insufficiency.* Brain 85:741, 1962.

342. WILLIAMS, S.: *Epidemic vertigo in children.* Med. J. Austr. 2:660, 1963.

343. WILPIZESKI, D.: *Effects of lead on the vestibular system: Preliminary findings.* Laryngoscope 160:821, 1974.

344. WILSON, W. H.: *Fungal derivatives as antigenic excitants of episodic vertigo.* Laryngoscope 84:1585, 1974.

345. WOLFF, D., ET AL.: *The pathology of Cogan's syndrome causing profound deafness.* Ann. Otol. Rhinol. Laryngol. 74:507, 1965.

346. WOLFF, H. G.: *Headache and Other Head Pain,* ed. 2. Oxford University Press, New York, 1963.

347. WRIGHT, A.: *Meniere's disease.* Proc. Roy. Soc. Med. 41:801, 1948.

348. YASSIN, A., BADRY, A., AND FATT-HI, A.: *The relationship between electrolyte balance and cochlear disturbances in cases of renal failure.* J. Laryngol. 84:429, 1970.

349. YOUNG, D., ELDRIDGE, R., AND GARDNER, W.: *Bilateral acoustic neuroma in a large kindred.* JAMA 214:347, 1970.

350. ZAJTCHUK, J., MATZ, G., AND LINDSAY, J.: *Temporal bone pathology in herpes oticus.* Ann. Otol. Rhinol. Laryngol. 81:331, 1972.

Index